T0191795

Mental Health in the Athlete

Eugene Hong • Ashwin L. Rao
Editors

Mental Health in the Athlete

Modern Perspectives and Novel Challenges
for the Sports Medicine Provider

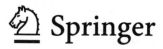 Springer

Editors
Eugene Hong
Department of Family Medicine
and Department of Orthopaedics
Medical University of South Carolina
Charleston, SC
USA

Ashwin L. Rao
Department of Family Medicine
University of Washington
Seattle, WA
USA

ISBN 978-3-030-44756-4   ISBN 978-3-030-44754-0   (eBook)
https://doi.org/10.1007/978-3-030-44754-0

© Springer Nature Switzerland AG 2020
This work is subject to copyright. All rights are reserved by the Publisher, whether the whole or part of the material is concerned, specifically the rights of translation, reprinting, reuse of illustrations, recitation, broadcasting, reproduction on microfilms or in any other physical way, and transmission or information storage and retrieval, electronic adaptation, computer software, or by similar or dissimilar methodology now known or hereafter developed.
The use of general descriptive names, registered names, trademarks, service marks, etc. in this publication does not imply, even in the absence of a specific statement, that such names are exempt from the relevant protective laws and regulations and therefore free for general use.
The publisher, the authors and the editors are safe to assume that the advice and information in this book are believed to be true and accurate at the date of publication. Neither the publisher nor the authors or the editors give a warranty, expressed or implied, with respect to the material contained herein or for any errors or omissions that may have been made. The publisher remains neutral with regard to jurisdictional claims in published maps and institutional affiliations.

This Springer imprint is published by the registered company Springer Nature Switzerland AG
The registered company address is: Gewerbestrasse 11, 6330 Cham, Switzerland

Preface

Mental Illness is an emerging concern in athletic circles, with good reason. As consumers, we are now, more than ever, aware of the personal lives of athletes, through media coverage, through published memories, or through various social media formats. As providers, however, we are woefully underprepared to help our own athletes manage the choppy waters of mental illness within the context of athletic participation. Today's societal appetite for sport is greater now than in any time in history, and with it, our awareness of the lives of our athletes has grown. Social media has allowed us to peer into the intimate details of their daily lives, and at times what we see surprises us. Media coverage has, in turn, raised questions about the relative risks of mental illness and related concerns in the athletic population.

There are numerous barriers faced by athletes hoping to secure mental health care within their communities. Mental health concerns are routinely stigmatized, and athletes may be unwilling to disclose their own battles with mental illness, fearing the consequences of disclosure to their personal identity and perception to various communities (coaches, teammates, public) important to them. To compound matters, coaches, administrators, and team medical providers are often unaware or underinformed about mental health concerns and remain reticent to discuss such issues, possibly fearing that the Pandora's box that entertaining such concerns may open. It was in this context that Dr. Hong and I began to discuss this book project, as a means of bridging the gap between providers and athletes through research, advocacy, legislation, and education.

Our first foray into mental health concerns among athletes was through research. Dr. Hong's research on depression in collegiate athletic communities began to answer the questions regarding prevalence of such symptoms among student athletes. Similarly, Dr. Rao's research, which came from compiling and evaluated data sets of sudden death among NCAA student athletes, identified suicide as a major contributor to all-cause mortality, and subsequent research focused on the incidence of suicide in this population. Our first collaboration came in the form of a theme edition of the *British Journal of Sports Medicine*, for which we served as guest editors for an entire issue focused on athlete mental health. This publication, the first of its kind for a peer-reviewed sports medicine journal, was well received and kindled the thought of future collaboration. In 2017, on the heels of podium presentations and moderated sessions focused on athlete mental health at annual meetings of the American Medical Society for Sports Medicine (AMSSM) and American College of Sports Medicine (ACSM), we were approached by Springer Health about developing a textbook focused on the topic of athlete mental health. This textbook is the product of our efforts.

Until now, sports medicine providers have not had a dedicated textbook in which to explore mental health topics relating specifically to athletes and their community. It is our sincere hope that this book serves as a resource to those who are interested in exploring this topic further. We have successfully secured the collaboration of a wide range of topic experts, ranging from leading researchers to thought leaders in the field of athletic mental health. We specifically sought contributors gifted with communication and leadership skills, to help guide the reader into challenging topics such as athletic suicide, risk-taking, depression, disordered eating, and more complex topics such as translational research, sports psychology, sports psychiatry, and sports legislation, to name a few. We also explore emerging topics such as performance-enhancing drugs, social media, exercise addiction, and sleep disruption. Our authors all share an uncommon comfort in engaging these topics with their own athletes, and we hope that you will find their chapters to be both informative and inspiring.

Ultimately, the purpose of this book is to engage and educate sports medicine providers about mental health concerns prevalent in athletic community. We intend to fill knowledge gaps common in the care of athletes in a sports medicine setting. We will present the limitations to the quality and quantity of data of the available evidence. We hope that you, the reader, use this book as a reference to deliver informed care to your athlete-patients. Athletes have begun to understand the importance of optimizing mental health for performance and for the betterment of their lives. As providers, we owe it to them to acknowledge and address their mental health concerns. Our hope is that this book provides you with a resource by which to do this.

Charleston, SC, USA   Eugene Hong
Seattle, WA, USA   Ashwin L. Rao

Contents

1 Overcoming the Stigma of Mental Health in Sport 1
Ashwin L. Rao and Eugene Hong

2 Screening for Mental Health Conditions in Athletes 11
Thomas H. Trojian

3 Depression in Athletes: Incidence, Prevalence, and
Comparisons with the Nonathletic Population. 25
Andrew T. Wolanin

4 Athletic Suicide 39
Ashwin L. Rao

5 Managing Psychiatric Disorders in Athletes 57
Claudia L. Reardon

6 Attention Deficit/Hyperactivity Disorder (ADHD) 69
Jason M. Matuszak

7 Risk-Taking Behaviors Among Athletes 85
Kyle Conley and Ashwin L. Rao

8 The Psychological Response to Injury and Illness. 95
Margot Putukian

9 Alcohol and Substance Abuse and Sport 103
Jason R. Kilmer, Cassandra D. Pasquariello, and Adrian J. Ferrera

10 Coping with Doping: Performance-Enhancing Drugs in
the Athletic Culture. 115
David M. Siebert

11 The Female Athlete Triad. 127
Andrea Kussman and Aurelia Nattiv

12 Mental Health Manifestations of Concussion................... 149
    Anthony P. Kontos, Raymond Pan, and Kouros Emami

13 Hazing and Bullying in Athletic Culture 165
    Aaron S. Jeckell, Elizabeth A. Copenhaver, and Alex B. Diamond

14 Impact of Social Media on Mental Health 181
    Steven K. Poon and Laura E. Sudano

15 Mental Health in the Pediatric Athlete 191
    Michele LaBotz

16 Pathological Exercise 203
    Jessica Knapp and Ashwin L. Rao

17 The Cellular and Physiological Basis of Behavioral
    Health After Mild Traumatic Brain Injury 211
    Laura L. Giacometti, Lauren A. Buck, and Ramesh Raghupathi

18 Mental Health Treatment Engagement of Athletes:
    Self-Determination Theory as a "Prescription for Excellence" 223
    Paul C. Furtaw

19 Mindfulness Approaches to Athlete Well-Being.................. 231
    Mike Gross

20 Administering Mental Health: Societal, Coaching, and
    Legislative Approaches to Mental Health...................... 245
    Emily Kroshus and Brian Hainline

21 Sport Psychology and Performance Psychology:
    Contributions to the Mental Health of Athletes................. 261
    David B. Coppel

22 Exercise as a Prescription for Mental Health................... 269
    Vicki R. Nelson and Irfan M. Asif

23 The Role of Sleep in Psychological Well-Being in Athletes........ 277
    Chad Asplund and Cindy J. Chang

Index... 291

Contributors

Irfan M. Asif, MD Prisma Health - Upstate and University of South Carolina School of Medicine – Greenville, Greenville, SC, USA

Chad Asplund, MD, MPH Department of Orthopaedics and Family Medicine, Mayo Clinic, Minneapolis, MN, USA

Lauren A. Buck, MS Department of Pharmacology and Physiology, College of Medicine, Drexel University, Philadelphia, PA, USA

Cindy J. Chang, MD, FACSM, FAMSSM Departments of Orthopaedics and Family & Community Medicine, University of California, San Francisco, San Francisco, CA, USA

Kyle Conley, BA University of Washington, Seattle, WA, USA

Elizabeth A. Copenhaver, MD, FAAP Vanderbilt University School of Medicine, Nashville, TN, USA

Program for Injury Prevention in Youth Sports, Monroe Carell Jr. Children's Hospital at Vanderbilt, Nashville, TN, USA

Department of Pediatrics, Vanderbilt University Medical Center, Nashville, TN, USA

David B. Coppel, PhD Department of Neurological Surgery, University of Washington, Seattle, WA, USA

Alex B. Diamond, DO, MPH, FAAP Vanderbilt University School of Medicine, Nashville, TN, USA

Program for Injury Prevention in Youth Sports, Monroe Carell Jr. Children's Hospital at Vanderbilt, Nashville, TN, USA

Department of Pediatrics, Vanderbilt University Medical Center, Nashville, TN, USA

Department of Orthopaedics and Rehabilitation, Vanderbilt University Medical Center, Nashville, TN, USA

Kouros Emami, PsyD UPMC Sports Medicine Concussion Program, Pittsburgh, PA, USA

Adrian J. Ferrera, PhD Auburn University, Auburn, AL, USA

Paul C. Furtaw, PsyD Department of Psychiatry, School of Osteopathic Medicine, Rowan University, Mt. Laurel, NJ, USA

Laura L. Giacometti, PhD Department of Pharmacology and Physiology, College of Medicine, Drexel University, Philadelphia, PA, USA

Mike Gross, PsyD Princeton University, Princeton, NJ, USA

Brian Hainline, MD Indiana University School of Medicine, Indianapolis, IN, USA

New York University School of Medicine, New York, NY, USA

Eugene Hong, MD, CAQSM, FAAFP Department of Family Medicine and Department of Orthopaedics, Medical University of South Carolina (MUSC), Charleston, SC, USA

Aaron S. Jeckell, MD Department of Psychiatry, Vanderbilt University Medical Center, Nashville, TN, USA

Vanderbilt University School of Medicine, Nashville, TN, USA

Program for Injury Prevention in Youth Sports, Monroe Carell Jr. Children's Hospital at Vanderbilt, Nashville, TN, USA

Jason R. Kilmer, PhD University of Washington, Psychiatry & Behavioral Sciences, School of Medicine, Seattle, WA, USA

Jessica Knapp, DO Sports Medicine MAHEC Family Medicine, Asheville, NC, USA

Anthony P. Kontos, PhD University of Pittsburgh, Department of Orthopaedic Surgery, Pittsburgh, PA, USA

UPMC Sports Medicine Concussion Program, Pittsburgh, PA, USA

Emily Kroshus, ScD, MPH Seattle Children's Research Institute, Center for Child Health, Behavior and Development, Seattle, WA, USA

University of Washington, Department of Pediatrics, Seattle, WA, USA

Andrea Kussman, MD Stanford University, Department of Orthopaedics, Stanford, CA, USA

Michele LaBotz, MD InterMed, Portland, ME, USA

Tufts University School of Medicine, Boston, MA, USA

Jason M. Matuszak, MD, FAAFP Excelsior Orthopaedics, Buffalo, NY, USA

University at Buffalo, School of Medicine, Buffalo, NY, USA

Aurelia Nattiv, MD UCLA Department of Family Medicine, Division of Sports Medicine, UCLA Department of Orthopaedics, Los Angeles, CA, USA

Vicki R. Nelson, MD Prisma Health - Upstate and University of South Carolina School of Medicine – Greenville, Greenville, SC, USA

Raymond Pan, MD University of Pittsburgh, Department of Psychiatry, Pittsburgh, PA, USA

Cassandra D. Pasquariello, PhD University of Wisconsin, Madison, WI, USA

Steven K. Poon, MD Sports Medicine Section, Arizona State University Health Services, Arizona State University Athletics, Tempe, AZ, USA

Margot Putukian, MD, FACSM Princeton University, Athletic Medicine, University Health Services, Princeton, NJ, USA

Rutgers-Robert Wood Johnson Medical School, University of Medicine and Dentistry of New Jersey, New Brunswick, NJ, USA

Ramesh Raghupathi, PhD Department of Neurobiology and Anatomy, College of Medicine, Drexel University, Philadelphia, PA, USA

Coatesville Veteran's Administration Medical Center, Coatesville, PA, USA

Ashwin L. Rao, MD Department of Family Medicine and Section of Sports Medicine, University of Washington, Seattle, WA, USA

UW Husky Athletics and Seattle Seahawks, Seattle, WA, USA

Claudia L. Reardon, MD University of Wisconsin School of Medicine and Public Health, Department of Psychiatry, Madison, WI, USA

David M. Siebert, MD Department of Family Medicine, Sports Medicine Section, Seattle, WA, USA

Laura E. Sudano, PhD, LMFT Collaborative Care, Family Medicine and Public Health, University of California, San Diego, San Diego, CA, USA

Thomas H. Trojian, MD, MMB, FACSM, FAMSSM Drexel University College of Medicine, Philadelphia, PA, USA

Andrew T. Wolanin, PsyD Wolanin Consulting and Assessment Inc., Bala Cynwyd, PA, USA

Chapter 1
Overcoming the Stigma of Mental Health in Sport

Ashwin L. Rao and Eugene Hong

Introduction

Mental illness has long carried a stigma in numerous social contexts [1]. Athletic culture, which champions resilience, toughness, and the goal of winning at any cost, has stigmatized mental illness, often labeling athletes harboring these conditions as weak, fragile, or inadequate. In other instances, the culture of athletics often fails to recognize mental health as a potential significant problem, conflating mental health concerns with other illness and thus failing to acknowledge the issue and adding to the burden of stigma. In truth, over 30% of individuals aged 18–25 experience serious mental health concerns, yet less than one-third of this cohort receive treatment targeting their mental well-being [2, 3]. Previous studies have demonstrated that the general population cohort aged 16–34 is the least likely group to seek mental health care, and this is largely the age range that constitutes the competitive athletic population [4, 5].

Athletes are seen as pillars of health and wellness within their communities, and many athletes adopt this idealized archetype, failing to recognize that such a perception creates its own burden [6]. Society, as a whole, associates success on the playing field with emotional fortitude and mental toughness, and thus, mental illness can be seen as contradictory to this perception. The perception of a mental

A. L. Rao (✉)
Department of Family Medicine and Section of Sports Medicine, Sports Medicine Fellowship, University of Washington, Seattle, WA, USA

UW Husky Athletics and Seattle Seahawks, Seattle, WA, USA
e-mail: ashwin@uw.edu

E. Hong
Department of Family Medicine and Department of Orthopaedics, Medical University of South Carolina (MUSC), Charleston, SC, USA
e-mail: hong@musc.edu

© Springer Nature Switzerland AG 2020
E. Hong, A. L. Rao (eds.), *Mental Health in the Athlete*,
https://doi.org/10.1007/978-3-030-44754-0_1

health concern as a sign of weakness may lead many athletes to limit disclosure. An athlete suffering from mental illness may thus fail to disclose their mental health concerns for fear that it may expose them to the risk of losing playing time, their role on the team, or gain the scorn of their teammates, coaches, family, and fans [1].

In recent years, a number of studies have aimed to evaluate the barriers and facilitators to improving mental health care in athletes, identifying that the stigma associated with mental health concerns is the primary barrier to care. While there is a paucity of evidence to develop strategies for overcoming these barriers, studies and expert opinions are beginning to reveal strategies for medical providers to better engage their athletes around the topic of mental health.

This chapter aims to review the concept of stigma as it pertains to the mental health of athletes. We will commence by defining stigma, reviewing athletic culture and the ways it impacts mental health and mental health care of athletes. We will consider the evidence around barriers and facilitators to care, and we will conclude with proposed interventions to overcome stigma and other barriers to mental health care.

Defining Stigma

Stigma is broadly defined as a mark of disgrace associated with a particular circumstance, quality, or person. Such circumstances may lead to social isolation and ostracism. In the context of health and wellness, stigma is defined as the manner in which someone is viewed in a negative way due a negatively perceived distinguishing characteristic. Stigma is a major barrier to the therapeutic goals of clinical psychology, as it may dissuade individuals from engaging in both self-care and seeking external sources of care. As a result, the stigma associated with mental health can have a profound impact on recovery. Stigma is driven by many factors, including one's social history and his or her own beliefs and expectations regarding identity and the exclusion of mental illness in one's conception of self, organizations, and associations that choose to ignore or acknowledge mental health concerns, expectations of relatives, and coaches and leadership, the risk of financial gain or loss for all involved, and media outlets who glorify success while critically appraising failure [1]. Further, culture, sport-type, and gender may all contribute to an athlete's willingness to disclose a mental health concern [7, 8].

Two forms of stigma have been identified in the medical context: public stigma and self-stigma [9]. Each can have an impact on both formal and informal help-seeking for those who might seek psychiatric or psychologic treatment. Public stigma describes the stereotypes, prejudice, and discrimination endorsed by the population as a whole. Essentially, public stigma refers to the negative attitudes held by members of the public about people with devalued characteristics. In contrast, self-stigma occurs when individuals internalize commonly held public attitudes and values, suffering negative consequences as a result. Self-stigma has often been equated with perceived stigma, a person's recognition that the others hold belief that will discriminate against them because of a mental illness label. Self-stigma has the capacity to impact self-esteem, self-confidence, and self-efficacy.

Mental Illness in the Sports World – A Brief Background

Over 30% of individuals aged 18–25 experience a serious mental health concern [2, 3]. Further, one in five individuals harbor a mental health condition that places them at an increased risk of suicide [10]. Despite the prevalence mental health disorders in the general population, only one-third of individuals impacted by mental illness receive treatment for their concern. In many sports, individuals are often at their peak athletic performance during a developmental period where the risk for mental health concerns is highest [5]. Notably, individuals aged 16–34, a demographic that encompasses a majority of competitive athletes, are the least likely cohort to seek care for a mental health concern, suggesting that athletes are relatively less likely to seek mental health care.

A wide range of studies demonstrate comparable rates of mental illness in the athletic population and general population. For example, recently published studies of US Collegiate athletes identified 19–25% of athletes who met symptomatic criteria for depression [11, 12]. Similarly, 21–27% of professional athletes met depression criteria, and in fact nearly 9% would meet criteria for a major depressive episode [13]. While depression is the most common mental illness in both the general population and among athletes, it is important to acknowledge the similar scope and range of mental health disorders that are prevalent in athletic communities and the general population alike. By virtue of competition and participation in athletic communities, athletes face a unique risk factor environment imposed by the demands and culture of their sports. For example, in certain athletic populations, particularly those involving aesthetic sports, disordered eating is more common than in the general population [14]. Athlete-specific risk factors for mood disorders include injuries that impact the ability to play or practice, intrinsic and extrinsic pressuress to perform, time demands, and loss of athletic identity (e.g., due to end of an athletic career) [15, 1].

Mental Health Versus Mental Toughness

Current perspectives suggest that mental toughness represents a collection of personal resources salient for goal-directed behavior in the setting of variable situational demands. The culture of most sports embraces the concept of "strive, survive, and thrive," and those who are perceived as mentally tough are felt to be more likely to succeed in this approach. Successful athletes are routinely expected to be "mentally tough" [16].

A recent commentary suggests that mental toughness and mental health are seen in contradictory terms in the world of elite performance [1]. The assumption derived from this supposition is that sports culture is not consistently amenable to respond to athletes seeking mental health treatment. In turn, athletes may feel that seeking help for such concerns may expose them to the risk of lost playing time, a loss of their status on the team or their capacity to compete. As a result, the incentive to ask for help and get better are outweighed by the negative consequences of appearing mentally fragile.

In truth, both mental health and mental toughness may have a more nuanced overlapping relationship than one that is truly oppositional [16]. In one sense, athletes who are mentally tough may remain vulnerable to mental illness, given the time and energy investment applied to the athlete lifestyle and identity. Success in their sport may not necessarily equate to success in their own mental health wellness. Such "successful" athletes may fail to find time to explore other aspects of their selves, acknowledge or properly manage competitive failure, contend with injury, or manage the emotional and physical separation from friends and family. Further, research in adolescents reveals an inverse relationship between self-reported mental toughness and measures of depression, stress, and anxiety, while conversely showing a positive association with affect. Collectively however, studies appear to show that athletes with higher measures of mental toughness report lower negative symptoms and higher positive mental health measures. In this manner, mental toughness may in fact be a facilitator for mental health in certain circumstances [16].

Barriers to Mental Health Care

Stigma associated with mental illness and mental health disorders appears to be the strongest barrier for athletes to seek mental health care [5]. A recent systematic review of perceived barriers to mental health help-seeking in young people identified stigma and embarrassment as the two principal impediments to help-seeking in this population [17]. In the athletic population, other notable barriers include: a lack of mental health literacy (e.g., not knowing about mental health disorder or important symptoms; not knowing when or where to seek help), negative past experiences with help-seeking, lack of familiarity with mental health care providers, lack of confidence in the professional opinion being sought, a culture of self-reliance, lack of awareness of a problem, financial cost of care, and perceived time constraints in which to acquire care. Male, black, US nationals, and younger-aged athletes were all demographics less likely to avail of mental health services [17].

Denial also plays an important role as a barrier in many athletes [5]. An absence of identifiable medical signs of disease may contribute to athletes' lack of knowledge, understanding, or willingness to consider mood disorders and other mental health concerns as an illness or condition that may benefit from appropriate medical attention. In one study, maladaptive escapism was used as a means of managing difficult emotional experiences, further establishing denial [18].

Perceptions held by coaches and teammates are often of great concern to athletes considering seeking help for their mental health concerns. Coaches and teammates who create a culture supporting disclosure, where consequences of such a disclosure are limited and potentially positive, may facilitate athletes to disclose their

concerns and work with a mental health care provider [1]. In contrast, team environments that shame mental illness may serve as a barrier by forcing athletes to hide
any potential vulnerability, and in turn could delay disclosure during periods of
subclinical illness, which may be more amenable to treatment.

Terminology may also have an impact on an athlete's willingness to engage. For
example, among male athletes, there was lesser stigma associated with the term
"sports psychologist" as opposed to "psychotherapist" [5].

Facilitators to Mental Health Care

A number of factors have recently been identified as facilitators for mental health
care in the athletic setting, though these factors are comparatively under-researched
when compared to barriers. Among young, elite athletes, encouragement to seek
care from others was a primary facilitator for seeking mental health care. Also
important are availability of mental health providers in the athletes' community, an
established relationship with a mental health care provider, pleasant prior interactions with providers, and positive attitudes of others, specifically family members,
coaches, and teammates [17]. Such findings suggest a role for familiarization of a
mental health care provider with members of an athletic community outside of the
clinical context. Coaches and support staff willing to facilitate care are vital to promoting a culture of disclosure and help-seeking to those in need.

Other important facilitators that have been reviewed include the availability of an
embedded mental health provider or care team, confidentiality and trust in the provider, education and awareness regarding mental health concerns, a perception of
the mental health concern as serious, positive attitudes toward seeking help, and the
ease of expressing emotion [5, 17]. Those with stronger positive coping skills are
more likely to seek care, suggesting a role for coping-skills training as part of orientation upon joining a team.

Recent Successes

Governing institutions and organizations within athletics have increasingly acknowledged the role of a mental health care team in the athletic setting. The International
Olympic Committee (IOC), National Collegiate Athletic Association (NCAA),
National Football League (NFL), and others have developed consensus statements
and other similar mental health initiatives aimed to support a culture of awareness
and help-seeking, while drafting guidelines by which care may be delivered to athletes. The NCAA's Mental Health Task Force has recently published a number of
documents, including an Inter-association consensus document, *Best Practices for
Understanding Student-Athlete Mental Wellness*, coming on the heels of their previously published *Mind, Body, and Sport* [19, 20]. The *Best Practices* document

stresses a collaborative process engaging the full complete of available resources on campus and within the community inhabited by athletes [19]. Resources that could compromise an interdisciplinary team include campus health services, a student-athlete advisory committee, a collegiate athletic department's own internal resources, campus counseling services, disability services, and community mental health agencies. Providers caring for athletes should be licensed to provide mental health care. Further, procedures to identify and refer student-athletes to qualified practitioners should be in place. The document goes on to stipulate that integration of such resources is crucial to a rapid and effective response to mental health concerns at all levels of immediacy.

In 2019, the IOC published its consensus statement reviewing *Mental Health in Elite Athletes*, suggesting that mental health disorders be reframed as a continuum of sport-related injury and illness as a means of reducing stigma [21]. Recently, the NFL and its players association, the NFLPA announced a joint initiative that requested every team to employ a mental health professional, such as a sports psychologist, to work onsite and be directly available to players. Others, such as the Federation Internationale de Football Association (FIFA), provide resources for interested parties to learn more about mental health topics important in athlete care.

By announcing and establishing ground rules and guidelines through these publications and initiatives, governing bodies have begun to embrace the importance of mental health care in the athletic setting and have provided some structural outlines on how to deliver more effective and comprehensive mental health care to athletes. Their efforts will be further guided by research in the area to better understand athletes' needs.

It is apparent that a culture change is occurring within sport with regard to athletes' willingness to disclose their struggles with mental illness, and in turn destigmatize this topic. In recent years, well-known athletes spanning a wide range of sports, including Michael Phelps (swimming, Olympics), Allison Schmitt (swimming, Olympian), Kevin Love (basketball), Mardy Fish (tennis), Zach Greinke (baseball), Imani Boyette (women's basketball), Brandon Marshall (Football), and DeMar DeRozen have all openly discussed their studies regarding their mental health and its impact on their sporting and personal lives. With such a climate of public disclosure and public acceptance, the burden of stigma may be reduced, and athletes may begin to find it easier to discuss their own struggles.

Interventions to Overcome the Stigma of Mental Health

There is a paucity of studies evaluating interventions to overcome the stigma of mental health in the athletic setting. In general, studies are beginning to show that improving mental health literacy, while destigmatizing mental health disorders, may have a limited impact on help-seeking within the general population.

Some studies have suggested that contact interventions (e.g. those involving exposure to individuals with mental illness) help destigmatize mental health disorders. Other studies have used educational interventions aimed to reduce stigma by providing information that contradict inaccurate stereotypes of mental illness. To date, studies utilizing contact and educational interventions have yielded only small to medium impacts in reducing stigmatizing attitudes.

Given the lack of clear research to guide interventions that destigmatize mental health in the athletic setting, a number of steps may be considered as means to promote a more accepting climate for mental health in the athletic setting. Both the IOC Consensus Statement and the NCAA *Best Practices* document offers some guidelines to help promote a culture of acceptance for mental health concerns as wells as a means for supporting and responding to concerns [19–21]. A number of steps have been considered as means to approach destigmatization of mental health, including (1) creating a culture of acceptance and accommodation for mental health concerns; (2) promoting awareness through educational intervention; (3) crafting a response to help mitigate stigma; (4) supporting individuals who are the targets of stigma and those who suffer from mental illness; and (5) conducting research to improve understanding.

Culture

Creating a culture in which athletes feel safe in disclosing mental health concerns is a first step towards the goal of overcoming stigma. Stakeholders, including team physicians and athletic trainers, team mental health providers, other licensed health care providers, and athletic administrators, may begin the process by approaching coaches about the importance of mental health in both wellness and performance and encouraging both dialogue and disclosure [19–21]. Administrations that grant time, effort, and resources to support mental health care are likely to see an increased awareness and response to mental health concerns disclosed by athletes. As more athletes begin to see positive outcomes of disclosure and management of their concerns, others may be willing to disclose their own concerns [1, 19–21]. Prior studies have demonstrated that familiarity with mental health providers is a primary facilitator for seeking care, and thus mental health care providers may seek opportunities to engage and interact with athletes outside of the clinical setting to gain familiarity and acceptance [5, 17]. Other strategies that have been proposed to combat mental health stigma include talking openly about mental health, encouraging equal perceptions of physical and mental illness, and choosing empowerment over shame [9].

Awareness

Awareness of mental health issues begins with education. Many athletes, coaches, and staff members are simply unaware of signs of mental health disorders or help-seeking for such disorders. Providing educational opportunities in which interested parties can learn about mental illness and its related signs and symptoms can be a valuable step in improving their mental health literacy, though there may be limits as to how effective this strategy is at increasing help-seeking [4, 5, 22]. Identification of mental health concerns and help-seeking in the clinical context can begin with asking an athlete about mental health concerns that they may harbor and providing athletes with a safe means of disclosure. Such opportunities exist on intake during the pre-participation evaluation process. Opportunities to screen for mental health concerns may also exist at other critical junctures, such as visits related to injury, illness, or inability to participate. Providers performing intake assessments should consider screening athletes for depression, anxiety, and other mood disorders using validated tools or questionnaires such as the PHQ-9, GAD-7, or other comparable tools. Providers should also be encouraged to ask openly about mental health concerns alongside any new or chronic physical concerns or illness. Athletes should also be made aware of resources by which they can openly or confidentially disclose their concerns, such as the presence of mental health providers on staff.

Response

Response to help-seeking is a critical piece to insure that athletes' mental health concerns are appropriately and effectively addressed, which in turn helps to destigmatize such concerns. As previously discussed, a coordinated and effective response may include recognition and coordination of community, campus, and team resources around mental health. Such responses may include treatment and triage protocols, emergency mental health action plans, and structured follow-up plans that hold both providers and athletes accountable for the follow-up process. Familiarity with resources and responses can bridge an awareness gap that often contributes to stigma [9, 21].

Support

Athletic organizations should enact measure to support athletes struggling with mental illness or mental health concerns [19–21]. Primary care providers and mental health providers should take steps to identify any public stigma harbored by members of the community and address these concerns [9]. Providers should also address self-stigma harbored by the athlete and attempt to understand and address the underlying factors for such beliefs. Support may involve utilization of team, departmental, and community resources appropriate to the needs of the athlete struggling with mental illness. Nonmedical staff, such as coaches and support personnel, should be aware of resources to which they can pass their concern about an athlete's mental wellness. Examples of such resources include team physicians and mental health providers, group meetings with similarly impacted athletes, and campus counseling services.

In encouraging a consistent and effective support strategy for athletes harboring mental health concerns informs them that the system believes their concern is important and not an issue that should be disregarded.

Research

The current state of evidence evaluating mental health in the athletic setting is limited. Retrospective studies, limited prospective research articles, and expert opinion papers largely form the current body of evidence in the medical literature, and numerous systematic reviews take note of the limits of the quality of data being analyzed to draw conclusions [5, 17, 21, 22]. The NCAA and others have acknowledged a research gap in mental health and are putting forth calls for research, along with support for those willing to pursue this area of inquiry [19].

Conclusion

Overcoming stigma in athletics remains a challenge. Athletes are similarly vulnerable to mental illness as the general population, and also face a number of population-specific risk factors for mental illness and stress. Athletic culture must continue to evolve to facilitate a climate where athletes may be more willing to disclose mental health concerns. Improving mental health literacy, dispelling both self-stigma and public stigma, and defining programs of care for athletes suffering from mental illness or anguish are all likely to promote a culture of acceptance in which stigma is diminished. The work of governing organizations, athletic departments, and national agencies are helping to facilitate these changes, and better research infrastructure is necessary to provide evidence-based recommendations for destigmatization.

References

1. Bauman NJ. The stigma of mental health in athletes: are mental toughness and mental health seen as contradictory in elite sport? Br J Sports Med. 2015;50(3):135–6.
2. Radloff L. The use of the center for epidemiologic studies depression scale in adolescents and young adults. J Youth Adolesc. 1991;20(2):149–66.
3. US Department of Health and Human Services, Substance Abuse and Mental Health Serrvices Administration. Results from a 2011 National Survey on Drug Use and Health. Mental Health Findings (NSDUH Series, H44, HHS Publication No (SMA) 12-473). Rockville, MD, 2012.
4. Rickwood D, Deane F, Wilson F. When and how do young people seek professional help for mental health problems? Med J Aust. 2007;187(7 Supple):S35–9.
5. Gulliver A, Griffiths KM, Christensen H. Barriers and facilitators to mental health help-seeking for young elite athletes: a qualitative study. BMC Psychiatry. 2012;12:157.

6. Markser VZ. Sports psychiatry and psychotherapy. Mental strains and disorders in professional sports. Challenge and answer to societal changes. Eur Arch Psychiatry Clin Neurosci. 2011;261(supple 2):S182–5.
7. Van Raalte J, Brewer D, Brewer B, et al. NCAA division II college football players' perceptions of an athlete who consults a sports psycholgosts. J Sport Exerc Psychol. 1992;14(3):273–82.
8. Martin SB, Lavallee D, Kellman M, et al. Attitudes toward sports psychology consult of adult athletes in the United States, United Kingdom, and Germany. Int J Sport Exerc Psychol. 2004;2(2):146–60.
9. Corrigan PW, Nieweglowski K. How does familiarity impact the stigma of mental illness. Clin Psych Rev. 2019;70:40–50.
10. Merikangas KR, He JP, Burstein M, et al. Lifetime prevalence of mental disorders in U.S. adolescents: results from the National Comorbidity Survey Replication V Adolescent Supplement (NCS-A). J Am Acad Child Adolesc Psychiatr. 2010;49:980Y9. Centers for Disease Control. Preventing suicide. 2018.
11. Yang J, Peek-Asa C, Corlette JD, et al. Prevalence of and risk factors associated with symptoms of depression in competitive collegiate student athletes. Clin J Sports Med. 2007;17(6):481–7.
12. Wolanin A, Hong E, Marks D, et al. Prevalence of clinically elevated depressive in college athletes and differences by gender and sport. BJSM. 2016;50:167–71.
13. Gulliver A, Griffiths KM, Mackinnon A, et al. The mental health of the Australian elite athletes. J Sci Sports Med. 2015;18(3):255–61.
14. Beable S, Fulcher M, Lee AC, et al. SHARPSports Mental Health Awareness Research Project; Prevalence and risk factors of depressive symptoms and life stress in elite athletes. J Sci Med Sport. 2017;20:1047–52.
15. Wolanin A, Gross M, Hong E. Depression in athletes: prevalence and risk factors. Curr Sports Med Rep. 2015;14:56–60.
16. Gucciardi DF, Hanton S, Fleming S. Are mental toughness and mental health contradictory concepts in elite sport? A narrative review of theory and evidence. J Sci Med Sport. 2017;20:307–11.
17. Castaldelli-Maia JM, Gallinaro JG, Falcao RS, et al. Mental health symptoms and disorders in elite athletes: a systemic review of cultural influencers and barriers to athletes seeking treatment. Br J Sports Med. 2019;53:707–21.
18. Wood S, Harrison LK, Kucharska J. Male professional footballers' experiences of mental health difficulties and help-seeking. Phys Sportsmed. 2017;45(2):120–8.
19. NCAA Mental Health Task Force. Interassociation Consensus Document; Mental Health Best Practices. Understand and supporting student-athlete mental wellness: NCAA Publications; 2017.
20. Brown GT, Hainline B, Kroshus E, Wilfert M. Mind, body and sport. Understanding and supporting student-athlete mental wellness: NCAA Publications; 2014.
21. Reardon CL, Hainline B, Aron CM, et al. Mental health in elite athletes: International Olympic Committee consensus statement. Br J Sports Med. 2019;53:667–99.
22. Gulliver A, Griffiths KM, Christensen H. Perceived barriers and facilitators to mental health help-seeking in young people: a systematic review. BMC Psychiatry. 2010;10(113):1–9.

Chapter 2
Screening for Mental Health Conditions in Athletes

Thomas H. Trojian

Introduction

Athletes experience mental health problems at rates comparable to the general population [1]. The Sports Medicine physician's role is to provide or direct preventive and restorative services for the athlete. This care includes the care of the mind, body, and psyche of the athlete. A crucial element of this care involves recognition that an athlete may have an active mental health concern. The NCAA Mental Health Taskforce recommends that the pre-participation exam (PPE) include mental health screening questionnaires [2]. The US Preventive Services Task Force (USPTF) also recommends mental health screening [3]. Both groups recommend that screening should be implemented with adequate systems in place to ensure accurate diagnosis, effective treatment, and appropriate follow-up [2, 3]. The American Association of Family Practice (AAFP) standard PPEn document does include a physician reminder to "consider additional questions on more sensitive issues" [4]. The National Athletic Trainers' Association (NATA) recommends that nine "mental well-being" questions be added to the pre-participation exam [2, 5, 6].

Despite these recommendations, a cross-sectional email survey study done in 2016 sent to all 1076 NCAA institutions demonstrated that only 39% of institutions had a "written plan related to identify student-athletes with mental health concerns" [7]. Less than 50% of institutions used screening tools for disordered eating, depression, or anxiety. Further, the strongest predictor of a mental health screening program was the presence of a written plan related to identifying student-athlete mental health concerns [7].

Athletics has its own unique stresses in life and athletic participation places these athletes at risk. For example, performance failure is significantly associated with

T. H. Trojian (✉)
Drexel University College of Medicine, Philadelphia, PA, USA
e-mail: tht34@drexel.edu

© Springer Nature Switzerland AG 2020
E. Hong, A. L. Rao (eds.), *Mental Health in the Athlete*,
https://doi.org/10.1007/978-3-030-44754-0_2

11

depression [8]. Depression prevalence among college athletes ranges from 15.6% to 25% [9]. Different subgroups of athletes have different rates of mental health problems and these should be considered during screening. Sexual orientation appears to have an independent impact on mental health outcomes in athletes [10]. Individuals with injury have a higher rate of depression or anxiety. High school students with orthopedic injuries are 3.8 (2.9–4.9) times more likely to have depression or anxiety [11]. High school students with concussion are 2.0 (1.5–2.6) times more likely to have depression or anxiety [11].

There is a growing concern about the impact of head injury on mental health in medical communities. NCAA recommends baseline neurocognitive testing, but the outcomes of such tests can be variable [12–14] due to factors such as baseline depression [15]. Symptoms of depression should be assessed as part of baseline neurocognitive assessments to help disentangle depression from concussion symptoms in post-concussion testing [15]. There has been growing concern that head injuries cause depression and suicides. In order to understand this question better and whether such a concern is valid, research to understand the contribution of underlying depression are necessary. Two studies highlight why depression screening is needed at concussion baseline, with the best predictor of post-concussion depression being baseline depression symptoms [16, 17]. Further, depression screening helps to increase the validity of baseline neurocognitive testing and help predict those student-athletes that will develop post-concussion depression.

Depression screening may be a beneficial strategy to predict recovery from future injuries in student-athletes. Galambo et al. showed that psychological measures have utility in predicting athletic injury, but since these measures are only able to partially explain the observed effect size, other factors must be considered [18]. Examples of other factors to consider in the injury prediction model include eating psychopathology (like the FAST, or EDQ [19]) since elevated levels serve as a potential risk factor for the development of depression in athletes in the next 6 months [20].

Mental health treatment services may be underutilized by athletes due to a myriad of variables such as time constraints and social stigma [21]. Recommendations for working with college and elite athletes include being flexible within reason about timing of sessions, involving family members when relationship issues are involved, and not compromising on delivering the appropriate treatment, including medications and hospitalizations [22]. As a team physician, it is important to meet with mental health providers to help coordinate referrals and assist them in understanding the difficulties athletes might have in seeking care.

The mechanics of screening for mental health concerns must be worked out prior to implementation if a screening program is to be successful [1]. The Chief Medical Officer of a team or organization must consider the following: (1) athlete availability, referral sources, and follow-up visit strategies prior to starting screening; (2) choice of disorder to be screened; (3) choice of screening tests and methodology; (4) lines of communication for informing athletes of a positive screen; (5) policies and procedures to manage athletes who decline further care upon notification; (6) triage and follow-up plan resources, including medications and counseling.

Regardless of the presence of a mental health screening program, all Sports Medicine providers should be attentive to behaviors that point towards a current or developing mental health disorder [23, 24].

Depression

Screening adults for depression is recommended in clinical practices that have systems in place to ensure accurate diagnosis, effective treatment, and follow-up [3, 25]. Depressive symptoms that do not meet the Diagnostic and Statistical Manual of Mental Disorders – V (DSM-V) criteria for depression may manifest from other psychological syndromes such as dysthymia, cyclothymic disorder, bipolar disorder, medical illness, substance abuse, or bereavement [26]. Bipolar disorder should be excluded as a manifestation of the patient's depression [25].

DSM-V criteria for major depressive disorder (see Table 2.1).

At least one study demonstrates that the rate of depression is significantly higher ($P = 0.03$) in current college student-athletes (about 17%) compared with former, graduated college student-athletes (8%), suggesting that current involvement in competitive sport at this level is a mental health stressor [27]. Other studies have identified female gender, low self-esteem, diminished social connectedness, and reduced sleep as independent predictors for depression [28]. Female student-athletes had 1.32 greater odds (95% CI, 1.01 to 1.73) of reporting symptoms of depression compared to male student-athletes. Freshmen have lesser social connectedness and 3.27 greater odds (95% CI, 1.63–6.59) of experiencing symptoms of depression than their more senior counterparts [29].

The United States Preventative Services Taskforce (USPSTF) recommends the use of one of the following: Patient Health Questionnaire – Depression Screener (PHQ-9), Beck Depression Inventory-II [BDI-II], or the Center for Epidemiologic Studies Depression Scale (CES-D). The PHQ-9 has 95% sensitivity and 88.3% specificity when scored with a threshold 11 [30]. The PHQ-9 assesses depressive symptoms equivalently across gender and racial/ethnic groups in a US college population [31]. The CES-D utilizes a ten-question survey and provides an 84% sensitivity, 60% specificity, and 77% positive predicted value using a threshold of 22 to evaluate for depression [32]. The BDI-II has been validated using college students, adult psychiatric outpatients, and adolescent psychiatric outpatients, yielding a good sensitivity, specificity, and test-test reliability [32]. The NCAA recommended the use of the depression screen HANDS [33] due to its relatively high sensitivity. When choosing one of these screening tools, a physician should examine each screening tool and determine which will work best in their screening program.

Depression screening is considered valuable in other populations. The USPSTF recommends screening for major depressive disorder (MDD) in adolescents aged 12–18 years [34]. In adolescent pediatric population (age 13–17), the PHQ-2 has sensitivity of 74% and specificity of 75% [35]. If PHQ-2 has a score of 3 or more, then the PHQ-9 should be used [36]. A PHQ-9 score of 11 or more had a sensitivity

Table 2.1 DSM 5 major depressive disorder

A. Five (or more) of the following symptoms have been present during the same 2-week period and represent a change from previous functioning; at least one of the symptoms is either (1) depressed mood or (2) loss of interest or pleasure. *Note:* Do not include symptoms that are clearly attributable to another medical condition.
1. Depressed mood most of the day, nearly every day, as indicated by either subjective report (e.g., feels sad, empty, hopeless) or observation made by others (e.g., appears tearful). (*Note:* In children and adolescents, can be irritable mood.)
2. Markedly diminished interest or pleasure in all, or almost all, activities most of the day, nearly every day (as indicated by either subjective account or observation).
3. Significant weight loss when not dieting or weight gain (e.g., a change of more than 5% of body weight in a month), or decrease or increase in appetite nearly every day. (*Note:* In children, consider failure to make expected weight gain.)
4. Insomnia or hypersomnia nearly every day.
5. Psychomotor agitation or retardation nearly every day (observable by others, not merely subjective feelings of restlessness or being slowed down).
6. Fatigue or loss of energy nearly every day.
7. Feelings of worthlessness or excessive or inappropriate guilt (which may be delusional) nearly every day (not merely self-reproach or guilt about being sick).
8. Diminished ability to think or concentrate, or indecisiveness, nearly every day (either by subjective account or as observed by others).
9. Recurrent thoughts of death (not just fear of dying), recurrent suicidal ideation without a specific plan, or a suicide attempt or a specific plan for committing suicide.
B. The symptoms cause clinically significant distress or impairment in social, occupational, or other important areas of functioning.
C. The episode is not attributable to the physiological effects of a substance or to another medical condition.
Note: Criteria A–C represent a major depressive episode.
Note: Responses to a significant loss (e.g., bereavement, financial ruin, losses from a natural disaster, a serious medical illness or disability) may include the feelings of intense sadness, rumination about the loss, insomnia, poor appetite, and weight loss noted in Criterion A, which may resemble a depressive episode. Although such symptoms may be understandable or considered appropriate to the loss, the presence of a major depressive episode in addition to the normal response to a significant loss should also be carefully considered. This decision inevitably requires the exercise of clinical judgment based on the individual's history and the cultural norms for the expression of distress in the context of loss.
D. The occurrence of the major depressive episode is not better explained by schizoaffective disorder, schizophrenia, schizophreniform disorder, delusional disorder, or other specified and unspecified schizophrenia spectrum and other psychotic disorders.
E. There has never been a manic episode or a hypomanic episode. *Note:* This exclusion does not apply if all of the manic-like or hypomanic-like episodes are substance-induced or are attributable to the physiological effects of another medical condition.

of 89.5% and a specificity of 77.5% for detecting youth who met the DSM- IV criteria for MDD [36].

Sexual assault is another concern impacting depression and related mental health concerns in student-athletes. The NCAA conducted a survey in which student-athletes were asked a series of questions regarding their mental health status within the past 30 days and 12 months [37]. The survey revealed that both male and female student-athletes who self-reported experiences of sexual assault were significantly more likely to experience hopelessness, mental exhaustion, depression, or suicidal thoughts. Those who indicated experiences of sexual assault within the past 12 months were three times more likely to have had recent suicidal thoughts than those who did not (13% vs. 4% for women, and 12% vs. 4% for men). The percent of female and male athletes reporting having experienced unwanted sexual touching or penetration in last 12 months in the NCHA survey is 9.1% and 4.6%, respectively. It is even higher in athletes diagnosed with depression; the NCHA survey noted the rate to be 1 in 8 females and 1 in 15 males who have been sexually victimized in last 12 months [2]. When addressing depression in athletes, it is important to address the possibility of sexual assault in both men and women. These student-athletes should also be referred to sexual assault response center, mental health provider and encouraged to contact law enforcement.

Injury history may play a role in long-term health and wellness of athletes both during and after career. While caring for former athletes, the sports medicine physician needs to remember that injuries suffered during competition may linger post-career and limit activity, thereby lowering their health-related quality of life [38, 39]. The combination of depression and pain in former athletes is strongly predictive of significant difficulties with sleep, social relationships, financial difficulties, and problems with exercise and fitness. A hypothesis explaining this association is that significant musculoskeletal disability and chronic pain interferes with physical activity and fitness during retirement and increases the risk of depression [40]. Very high physical activity has a significant protective effect against depression [41].

Screening for depression should be recognized as a screen of depressive symptoms. Those receiving a concerning score on a mental health screen must have a follow-up visit to determine if the positive screen is depression or another disorder. Although those who screen high on the CES-D or PHQ-9 are most commonly psychiatric in nature, other illnesses can present with depressive symptoms. Depression was found to be the most common affective prodromal of medical disorders and was consistently reported in Cushing's syndrome, hypothyroidism, hyperparathyroidism, pancreatic and lung cancer, myocardial infarction, Wilson's disease, and AIDS [42]. There is also an association between depression and decreased ferritin levels before the occurrence of anemia [43, 44]. Athletes with suspected depression should be tested for iron-deficiency (ferritin) [43], subclinical thyroid (TSH, free T4) [45], and vitamin D deficiency (Vitamin D 25-OH) [46–48].

Anxiety Disorder

Anxiety disorders are prevalent across populations [49]. As with depression, anxiety disorder must be distinguished from anxiety symptoms, which can be attributed to a wider array of mental and physical health conditions (see Tables 2.2 and 2.3). Notably, approximately 30% of athletes experience anxiety symptoms, the prevalence of anxiety disorder is 4.7% [49, 50].

Table 2.2 General anxiety disorder

The diagnostic and statistical manual of mental disorders, fifth edition
When assessing for GAD, clinical professionals are looking for the following:
1. The presence of excessive anxiety and worry about a variety of topics, events, or activities. Worry occurs more often than not for at least 6 months and is clearly excessive.
2. The worry is experienced as very challenging to control. The worry in both adults and children may easily shift from one topic to another.
3. The anxiety and worry are accompanied with at least three of the following physical or cognitive symptoms

Table 2.3 DSM-5 criteria for generalized anxiety disorder

Signs and symptoms of an anxiety disorder
Edginess or restlessness
Tiring easily; more fatigued than usual
Impaired concentration or feeling as though the mind goes blank
Irritability (which may or may not be observable to others)
Increased muscle aches or soreness
Difficulty sleeping (due to trouble falling asleep or staying asleep, restlessness at night, or unsatisfying sleep)

The Generalized Anxiety Disorder – 7 Index (GAD-7) [51, 52] has been validated in the general population and has the best evidence in the primary care setting. It has 89% sensitivity and 82% specificity [52]. However, there is a paucity of data about screening athletes for GAD. In one study of German women soccer players, the GAD-7 score indicated GAD in 8.3% players [53]. The prevalence of GAD was no different when compared to the female general population of similar age.

The State-Trait Anxiety Inventory (STAI) is another index that is useful in evaluating anxiety symptoms, using a 20-question index that utilizes a Likert scale and with different population-specific thresholds [51]. One study using the STAI found that 28% of athletes presented with pre-season anxiety symptoms [50]. The relatively low sensitivity and specificity of the STAI likely underestimates the number of athletes with true anxiety disorder [54].

The Sport Anxiety Scale (SAS) is a reliable and validated tool for Sport Performance Anxiety. The SAS includes 21 questions to measure cognitive and somatic sport performance anxiety. SAS-2 was developed from the SAS and is validated in younger children [55]. As athletes are at risk for a variety of different types of anxiety that may not meet criteria for GAD, further research needs to be done to evaluate anxiety-screening inventories in this population.

Eating Disorder

Athletic participation in certain situations can be protective against eating problems; however, female athletes have a higher incidence of eating problems than the general population. This includes a higher prevalence of eating disorders and sub-clinical eating disorders in female athletes compared to the general adult popula-tion, with the latter found in up to 50% of high school female athletes [5]. It is important to have athlete-specific screening tools as many behaviors that an athlete may have (perfectionism, calorie counting, prolonged exercise) may overlap with diagnostic criteria of eating disorders in the general population without being patho-logic in the athletic population [19].

The standard AAFP PPE includes various questions related to eating disorders (see Questions 47–50 and 52–54); however, there is currently no validated tool spe-cifically for screening for eating disorders in all athletes. Despite this, the ACSM, NATA, and IOC recommend screening for eating disorders in athletes. The Eating Disorder Examination (EDE) is the gold standard in eating disorder diagnosis but has not been validated in athletes [19]. Knapp et al. looked at the evidence for screening tools for eating disorders in athletes and found that there were three vali-dated screening tools for athletes: the Athletic Milieu Direct Questionnaire (AMDQ), Brief Eating Disorders in Athletes Questionnaire (BEDA-Q), and Female Athlete Screening Tool (FAST) [19].

The FAST was not only a validated tool within DI and DIII NCAA but addition-ally could identify those at risk for developing an eating disorder [56]. The AMDQ is a self-reported questionnaire comprised of a nine-question inventory with high sensitivity and specificity [57]. The BEDA-Q was developed for elite high school female athletes and is the newest of the three. The questionnaire was developed in three phases and one of the versions (a nine-question version) had a sensitivity of 82.1% and specificity of 84.6%. All three screenings would be reasonable screening tools for female athletes. No tools have been validated in male athletes. Of note, none of these tools has as yet been modified to the most recent DSM-V criteria for eating disorder [19].

Injured Athlete – Fear Avoidance and Pain Catastrophe

In any injured athlete, particularly in seriously injured athletes, there is often accom-panying depression, anger, and low self-esteem. Studies have revealed that both con-cussion and musculoskeletally injured athletes experience emotional disturbance after injury [58]. Younger athletes may be particularly sensitive to injury-related stim-uli, which augment injury-related distress [59]. In injured athletes, there are two par-ticular features that should be screened. Fear avoidance is independently associated with decreased physical function. On the other hand, catastrophizing pain may be associated with increased pain intensity [60]. Fear and depression have been identi-fied as factors that should be targeted in low back pain patients to reduce back-pain-related disability [60]. Pain catastrophizing at 4 weeks was associated with pain intensity and pain interference [61]. Athletes experience significant mood changes throughout rehabilitation, which may hinder rehabilitation early in the process [62, 63]. Catastrophizing behavior patterns and depressive symptoms are associated with more severe pain and worse function after traumatic lower extremity injury. Depressive symptoms at 4 weeks were associated with pain intensity, pain interference, and physical health at 1 year [61]. Therefore, athletes with high fear of reinjury may benefit from a psychologically informed practice approach to improve rehabilitation outcomes through destigmatizing and decatastrophizing the impact of injury [63, 64].

Much has been made of the link between concussion and depression. However, athletes with ACL injury reported higher levels of depressive symptoms for a longer duration than athletes with concussion [65]. This finding highlights that any significant injury can trigger mental health concerns.

The process of rehabilitation is an important time during which mental health concerns may be identified and addressed. Athletic trainers have routine contact with athletes recovering from injury and are well positioned to monitor the mental well-being of the injured athlete [66]. Mood disturbance can associate with the athlete's perceived progress in rehabilitation and, poor outlook and mood has been shown to negatively relate to adherence to a rehabilitation program [62, 67]. Current studies suggest that mental health screening in this setting should be undertaken carefully, gently, and longitudinally through the entire injury recovery process [68]. Each athlete has their own unique nature of pain perception and coping strategies, but clinicians should consider screening for pain catastrophizing for athletes not following an expected recovery process [69].

For patients with acute low back pain, the Fear-Avoidance Beliefs Questionnaire (FAB-Q) screen is an independent outcome factor predicting recovery [70, 71]. General assessment of fear-avoidance beliefs using the FABQ-PA can be appropriate for use in patients with various musculoskeletal pain conditions [72]. While the FAB-Q and the FABQ-PA are useful questionnaires, another questionnaire with good internal and external validity is the Athlete Fear Avoidance Questionnaire (AFAQ) [73]. The AFAQ is a scale that measures sport-injury-related fear avoidance in athletes and could be used to identify potential psychological barriers to rehabilitation. AFAQ has high internal consistency with a Cronbach α coefficient of 0.805 [73]. The AFAQ benefits from having been designed specifically for the injured athlete population.

In injured athletes with high fear avoidance or pain catastrophizing, interventions such as positive self-talk, relaxation, goal setting and healing imagery can be appropriate to assist them in coping with injury [74, 75]. Using optimism can decrease the negative influence of pain catastrophizing in athletes, but optimism does not alter the influence of fear-avoidance beliefs [76]. Short mindfulness video exercise may be effective in improving momentary pain, anxiety, depression, and fear avoidance in the injured population.

Substance Abuse

Substance use is the most common health risk behavior among adolescents [77]. Substance use is an increasing concern in high school, college athletes, and of course professional athletes. Universal screening of adolescents can be useful in identifying substance use early, before further problems develop and when treatment is more likely to be effective. Screening in and of itself may have some therapeutic effect [77]. Screening can be difficult as the fear of punishment and stigma of substance use may preclude an athlete from being honest when screened. In fact, most athletes prefer that providers not directly ask about substance use [78]. Random drug testing is often the only screening tool utilized in college, professional, and Olympic athletes [79]. There is a lack of high-quality research on screening athletes for recreational drug use and other substance abuse. Most athletic institutions do screenings by large-scale surveys of the entire student body to develop prevention strategies.

Alcohol Abuse

Unlike for performance enhancing or recreational drugs, no collegiate or professional associations employ blood testing for alcohol abuse in athletes. Thus, providers have to rely on screening tools and a willingness of athletes to discuss their alcohol intake. Athletes at many levels are at high risk for alcohol abuse [80]. The National Institute on Alcohol Abuse and Alcoholism (NIAAA) recommends the Alcohol Use Disorders Identification Test (AUDIT) to screen a general adult population for alcohol abuse [81]. The AUDIT is comprised of ten questions and a score of 8 or above is considered a positive screen. The single question screen asks, "How many times in the past year have you had X or more drinks in a day?" where $X = 5$ for men and 4 for women. A response of 1 or more was considered a positive test [80]. A three-item version of the AUDIT, called the AUDIT-C, may also be used as a brief screening tool [82, 83].

Majka et al. compared the use of AUDIT to a single question screen in 225 athletes from the College of Charleston [80]. They found that the sensitivity and specificity of the single-question screen compared to the AUDIT was 92% and 55%. The negative predictive value (NPV) of single-question screen compared to the AUDIT was 95%. When stratified by gender, the single-question screen had a higher sensitivity in males and a higher specificity in females, while the NPV was similar in both genders (92.4% in females and 100% in males). Therefore, this one-question screen may be useful in ruling out alcohol abuse, while a positive screen can prompt a more thorough evaluation with the AUDIT.

Drug Use

It is rare for athletes to voluntarily disclose recreational or performance enhancing drug use, and hence anonymous surveys and self-reportings have been the mainstay in reviewing substance abuse in the athletic population [84]. There is no validated screening tool for drug use specifically in athletes and no brief validated tools for screening for drug use in the general population [85]. In addition, the USPSTF has stated that there is insufficient evidence to screen for drug abuse. However, the NCAA does mention the use of the Cannabis Use Disorder Identification Test (CUDIT-R) as a useful screening tool [86]. In addition, the Tobacco, Alcohol, Prescription Medication, and other Substance Use Tool (TAPS) has been studied in primary care offices as a brief screening tool with positive results [85]. More studies are needed to develop and validate appropriate screening strategies for substance use in athletes [87].

Conclusion

Mental health screening has shown promise and value in the athletic population, though much work remains to validate such tools for the athletic population. Screening and subsequent discussion regarding mental health concerns should be considered by the team physician and allied health professionals, including staff psychologists and team athletic trainers. Ideally, screening would take place on intake and following injury, and testing should be considered for depression, anxiety, sexual abuse, and alcohol and drug use in the appropriate context, particularly for at-risk athletes or for those athletes not following predictable recovery courses following injury.

References

1. Trojian T. Depression is under-recognised in the sport setting: time for primary care sports medicine to be proactive and screen widely for depression symptoms. Br J Sports Med. 2016;50(3):137–9.
2. Brown GT, Hainline B, Kroshus E, Wilfert M. Mind, body and sport: understanding and supporting student-athlete mental wellness. Indianapolis, IN: NCAA; 2014.
3. Siu AL, Bibbins-Domingo K, Grossman DC, Baumann LC, Davidson KW, Ebell M, et al. Screening for depression in adults: US preventive services task force recommendation statement. JAMA. 2016;315(4):380–7.
4. Mirabelli MH, Devine MJ, Singh J, Mendoza M. The preparticipation sports evaluation. Am Fam Physician. 2015;92(5):371–6.
5. Bonci CM, Bonci LJ, Granger LR, Johnson CL, Malina RM, Milne LW, et al. National athletic trainers' association position statement: preventing, detecting, and managing disordered eating in athletes. J Athl Train. 2008;43(1):80–108.
6. Conley KM, Bolin DJ, Carek PJ, Konin JG, Neal TL, Violette D. National Athletic Trainers' Association position statement: preparticipation physical examinations and disqualifying conditions. J Athl Train. 2014;49(1):102–20.
7. Kroshus E. Variability in institutional screening practices related to collegiate student-athlete mental health. J Athl Train. 2016;51(5):389–97.
8. Hammond T, Gialloreto C, Kubas H, Hap Davis H. The prevalence of failure-based depression among elite athletes. Clin J Sport Med. 2013;23(4):273–7.
9. Wolanin A, Hong E, Marks D, Panchoo K, Gross M. Prevalence of clinically elevated depressive symptoms in college athletes and differences by gender and sport. Br J Sports Med. 2016;50(3):167–71.

10. Kroshus E, Davoren AK. Mental health and substance use of sexual minority college athletes. J Am Coll Heal. 2016;64(5):371–9.
11. Roiger T, Weidauer L, Kern B. A longitudinal pilot study of depressive symptoms in concussed and injured/nonconcussed National Collegiate Athletic Association Division I student-athletes. J Athl Train. 2015;50(3):256–61.
12. Nelson LD, Pfaller AY, Rein LE, McCrea MA. Rates and predictors of invalid baseline test performance in high school and collegiate athletes for 3 computerized neurocognitive tests: ANAM, axon sports, and ImPACT. Am J Sports Med. 2015;43(8):2018–26.
13. Silverberg ND, Berkner PD, Atkins JE, Zafonte R, Iverson GL. Relationship between short sleep duration and preseason concussion testing. Clin J Sport Med. 2016;26(3):226–31.
14. Yengo-Kahn AM, Solomon G. Are psychotropic medications associated with differences in baseline neurocognitive assessment scores for young athletes? A pilot study. Phys Sportsmed. 2015;43(3):227–35.
15. Covassin T, Elbin RJ 3rd, Larson E, Kontos AP. Sex and age differences in depression and baseline sport-related concussion neurocognitive performance and symptoms. Clin J Sport Med. 2012;22(2):98–104.
16. Vargas G, Rabinowitz A, Meyer J, Arnett PA. Predictors and prevalence of postconcussion depression symptoms in collegiate athletes. J Athl Train. 2015;50(3):250–5.
17. Yang J, Peek-Asa C, Covassin T, Torner JC. Post-concussion symptoms of depression and anxiety in division I collegiate athletes. Dev Neuropsychol. 2015;40(1):18–23.
18. Galambos SA, Terry PC, Moyle GM, Locke SA, Lane AM. Psychological predictors of injury among elite athletes. Br J Sports Med. 2005;39(6):351–4; discussion −4.
19. Knapp J, Aerni G, Anderson J. Eating disorders in female athletes: use of screening tools. Curr Sports Med Rep. 2014;13(4):214–8.
20. Shanmugam V, Jowett S, Meyer C. Eating psychopathology as a risk factor for depressive symptoms in a sample of British athletes. J Sports Sci. 2014;32(17):1587–95.
21. Wippert P-M, Wippert J. The effects of involuntary athletic career termination on psychological distress. J Clin Sport Psychol. 2010;4(2):133–49.
22. Glick ID, Stillman MA, Reardon CL, Ritvo EC. Managing psychiatric issues in elite athletes. J Clin Psychiatry. 2012;73(5):640–4.
23. Neal TL, Diamond AB, Goldman S, Liedtka KD, Mathis K, Morse ED, et al. Interassociation recommendations for developing a plan to recognize and refer student-athletes with psychological concerns at the secondary school level: a consensus statement. J Athl Train. 2015;50(3):231–49.
24. Neal TL, Diamond AB, Goldman S, Klossner D, Morse ED, Pajak DE, et al. Inter-association recommendations for developing a plan to recognize and refer student-athletes with psychological concerns at the collegiate level: an executive summary of a consensus statement. J Athl Train. 2013;48(5):716–20.
25. Maurer DM. Screening for depression. Am Fam Physician. 2012;85(2):139–44.
26. Maurer DM, Raymond TJ, Davis BN. Depression: screening and diagnosis. Am Fam Physician. 2018;98(8):508–15.
27. Weigand S, Cohen J, Merenstein D. Susceptibility for depression in current and retired student athletes. Sports Health. 2013;5(3):263–6.
28. Armstrong S, Oomen-Early J. Social connectedness, self-esteem, and depression symptomatology among collegiate athletes versus nonathletes. J Am Coll Heal. 2009;57(5):521–6.
29. Yang J, Peek-Asa C, Corlette JD, Cheng G, Foster DT, Albright J. Prevalence of and risk factors associated with symptoms of depression in competitive collegiate student athletes. Clin J Sport Med. 2007;17(6):481–7.
30. Patten SB, Burton JM, Fiest KM, Wiebe S, Bulloch AG, Koch M, et al. Validity of four screening scales for major depression in MS. Mult Scler (Houndmills, Basingstoke, England). 2015;21(8):1064–71.
31. Keum BT, Miller MJ, Inkelas KK. Testing the factor structure and measurement invariance of the PHQ-9 across racially diverse U.S. college students. Psychol Assess. 2018;30(8):1096–106.

32. Smarr KL, Keefer AL. Measures of depression and depressive symptoms: Beck Depression Inventory-II (BDI-II), Center for Epidemiologic Studies Depression Scale (CES-D), Geriatric Depression Scale (GDS), Hospital Anxiety and Depression Scale (HADS), and Patient Health Questionnaire-9 (PHQ-9). Arthritis Care Res (Hoboken). 2011;63 Suppl 11:S454–66.
33. Baer L, Jacobs DG, Meszler-Reizes J, Blais M, Fava M, Kessler R, et al. Development of a brief screening instrument: the HANDS. Psychother Psychosom. 2000;69(1):35–41.
34. Siu AL. Screening for depression in children and adolescents: US preventive services task force recommendation statement. Pediatrics. 2016;137(3):e20154467.
35. Richardson LP, Rockhill C, Russo JE, Grossman DC, Richards J, McCarty C, et al. Evaluation of the PHQ-2 as a brief screen for detecting major depression among adolescents. Pediatrics. 2010;125(5):e1097–103.
36. Richardson LP, McCauley E, Grossman DC, McCarty CA, Richards J, Russo JE, et al. Evaluation of the patient health questionnaire-9 item for detecting major depression among adolescents. Pediatrics. 2010;126(6):1117–23.
37. Bell L, Wilfert M. Interpersonal violence and the student-athlete population. In: Brown G, editor. Mind, body and sport: understanding and supporting student-athlete mental wellness. 1. www.ncaa.org: National Collegiate Athletic Association; 2014. pp 84–95.
38. Kamm RL. Interviewing principles for the psychiatrically aware sports medicine physician. Clin Sports Med. 2005;24(4):745–69.. vii
39. Simon JE, Docherty CL. Current health-related quality of life is lower in former Division I collegiate athletes than in non-collegiate athletes. Am J Sports Med. 2014;42(2):423–9.
40. Schwenk TL, Gorenflo DW, Dopp RR, Hipple E. Depression and pain in retired professional football players. Med Sci Sports Exerc. 2007;39(4):599–605.
41. Backmand H, Kaprio J, Kujala U, Sarna S. Influence of physical activity on depression and anxiety of former elite athletes. Int J Sports Med. 2003;24(8):609–19.
42. Cosci F, Fava GA, Sonino N. Mood and anxiety disorders as early manifestations of medical illness: a systematic review. Psychother Psychosom. 2015;84(1):22–9.
43. Vahdat Shariatpanaahi M, Vahdat Shariatpanaahi Z, Moshtaaghi M, Shahbaazi SH, Abadi A. The relationship between depression and serum ferritin level. Eur J Clin Nutr. 2007;61(4):532–5.
44. Trojian TH. To screen or not to screen: commentary and review on screening laboratory tests in elite athletes. Curr Sports Med Rep. 2014;13(4):209–11.
45. Demartini B, Ranieri R, Masu A, Selle V, Scarone S, Gambini O. Depressive symptoms and major depressive disorder in patients affected by subclinical hypothyroidism: a cross-sectional study. J Nerv Ment Dis. 2014;202(8):603–7.
46. Annweiler C, Rastmanesh R, Richard-Devantoy S, Beauchet O. The role of vitamin D in depression: from a curious idea to a therapeutic option. J Clin Psychiatry. 2013;74(11):1121–2.
47. Black LJ, Jacoby P, Allen KL, Trapp GS, Hart PH, Byrne SM, et al. Low vitamin D levels are associated with symptoms of depression in young adult males. Aust N Z J Psychiatry. 2014;48(5):464–71.
48. Ju SY, Lee YJ, Jeong SN. Serum 25-hydroxyvitamin D levels and the risk of depression: a systematic review and meta-analysis. J Nutr Health Aging. 2013;17(5):447–55.
49. Bitsko RH, Holbrook JR, Ghandour RM, Blumberg SJ, Visser SN, Perou R, et al. Epidemiology and impact of health care provider-diagnosed anxiety and depression among US children. J Dev Behav Pediatr. 2018;39(5):395–403.
50. Li H, Moreland JJ, Peek-Asa C, Yang J. Preseason anxiety and depressive symptoms and prospective injury risk in collegiate athletes. Am J Sports Med. 2017;45(9):2148–55.
51. Julian LJ. Measures of anxiety: State-Trait Anxiety Inventory (STAI), Beck Anxiety Inventory (BAI), and Hospital Anxiety and Depression Scale-Anxiety (HADS-A). Arthritis Care Res. 2011;63 Suppl 11(0 11):S467–S72.
52. Spitzer RL, Kroenke K, Williams JB, Lowe B. A brief measure for assessing generalized anxiety disorder: the GAD-7. Arch Intern Med. 2006;166(10):1092–7.
53. Junge A, Prinz B. Depression and anxiety symptoms in 17 teams of female football players including 10 German first league teams. Br J Sports Med. 2019;53(8):471–7.

54. Kabacoff RI, Segal DL, Hersen M, Van Hasselt VB. Psychometric properties and diagnostic utility of the Beck Anxiety Inventory and the State-Trait Anxiety Inventory with older adult psychiatric outpatients. J Anxiety Disord. 1997;11(1):33–47.
55. Grossbard JR, Smith RE, Smoll FL, Cumming SP. Competitive anxiety in young athletes: differentiating somatic anxiety, worry, and concentration disruption. Anxiety Stress Coping. 2009;22(2):153–66.
56. McNulty KY, Adams CH, Anderson JM, Affenito SG. Development and validation of a screening tool to identify eating disorders in female athletes. J Am Diet Assoc. 2001;101(8):886–92; quiz 93–4.
57. Wagner AJ, Erickson CD, Tierney DK, Houston MN, Bacon CE. The diagnostic accuracy of screening tools to detect eating disorders in female athletes. J Sport Rehabil. 2016;25(4):395–8.
58. Hutchison M, Mainwaring LM, Comper P, Richards DW, Bisschop SM. Differential emotional responses of varsity athletes to concussion and musculoskeletal injuries. Clin J Sport Med. 2009;19(1):13–9.
59. Newcomer RR, Perna FM. Features of posttraumatic distress among adolescent athletes. J Athl Train. 2003;38(2):163–6.
60. Fischerauer SF, Talaei-Khoei M, Bexkens R, Ring DC, Oh LS, Vranceanu AM. What is the relationship of fear avoidance to physical function and pain intensity in injured athletes? Clin Orthop Relat Res. 2018;476(4):754–63.
61. Archer KR, Abraham CM, Obremskey WT. Psychosocial factors predict pain and physical health after lower extremity trauma. Clin Orthop Relat Res. 2015;473(11):3519–26.
62. Morrey MA, Stuart MJ, Smith AM, Wiese-Bjornstal DM. A longitudinal examination of athletes' emotional and cognitive responses to anterior cruciate ligament injury. Clin J Sport Med. 1999;9(2):63–9.
63. Psychological issues related to illness and injury in athletes and the team physician: a consensus statement-2016 update. Med Sci Sports Exerc. 2017;49(5):1043–54.
64. Hsu CJ, Meierbachtol A, George SZ, Chmielewski TL. Fear of reinjury in athletes. Sports Health. 2017;9(2):162–7.
65. Mainwaring LM, Hutchison M, Bisschop SM, Comper P, Richards DW. Emotional response to sport concussion compared to ACL injury. Brain Inj. 2010;24(4):589–97.
66. Trojian TH, Cracco A, Hall M, Mascaro M, Aerni G, Ragle R. Basketball injuries: caring for a basketball team. Curr Sports Med Rep. 2013;12(5):321–8.
67. Baranoff J, Hanrahan SJ, Connor JP. The roles of acceptance and catastrophizing in rehabilitation following anterior cruciate ligament reconstruction. J Sci Med Sport. 2015;18(3):250–4.
68. Arvinen-Barrow M, Massey WV, Hemmings B. Role of sport medicine professionals in addressing psychosocial aspects of sport-injury rehabilitation: professional athletes' views. J Athl Train. 2014;49(6):764–72.
69. Sciascia A, Waldecker J, Jacobs C. Pain catastrophizing in collegiate athletes. J Sport Rehabil. 2018:1–20.
70. George SZ, Fritz JM, McNeil DW. Fear-avoidance beliefs as measured by the fear-avoidance beliefs questionnaire: change in fear-avoidance beliefs questionnaire is predictive of change in self-report of disability and pain intensity for patients with acute low back pain. Clin J Pain. 2006;22(2):197–203.
71. Werneke MW, Hart DL, George SZ, Stratford PW, Matheson JW, Reyes A. Clinical outcomes for patients classified by fear-avoidance beliefs and centralization phenomenon. Arch Phys Med Rehabil. 2009;90(5):768–77.
72. George SZ, Stryker SE. Fear-avoidance beliefs and clinical outcomes for patients seeking outpatient physical therapy for musculoskeletal pain conditions. J Orthop Sports Phys Ther. 2011;41(4):249–59.
73. Dover G, Amar V. Development and validation of the athlete fear avoidance questionnaire. J Athl Train. 2015;50(6):634–42.
74. Smith AM. Psychological impact of injuries in athletes. Sports Med (Auckland, NZ). 1996;22(6):391–405.

75. Nippert AH, Smith AM. Psychologic stress related to injury and impact on sport performance. Phys Med Rehabil Clin N Am. 2008;19(2):399–418.. x
76. Coronado RA, Simon CB, Lentz TA, Gay CW, Mackie LN, George SZ. Optimism moderates the influence of pain catastrophizing on shoulder pain outcome: a longitudinal analysis. J Orthop Sports Phys Ther. 2017;47(1):21–30.
77. Harris SK, Louis-Jacques J, Knight JR. Screening and brief intervention for alcohol and other abuse. Adolesc Med State Art Rev. 2014;25(1):126–56.
78. Carek PJ, Futrell M. Athletes' view of the preparticipation physical examination. Attitudes toward certain health screening questions. Arch Fam Med. 1999;8(4):307–12.
79. Hadland SE, Levy S. Objective testing: urine and other drug tests. Child Adolesc Psychiatr Clin N Am. 2016;25(3):549–65.
80. Majka E, Graves T, Diaz VA, Player MS, Dickerson LM, Gavin JK, et al. Comparison of alcohol use disorder screens during college athlete pre-participation evaluations. Fam Med. 2016;48(5):366–70.
81. Stewart SH, Connors GJ. Screening for alcohol problems: what makes a test effective? Alcohol Res Health. 2004;28(1):5–16.
82. Garcia Carretero MA, Novalbos Ruiz JP, Martinez Delgado JM, O'Ferrall GC. Validation of the alcohol use disorders identification test in university students: AUDIT and AUDIT-C. Adicciones. 2016;28(4):194–204.
83. Campbell CE, Maisto SA. Validity of the AUDIT-C screen for at-risk drinking among students utilizing university primary care. J Am Coll Heal. 2018;66(8):774–82.
84. Terry-McElrath YM, Patrick ME. Simultaneous alcohol and marijuana use among young adult drinkers: age-specific changes in prevalence from 1977 to 2016. Alcohol Clin Exp Res. 2018;42(11):2224–33.
85. Gryczynski J, McNeely J, Wu LT, Subramaniam GA, Svikis DS, Cathers LA, et al. Validation of the TAPS-1: a four-item screening tool to identify unhealthy substance use in primary care. J Gen Intern Med. 2017;32(9):990–6.
86. Bonn-Miller MO, Heinz AJ, Smith EV, Bruno R, Adamson S. Preliminary development of a brief Cannabis use disorder screening tool: the Cannabis use disorder identification test short-form. Cannabis Cannabinoid Res. 2016;1(1):252–61.
87. Saitz R. Screening and brief intervention for unhealthy drug use: little or no efficacy. Front Psych. 2014;5:121.

Chapter 3
Depression in Athletes: Incidence, Prevalence, and Comparisons with the Nonathletic Population

Andrew T. Wolanin

Introduction

Mental health has become an increasingly important issue relevant to the care of athletes in the context of sports medicine practices. Increasingly, mental health concerns are highly prevalent in the general population and recent research points to similar prevalence in athletic populations. For example, Rice et al. [1] completed a systematic review of literature published on the mental health of athletes and offered that elite athletes have a similar risk of mental health disorders as the general population. In research conducted by the National Institute of Mental Health, 17.9% of American adults reported a diagnosable mental illness in the preceding year [2], showing the level of prevalence and the required attention and focus on mental health concerns. The last decade has witnessed an increase in research and attention on mental health issues in athletes, and there has been a noticeable increase in media exposure and public disclosures of mental health challenges by elite professional and collegiate athletes. This has led to policy development, such as the National Collegiate Athletic Association (NCAA) Mental Health Best Practices manual, which details guidelines for the screening, evaluation, on provision of mental health services for NCCA student athletes [3]. Among mental health concerns, depressive disorders are one of the most prevalent conditions that sports medicine professionals will encounter and manage, and this chapter will provide a review of the prevalence and risk factors of depression in athletes to guide sports medicine decision making and practice.

A. T. Wolanin (✉)
Wolanin Consulting and Assessment Inc., Bala Cynwyd, PA, USA
e-mail: andrew@wolaninconsulting.com

© Springer Nature Switzerland AG 2020
E. Hong, A. L. Rao (eds.), *Mental Health in the Athlete*,
https://doi.org/10.1007/978-3-030-44754-0_3

Prevalence

Studies on prevalence rates of depression in the general adult population have found that approximately between 16% and 20% of American adults have had at least one major depressive episode in their lifetime [4–6]. This rate of depression appears to be trending upward, with noted increases in prevalence of depression among younger Americans [7]. Of particular interest for sports medicine professionals is the prevalence of depression in athletes and particular risk factors that may help guide and manage evidence-based care of mental health issues in athletes. Research to date suggests that rates of depressive disorders and other mental health concerns may be higher or equal among athletes compared to the general population [1, 8–11]; however, there are likely differences between subgroups of athletes as well as degree of athletic participation (i.e., high school, college, or professional).

Prevalence rates for depression among athlete populations vary based on the exact nature of the population and the manner in which the prevalence rates are measured and estimated. Published in 2016, Wolanin, Hong, Marks, et al. [12] conducted a study investigating rates of depressive symptoms as measured by the Center for Epidemiological Studies Depression Scale (CES-D) and found that in a sample of 465 collegiate athletes, there was a 23.7% rate of clinically elevated depressive symptoms and a 6.3% rate of moderate depressive symptoms. This general level of depressive symptoms tends to be consistent across other recent research studies. For example, these findings are consistent with depression prevalence rates found by Yang et al. [13], who reported that 21% of college student athletes reported depressive symptoms. Likewise, Li et al. [14] measured depressive symptoms with the CES-D in athletes during the preseason period and found that 21% of athletes reported elevated depressive symptoms during this timeframe. Additionally, Beable et al. [15] conducted an Internet-based anonymous survey measuring depressive symptoms of New Zealand athletes using the CESD-R and 21% of participants in this sample reported symptoms consistent with clinical depression.

While most recent studies indicate that there are likely comparable rates of depression between athletes and nonathletes, some studies suggest that there may be protective factors for athletes for reduced depressive symptoms compared to the general population. For example, Armstrong and Oomen-Early [16] reported that a sample of college athletes across sports reported lower levels of depression than nonathletes and hypothesized that team support and the social nature of athletics may safeguard college athletes from developing depression. Furthermore, there is a foundation of studies and research that indicated that regular exercise serves as a protective factor against depressive symptoms [17, 18]. Factors such as these may provide explanation for studies such as the Proctor and Boan-Lenzo [19] study of college athletes and depression who found that male athletes baseball players reported fewer depressive symptoms compared to male nonathletes and nonathletes reported higher levels of depression (29.4%) versus the 15.6% of the athletes who met symptom criteria for a potential diagnosis of clinical depression.

   Mental health comorbidities are also a likely factor in the risk for depression, both in the general population [20], and also with emerging evidence in athletes. For example, Steven et al. [21] used CES-D data with athletes who had either a history of attention-deficit hyperactivity disorder, a history of concussion, or a history of ADHD and concussion, and a history of neither ADHD nor concussion. Their findings were that depression scores were significantly higher for athletes with a history of both ADHD and concussion than any of the other groups. Taken together, the general prevalence rate of depressed athletes is generally likely to be approximately 20%, consistent with the prevalence of the general adult population; however, there are unique environmental stressors and possible protective factors that may result in varied rates and severity of depression in athletes over the course of a season or career.

Gender Difference

Consistent with gender differences in depression in most populations [22], female athletes appear to have high prevalence of depressive symptoms compared to male athletes. Wolanin et al. [12] found that female athletes were 1.84 times more likely to experience clinically elevated depressive symptoms than male athletes, and Yang et al. [13] found that female student athletes were more likely (1.32 times) than male student athletes to report significant depressive symptoms. Storch et al. [23] also compared rates of depressive symptoms in athletes and found that female athletes reported experiencing depressive symptoms, social anxiety, and nonsupport to a greater extent than male athletes. More recently, Gorczynski, et al. [24] reported that in high-performing athletes, males were 52% less likely to report mild or more severe depressive symptoms compared to females. In contrast to most findings, a moderate-sized study of elite and amateur German athletes found that 19% endorsed depressive symptoms on the CESD consistent with a diagnosis of MDD (CES-D score of 22 or higher) with no significant gender differences [25]. In general, female athletes have higher rates of depressive disorders compared to male athletes, which is consistent with the general difference in the normal population; however, there may be situational or cultural factors that alter the gender difference in particular populations.

Risk Factors

Other than age and gender, there are risk factors for depression that are more unique to athletes and may increase the likelihood of depression. While these factors may differ between type of sport, culture, and even a particular coach or team environment, the four primary risk factors for athletes are level and type of sport, injury, career termination/retirement, and performance concerns.

Level of Athletic Performance

The type, level, and stage of career related to athletic performance appear to have differing influences on depressive symptomatology in athletes. Gorczynski et al. [24] conducted a study comparing levels of depressive symptoms based on level of athletic performance and participation. They concluded that female high-performance athletes and nonathletes have similar rates of depressive symptoms and that male high-performance athletes have comparable rates of depression to male nonathletes. Nixdorf et al. [25] found that 29% of amateur athletes endorsed significant depressive symptoms compared to 15% of elite athletes. In this study, those who were contemplating retirement, less than 25 years old, and participating in an individual sport had significantly increased risk of reporting depression. This study also demonstrated a significant correlation between general life stress and depressive symptoms.

Type of Sport

The type of sport may also be a factor in depression risk. Wolanin and colleagues [12] reported that track and field college athletes endorsed a statistically significant higher rate of clinical depression symptoms than those in team-based sports. Lacrosse players in this study had the lowest level of reported depressive symptoms, and there was variability among other sports. The authors noted that in an individual-based sport such as track there is only one fully successful athlete in any given event, while in a team-based sport half the participants are able to record a win. Age of specialization is also hypothesized [26] to be a factor in differences of burnout and depression rates between types of sports. While there is a paucity of research into the link between specialization and depression in athletes, there is research into burnout [27] and injury risk [28] based on early specialization.

Stage of career may be an important variable in determining depression rates in athletes compared to the general population. Yang et al. [13] used the CES-D in a large sample of college athletes and found that Freshman athletes with pain symptoms also reported more depressive symptoms. However, Wolanin et al. [12] without considering pain as a factor, found no statistical differences in level of depressive symptoms based on year of academic study in college athletes.

Injury

There is a complex and ongoing relationship between injury, performance, and depression or other psychopathology in athletes [1, 29]. For sports medicine professionals, this is a key interaction that should be attended to and understood in order to effectively provide services to athletes. Competitive athletics has elevated performance stress and numerous other stressors that may increase the prevalence of injury, trigger mental health concerns, or exacerbate depression of athletes who are prone to mental health issues [30–33]. Furthermore, after an injury occurs, the athlete's psychological response to the injury and the rehabilitation process may trigger depression or other mental health concerns, as well as reveal disorders including depression and other psychological or substance use disorders [16, 34, 35]. Brewer and Petrie [36] compared depression symptoms in a large sample of NCAA Division I college football players who had and had not experienced injuries. They found that athletes who experienced an injury during the previous year reported significantly higher depressive symptoms after the injury compared to a control group of noninjured football players. Interestingly, this research also reported that both groups of college football players reported high levels of depression symptoms, as 33% of athletes with an injury history and 27% of noninjured athletes could likely be identified as clinically significant depression on the CES-D. In another study, Leddy et al. [37] investigated depression symptoms in athletes following injury, and found that over half of the athletes (51%) who sustained an injury during the course of the research study reported mild-to-severe depression symptoms.

A limitation in the injury and depression research has been the use of self-report measures to gauge depression. Appaneal et al. [38] aimed to address this limitation by including two measures (semi-structured interview and self-report) of depression in their study examining NCAA Division I, NCAA Division II, and high school level athlete's postinjury depression symptoms. Their findings indicated that depression symptoms of injured athletes were elevated on semi-structured interview 1-week postinjury and continued for 1 month after injury when compared with healthy controls, while no significant differences between groups were found on the self-report measure.

There has been a recent popular and research-based discussion of evidence suggesting that sports-related concussions can lead to changes in emotional state and possible mental health concerns [39, 40]. Furthermore, there is some evidence to indicate that sports concussions may be associated with long-term mental health issues, specifically depressive symptoms, in certain specific athletic subgroups. In a self-report survey of a large sample of retired National Football League (NFL) players, the researchers found that the 9-year risk of a depression diagnosis increased with the number of self-reported concussions [41]. According to this self-report study, retired athletes who identified having three or more concussions were three times more likely to report also being diagnosed with lifetime depression compared to athletes with no self-reported history of concussions.

Strain et al. [42] conducted a study on a small sample of retired NFL athletes who underwent a magnetic resonance imaging technique known as diffusion tensor imaging scanning. Their findings indicated that specific brain areas were positively and negatively correlated with depression scores. They also identified measurement of brain differences and abnormalities that differentiated depressed from nondepressed athletes with 100% sensitivity and 95% specificity, and offered that diffusion tensor imaging is a promising biomarker predictor of depression symptoms.

Similarly, Hart et al. [43] conducted a neuro-imaging study measuring cognitive impairment and depression in a small sample of retired NFL players and reported a 23.5% prevalence of depression and a high rate of cognitive deficits compared with a control group. They concluded that cognitive deficits and depression symptoms appear to be more prevalent in retired NFL players when compared with those in a healthy control group.

While the correlation between concussion and depression warrants continued investigation, there is limited evidence to date identifying a causal relationship between concussions and depression as well as the difference between concussions and other sports injuries on depressive symptoms. For example, Mainwaring et al. [44] conducted a study to compare the differences between emotional response of athletes who had suffered a concussion compared with anterior cruciate ligament (ACL) injury. They found that athletes with ACL injuries had more severe levels of depressive symptoms and a longer duration of these symptoms compared to athletes who suffered a concussion. They concluded that athletes with an acute knee injury have a higher prevalence of depressive symptoms compared to concussed athletes. This research highlights the potential emotional impact of all types of injuries on athletes and underscores the need for sports medicine professionals to be in tune to the possibility of a depressive reaction to a various sport injury.

While mental health reaction to injury has been relatively well researched, preinjury depression may conversely be a risk factor for injury. For example, Li et al. [14] found that preseason depressive symptoms alone at preseason did not predict increased risk for injury during the season; interestingly, they reported that male athletes with symptoms of both depression and anxiety had a greater risk for injury than male athletes without co-occurring symptoms. It is possible that untreated depression and comorbid symptoms such as anxiety could result in symptoms such as concentration difficulties or poor self-care (i.e., fitness, nutrition, etc.) that could increase an athlete's risk of injury. This finding illustrates that need for consistent mental health screening in sports medicine practices prior to injury occurrence.

Career Termination

Career Termination is a major life transition for an athlete that can disrupt their interpersonal relationships, roles, and daily routines [45]. While this is a significant life change for many athletes, it does not inevitably result in psychological distress. For some individuals, athletic retirement is done effectively where they use the life skills developed as athletes to engage in new life opportunities and occupational endeavors. However, for other athletes, the lack of competitive sport participation and post athletic retirement stressors have been linked to behavioral difficulties and emotional distress [46]. For example, competitive athletic career termination has been correlated with depression, anxiety, increased hostility and anger, dysfunctional coping strategies, and substance abuse across multiple studies and samples [45, 47–49].

There are factors that sports medicine professionals should recognize in order to understand an athlete's psychological response to career termination. The first factor for attention is to understand if the athletic retirement is voluntary (i.e., individual decision to retire) versus involuntary (i.e., injury, contract isn't renewed) career termination. Involuntary career termination is more likely to negatively impact an athlete's mental health compared to voluntary career termination [50], and Wippert and Wippert [49] found that involuntary career termination of skiers was associated with significantly greater mental health symptoms, including depressive symptomatology. While depressive symptoms increased immediately following involuntary athletic career termination, the mental health symptoms decreased over time, suggesting that as athletes adapt to changes associated with career termination they experience a reduction in psychological distress. Alfermann et al. [51] found consistent findings in their research of a large sample of amateur athletes regarding the mental health effects of career termination, and reported that a planned retirement from sports was associated with fewer mental health symptoms (including sadness) when compared with those who had an involuntary and unplanned retirement.

A person's athletic identity, that is, the degree to which athletes define themselves in an athletic role, is an additional factor to understand in relation to the mental health impact of retiring from sports [52]. Brewer [52] found that athletes with a high level of athletic identity reported higher depressive reactions when responding to hypothetical career-ending injuries. Baillie and Danish [53] found that athletes rating high in athletic identity were prone to experiencing emotional and social adjustment issues after they ended their sports career and a high level of athletic identity also has been associated with elevated stress and anxiety following sports career termination [47]. Taken together, the stronger the athletic identity, and the higher is the risk of mental health concerns with high intensity and duration following retirement from sports [47, 51, 53].

While retirement from sports may be a stressor for many athletes, it may also serve as a reduction of stressors such as performance, injury, schedule, etc. that allows the individual to function well in life. Weigand et al. [34] found that depression consistent with a diagnosis was significantly higher among current athletes when compared to retired athletes, with 17% of current college athletes meeting the criteria for depression compared to 8% of retired college athletes. These findings indicate that voluntary sports career retirement for the college athlete does not necessarily put the athlete at higher risk for depression, but the findings may or may not be applicable to the athlete whose career is involuntarily terminated by injury or due to other causes.

Performance

It is not uncommon to observe significant emotional reactions from athletes after they experience a loss of the field or court. Depressive symptoms may develop at the end of a season or event as a result of a decrease in external reinforcement (i.e., money, endorsements, attention), behavioral deactivation (i.e., staying home), negative self-perceptions and evaluations, and feeling of helplessness or hopelessness about their future performances and career. Furthermore, athletes may be prone to experience depression symptoms when they suffer a catastrophic ("choking") athletic performance or when they have a slow decline in performance that results in less playing time or fewer opportunities to perform. Hammond et al. [10] examined the prevalence of performance-failure-based depression in a moderate-sized sample of elite swimmers, and found that 34% of the athletes had clinically elevated depression scores after athletic competition, but that the top quartile of elite performers had twice the rate of elevated depression scores. This study highlights that some high-performing athletes actually may be more prone to depressive symptoms when their performance outcomes are below expectation. Sports medicine professionals should be cognizant of the psychological consequences of losing or personally failing during competition and should understand that the expectations for athletic performance are likely influenced by the athletic environment, teammates, coaches, and family.

Social Desirability and Underreporting of Depressive Symptoms

A complicating factor in the assessment and management of depression in athletes for sports medicine professionals is the engagement in impression management by the athletes during sports medicine interactions and screenings. Many athletes are likely to portray themselves in a positive light as they believe that endorsing a mental health concern may result in a reduction of playing time or negative evaluation by a coach or other players. When athletes are administered self-report measures of depression or other mental health conditions, there are instances in which the positive endorsement rate is well below what would be expected [54] based on known prevalence data. In a large sample of Division I and Division III athletes, Gross et al. [55] found that 25% of athletes engaged in impression management during an anonymous depression screening. They further reported that the mean impression management score of athletes was similar to a forensic sample [56] who were trying to appear well adjusted as well as a pre-hire police candidate sample [57] who were being assessed for mental health concerns prior to working in law enforcement. These findings illustrate that athletes may view reporting depressive symptoms as undesirable due to the potential perceived cost to their athletic career, and the complicated nature of assessing depressive symptoms in sports medicine contexts.

Treatment Approaches

After navigating the process of identifying depressive symptoms in athletes, sport medicine providers are tasked with determining the level and type of treatment or referral that is best suited for the athlete in the context of their particular environment. While sports medicine must be vigilant to identifying depression in athletes, they must also cognizant of understanding the difference between a clinical condition and a normal performance concern for an athlete. For the athlete with clinical depression, there should be a multi-disciplinary team approach; this team may include a mental health provider familiar with athletes, a team physician or primary care provider, an athletic trainer, and if appropriate the family and coach and other professional support staff. This team approach is particularly relevant for athletes as depression may impact with recovery from an injury, delay return to play and result in a cyclical relationship between depression and chronic injury.

Cognitive behavioral therapy (CBT), acceptance-based therapy, and mindfulness approaches have all been used to treat athletes. Psychological treatment should be designed for the particular athlete and context of their particular sports and environment. CBT for depression in athletes focuses on the relationship between depressive symptoms, cognitions, and physiological states. For example, hopeless cognitions in athletes are the foundation of believing that they don't have the ability to achieve a goal or an outcome [58]. Many of these beliefs are identified as "cognitive distortions," which are distorted beliefs about one's self, the world, and future outcomes [59]. More contemporary cognitive-behavioral models of acceptance-based therapy, and mindfulness approaches focus on the relationship that a person has with their thoughts and emotions and that avoidance of the content of particular cognition results in reduced adaptive behaviors [60, 61]. To date, there are limited studies of randomized controlled trials of psychological interventions with athletes.

Psychotropic medications are often used as stand-alone treatment or in conjunction with psychological treatments. Prescribing practitioners should pay considerable attention to the potential side effects of psychotropic medications for depression that may hinder athletic performance. While there is limited research of outcome studies of various medications with athletes in the treatment of depression, an international survey of sports psychiatrists revealed that bupropion was the most often prescribed medication for athletes with depression without comorbid anxiety due to minimal weight gain and activating nature of the medication [62]. Selective serotonin reuptake inhibitors are also often prescribed to treat depression in athletes, and fluoxetine in particular has not shown to have a negative impact on athletic performance [63–65]. Other psychotropic medications for depression have limited research into their effects on athletes, and sports medicine professionals should consult with psychiatrists due to potential complications or side effects that may occur with other medication classes [66]. Psychiatric medication use in athletes is discussed further elsewhere in this book.

Conclusions and Future Directions

Sports medicine professionals need to recognize that approximately one-fifth of all athletes that they are providing services to may experience clinically significant depressive symptoms at some point. This mental health condition not only has an impact on the athlete's quality of life and well-being, but is also relevant to athletic performance and response to injury prevention and injury rehabilitation. While knowledge about the prevalence of depression is important, there is considerable research and applied work to be done to increase accurate identification of depression in athletes, and as importantly to deliver interventions to athletes that improve quality of life and help the athlete function as effectively as possible in an athletic arena. The last decade has yielded more empirical studies that have investigated the prevalence of depression in athletes; however, continued research is needed to identify subgroups of athletes that may be more prone to depression and temporal or developmental periods that may be high risk for athlete depression. There are likely certain events in athletics, particular sports, and windows of time during a season in which depression may be more prevalent and can guide allocation of personnel and resources to screen for depressive symptoms. More research is needed into the link between injury and depression, and how different types of injuries (i.e., concussion versus ACL) may have varied acute or chronic mental health consequences. While screening the right athletes at the right time is important, one of the biggest challenges of mental health in athletes is the difficulty in effectively screening athletes with face-to-face interview or self-report measures. As discussed in this chapter, impression management by athletes may render the many well-intentioned screening methods less useful since there tends to be a high degree of denial of any mental health symptomology in the athlete population. Consequently, sports medicine professionals need continued training and experience in understanding behavioral indicators of depression, rather than relying on the athlete to self-disclose their mental health symptoms. Further research is called for in the optimal evaluation, diagnosis, and management of depression in athletes.

References

1. Rice SM, Purcell R, De Silva S, Mawren D, McGorry PD, Parker AG. The mental health of elite athletes: a narrative systematic review. Sports Med. 2016;46(9):1333–53.
2. National Institute of Mental Health. The NIMH Depression Page. Available from: http://www.nimh.nih.gov/health/topics/depression/index.shtml. Accessed 6 June 2019.
3. National Collegiate Athletic Association. Interassociation consensus document: understanding and supporting student-athlete mental wellness. Mental Health Best Practices. http://www.ncaa.org/sites/default/files/SSI_MentalHealthBestPractices_Web_20170921.pdf. Accessed 39 July 2019.
4. Andrade L, Caraveo-anduaga JJ, Berglund P, Bijl RV, Graaf RD, Vollebergh W, et al. The epidemiology of major depressive episodes: results from the International Consortium of Psychiatric Epidemiology (ICPE) surveys. Int J Methods Psychiatr Res [Internet]. Wiley; 2003;12(1):3–21. Available from: https://doi.org/10.1002/mpr.138
5. Kessler RC, Berglund P, Demler O, Jin R, Koretz D, Merikangas KR, et al. The epidemiology of major depressive disorder: results from the National Comorbidity Survey Replication (NCS-R). J Am Med Assoc. 2003;289:3095–105.

6. Shim RS, Baltrus P, Ye J, Rust G. Prevalence, treatment, and control of depressive symptoms in the United States: results from the National Health and Nutrition Examination Survey (NHANES), 2005–2008. J Am Board Fam Med. 2011;24(1):33–8. https://doi.org/10.3122/jabfm.2011.01.100121.
7. Weinberger A, Gbedemah M, Martinez A, Nash D, Galea S, Goodwin R. Trends in depression prevalence in the USA from 2005 to 2015: widening disparities in vulnerable groups. Psychol Med. 2018;48(8):1308–15. https://doi.org/10.1017/S0033291717002781.
8. Bär K-J, Markser V. Sport specificity of mental disorders: the issue of sport psychiatry. Eur Arch Psychiatry Clin Neurosci. 2013;263 https://doi.org/10.1007/s00406-013-0458-4.
9. Frank R, Nixdorf I, Beckmann J. Depression among elite athletes: prevalence and psychological factors. Deutsche Zeitschrift Fur Sportmedizin [German J Sport Med]. 2013;64:320–6.
10. Hammond T, Gialloreto C, Kubas H, et al. The prevalence of failure-based depression among elite athletes. Clin J Sport Med. 2013;23:273–7.
11. Reardon CL, Factor RM. Considerations in the use of stimulants in sport. Sports Med. 2016;46(5):611–7.
12. Wolanin A, Hong E, Marks D, et al. Prevalence of clinically elevated depressive symptoms in college athletes and differences by gender and sport. Br J Sports Med. 2016;50(3):167–71.
13. Yang J, Peek-Asa C, Corlette JD. Prevalence of and risk factors associated with symptoms of depression in competitive collegiate student athletes. Clin J Sports Med. 2007;17(6):481–7.
14. Li H, Moreland JJ, Peek-Asa C, Yang J. Preseason anxiety and depressive symptoms and prospective injury risk in collegiate athletes. Am J Sports Med. 2017;45(9):2148–55.
15. Beable S, Fulcher M, Lee AC, Hamilton B. SHARPSports mental health awareness research project: prevalence and risk factors of depressive symptoms and life stress in elite athletes. J Sci Med Sport. 2017;20(12):1047–52.
16. Armstrong S, Oomen-Early J. Social connectedness, self-esteem, and depression symptomatology among collegiate athletes versus nonathletes. J Am Coll Heal. 2009;57:521–6.
17. Harvey SB, Øverland S, Hatch SL. Exercise and the prevention of depression: results of the HUNT cohort study. Am J Psychiatry. 2018;175:28–36.
18. Teychenne M, Ball K, Salmon J. Physical activity and likelihood of depression in adults: a review. Prev Med. 2008;46:397–411.
19. Proctor SL, Boan-Lenzo C. Prevalence of depressive symptoms in male intercollegiate student-athletes and nonathletes. J Clin Sport Psychol. 2010;4:204–20.
20. Lai HMX, Michelle C, Sitharthan T, Hunt G. Prevalence of comorbid substance use, anxiety and mood disorders in epidemiological surveys, 1990–2014: a systematic review and meta-analysis. Drug Alcohol Depend. 2015;154 https://doi.org/10.1016/j.drugalcdep.2015.05.031.
21. Steven GB, James MKJ, Toni TM, Davis M. Attention deficit hyperactivity disorder increases anxiety and depression in concussed college athletes. Neurology. 2018;91(23 Supplement 1):S27–8.
22. Piccinelli M, Wilkinson G. Gender differences in depression: critical review. Br J Psychiatry. 2001;177:486–92. https://doi.org/10.1192/bjp.177.6.486.
23. Storch EA, Storch JB, Killiany EM, Roberti JW. Self-reported psychopathology in athletes: a comparison of intercollegiate student-athletes and non-athletes. J Sport Behav. 2005;28:86–98.
24. Gorczynski PF, Coyle M, Gibson K. Depressive symptoms in high-performance athletes and non-athletes: a comparative meta-analysis. Br J Sports Med. 2017;51(18):1348–54.
25. Nixdorf I, Frank R, Hautzinger M, Beckmann J. Prevalence of depressive symptoms and correlating variables among German elite athletes. J Clin Sport Psychol. 2013;7:313–26.
26. Myer G, Jayanthi N, Difiori JP, Faigenbaum A, Kiefer A, Logerstedt D, Micheli L. Sport specialization, part I: does early sports specialization increase negative outcomes and reduce the opportunity for success in young athletes? Sports Health. 2015;7 https://doi.org/10.1177/1941738115598747.
27. Wall M, Côté J. Developmental activities that lead to dropout and investment in sport. Phys Educ Sport Pedagogy. 2007;12:77–87.

28. Jayanthi NA, Dechert A, Durazo R, Luke A. Training and specialization risks in junior elite tennis players. J Med Sci Tennis. 2011;16(1):14–20.
29. Putukian M. The psychological response to injury in student athletes: a narrative review with a focus on mental health. Br J Sports Med. 2015;50:1–5. https://doi.org/10.1136/bjsports-2015-095586.
30. Ivarsson A, Johnson U, Podlog L. Psychological predictors of injury occurrence: a prospective investigation of professional Swedish soccer players. J Sport Rehabil. 2013;22(1):19–26.
31. Ivarsson A, Johnson U, Anderson MB, et al. Psychosocial factors and sport injuries: meta-analyses for prediction and prevention. Sports Med. 2017;47:353–65.
32. Ardern CL, Taylor NF, Feller JA, et al. A systematic review of the psychological factors associated with returning to sport following injury. Br J Sport Med. 2013;47(17):1120–6.
33. Nippert AH, Smith AM. Psychological stress related to injury and impact on sport performance. Phys Med Rehabil Clin N Am. 2008;19(2):399–418.
34. Weigand S, Cohen J, Merenstein D. Susceptibility for depression in current and retired student athletes. Sports Health. 2013;5(3):263–6.
35. Wolanin A, Gross M, Hong E. Depression in athletes: prevalence and risk factors. Curr Sports Med Rep. 2015;14:56–60.
36. Brewer BW, Petrie TA. A comparison between injured and uninjured football players on selected psychosocial variables. Acad Athl J. 1995;10:11–8.
37. Leddy MH, Lambert MJ, Ogles BM. Psychological consequences of athletic injury among high-level competitors. Res Q Exerc Sport. 1994;65:347–54.
38. Appaneal RN, Levine BR, Perna FM, Roh JL. Measuring postinjury depression among male and female competitive athletes. J Sport Exerc Psychol. 2009;31:60–76.
39. Hutchison M, Mainwaring LM, Comper P, Richards DW, Bisschop SM. Differential emotional responses of varsity athletes to concussion and musculoskeletal injuries. Clin J Sport Med. 2009;19:13–9.
40. Mainwaring L, Bisschop SM, Green R, Antoniazzi M, Comper P, Kristman V, Provvidenza C, Richards D. Emotional reaction of varsity athletes to sport-related concussion. J Sport Exerc Psychol. 2004;26:119–35. https://doi.org/10.1123/jsep.26.1.119.
41. Kerr ZY, Marshall SW, Harding HP, Guskiewicz KM. Nine-year risk of depression diagnosis increases with increasing self-reported concussions in retired professional football players. Am J Sports Med. 2012;40(10):2206–12.
42. Strain J, Didehbani N, Cullum CM, Mansinghani S, Conover H, Kraut MA, et al. Depressive symptoms and white matter dysfunction in retired NFL players with concussion history. Neurology. 2013;81:25–32.
43. Hart JJ, Kraut MA, Womack KB, Strain J, Didehbani N, Bartz E, et al. Neuroimaging of cognitive dysfunction and depression in aging retired National Football League players: a cross-sectional study. JAMA Neurol. 2013;70:326–35. https://doi.org/10.1001/2013.jamaneurol.340.
44. Mainwaring LM, Hutchison M, Bisschop SM, Comper P, Richards DW. Emotional response to sport concussion compared to ACL injury. Brain Inj. 2010;24:589–97. https://doi.org/10.3109/02699051003610508.
45. Stephan Y, Bilard J, Ninot G, Delignieres D. Repercussions of transition out of elite sport on subjective well-being: a one-year study. J Appl Sport Psychol. 2003;15:354–71.
46. Murphy SM. Transitions in competitive sport: maximizing individual potential. In: Murphy SM, editor. Sport psychology interventions. Champaign, IL: Human Kinetics; 1995. p. 331–46.
47. Grove JR, Lavallee D, Gordon S. Coping with retirement from sport: the influence of athletic identity. J Appl Sport Psychol. 1997;9:191–203.
48. Wippert PM, Wippert J. Perceived stress and prevalence of traumatic stress symptoms following athletic career termination. J Clin Sport Psychol. 2008;2:1–16.
49. Wippert PM, Wippert J. The effects of involuntary athletic career termination on psychological distress. J Clin Sport Psychol. 2010;4:133–49.
50. Erpic SC, Wylleman P, Zupancic M. The effect of athletic and non-athletic factors on sports career termination process. Psychol Sport Exerc. 2004;5:45–59.

51. Alfermann D, Stambulova N, Zemaityte A. Reactions to sport career termination: a cross national comparison of German, Lithuanian, and Russian athletes. Psychol Sport Exerc. 2004;5:61–75.
52. Brewer BW. Self-identity and specific vulnerability to depressed mood. J Pers. 1993;61:343–64.
53. Baillie PH, Danish SJ. Understanding the career transition of athletes. Sport Psychol. 1992;6(1):77–98.
54. DiPasquale LD, Petrie TA. Prevalence of disordered eating: a comparison of male and female collegiate athletes and nonathletes. J Clin Sport Psychol. 2013;7:186–97. https://doi.org/10.1123/jcsp.7.3.186.
55. Gross M, Moore ZE, Gardner FL, Wolanin AT, Pess R, Marks D. An empirical examination comparing the mindfulness-acceptance-commitment approach and psychological skills training for the mental health and sport performance of female student athletes. Int J Sport Exerc Psychol. 2016:1–21. https://doi.org/10.1080/1612197X.2016.1250802.
56. Andrews P, Meyer RG. Marlowe-Crowne social desirability scale and short form-C: forensic norms. J Clin Psychol. 2003;59(4):483–92. https://doi.org/10.1002/jclp.10136.
57. Greenberg B, Weiss PJ. Validation of a short form of the Marlowe-Crowne for use with law enforcement personnel. J Police Crim Psychol. 2012;27(2):123–8. https://doi.org/10.1007/s11896-012-9100-z.
58. Abramson LY, Metalsky GI, Alloy LB. Hopelessness depression: a theory-based subtype of depression. Psychol Rev. 1989;96:358–72. https://doi.org/10.1037/0033-295X.96.2.358.
59. Beck AT, Rush AJ, Shaw BF, Emery G. Cognitive therapy of depression. New York, NY: Guilford; 1979.
60. Hayes SC, Strosahl KD, Wilson KG. Acceptance and commitment therapy: the process and practice of mindful change. 2nd ed. New York, NY: Guilford; 2011.
61. Segal ZV, Williams JMG, Teasdale JD. Mindfulness-based cognitive therapy for depression. 2nd ed. New York, NY: Guilford Press; 2012.
62. Reardon CL, Creado S. Psychiatric medication preferences of sports psychiatrists. Phys Sportsmed. 2016;44:397–402.
63. Parise G, Bosman MJ, Boecker DR, et al. Selective serotonin reuptake inhibitors: their effect on high-intensity exercise performance. Arch Phys Med Rehabil. 2001;82:867–71.
64. Glick ID, Stillman MA, Reardon CL, et al. Managing psychiatric issues in elite athletes. J Clin Psychiatry. 2012;73:640–4.
65. Johnston A, McAllister-Williams RH. Psychotropic drug prescribing. In: Currie A, Owen B, editors. Sports psychiatry. Oxford: Oxford University Press; 2016. p. 133–43.
66. Reardon CL. The sports psychiatrist and psychiatric medication. Int Rev Psychiatry. 2016;28:606–13.

Chapter 4
Athletic Suicide

Ashwin L. Rao

Introduction

Suicide is a global health problem affecting countless communities and impacting individuals of all backgrounds. A person dies from suicide every 40 s, and many more make suicide attempts [1]. By no means are athletic communities immune to these tragic events. When an athlete dies from suicide, there is an inevitable sense of preventable loss, grief, and surprise among friends, family, coaches, teammates, staff, and the communities in which they had lived and interacted. Unfortunately, explaining why any individual would take his or her life is difficult. Athletes are perceived as among the healthiest members of their communities, and they are regularly perceived as models of health and wellness worthy of role-model status among their peers. It is thus challenging to reconcile this identity against the vulnerability to mental health concerns that many athletes experience.

Media reports covering these tragedies broaden and magnify the impact of these tragedies to even larger communities while attempting to provide closure and an explanation. In recent years, the suicide deaths of such prominent athletes as Junior Seau (Football), Dave Mirra (X-sports/BMX), Wade Belak (Hockey), Ryan Freel (baseball), Tyler Hilinski (NCAA), Maddie Holleran (Track and Field), and Giulia Albini (handball) have demonstrated suicide as a growing concern in athletic communities [2–8]. These prominent deaths also suggest that no sport, culture, gender, identity, or ethnicity is spared from the threat of suicide. The stories also suggest that many athletes wrestle with mental health in the shadows. In some instances, their struggles are complicated by substance abuse, violent behavior, financial

A. L. Rao (✉)
Department of Family Medicine and Section of Sports Medicine, Sports Medicine Fellowship, University of Washington, Seattle, WA, USA

UW Husky Athletics and Seattle Seahawks, Seattle, WA, USA
e-mail: ashwin@uw.edu

© Springer Nature Switzerland AG 2020
E. Hong, A. L. Rao (eds.), *Mental Health in the Athlete*,
https://doi.org/10.1007/978-3-030-44754-0_4

hardship, and deviant behavior, but in other instances, athletes die from suicide without clear explanation. This lack of certainly has led many media reports to attribute suicidal behavior to tangible problems, in particular brain injury. In turn, youth participation in contact sports such as football has dropped due to fears regarding player safety [9, 10]. Whether or not these associations will be supported by clear causal attribution remains to be seen, but until then, these attributions will continue to impact how athletic suicide is perceived.

A number of studies have begun to ask whether athletes are at the same, greater or lesser risk of suicide than their nonathletic peers [11–15]. Regardless of risk, the growing recognition of mental health concerns in athletes has led the medical profession to suggest that mental health be given its on platform for consideration, discussion, and management. Athletic departments are increasingly providing resources, including staff psychologists and mental health professionals equipped with the skills to manage athletes suffering mental health disorders or crises [16, 17]. While physicians remain reticent to discuss mental health issues with athletes, increased suicide awareness has promoted a greater effort to screen athletes entering and existing within athletic communities at all levels.

Defining Suicide

The CDC defines suicide as death caused by self-directed injurious behavior with intent to die as a result of that behavior [18]. A suicide attempt involves a nonfatal, self-directed, potential injurious event with intent to die as a result of that behavior, which may or may not incur injury. Suicide may include the following contexts: (1) the death of a person who intended to only injure themselves but died as a result of their attempt; (2) individuals who initially planned to kill themselves, changed their mind, but died as a result of an attempt; (3) deaths associated with risk-taking behavior unintended to inflict death, but with associated high risk of death; (4) suicides that occurred while under the influence of drugs or alcohol taken voluntarily; (5), suicide that occurred under the influence of a mental illness; and (6) suicides involving another person who provides passive assistance. The following ICD-10 codes may be used to define suicide X60-X84, Y87.0, and U03 [19].

Suicidal ideation involves the thought, consideration, and/or planning of a suicide attempt. Not all self-inflicted deaths are suicides. For example, accidental drowning, without the intent to take one's own life, would not qualify as suicide. Thus, non-suicidal self-injury may be defined as behavior that is self-directed and deliberately results in injury, without suicidal intent.

Scope of Suicide

One in five people harbor a severe mental health condition that places them at greatest risk for suicide [20]. In the United States alone, suicide is the tenth overall leading cause of death [21]. In 2016, there were 44,965 reported suicide deaths (123/day). For every suicide death, there are 12 suicide attempts [22]. Males are over three times as likely to die from suicide as females, though females are more likely to attempt suicide [SOURCE]. Males are in fact more likely to utilize a firearm in suicide attempts than women, imparting a higher suicide rate in males through the use of lethal means [23, 24]. Firearm fatalities account for 51% of all suicide deaths [25].

The highest rates of suicide occur in adults in middle age (ago 45–54; 19.7/100,000), while the second highest age-specific risk group is the elderly (age 85 or older, 19.0) [26]. A 2016 National Survey of Drug Use and Mental Health estimates that 0.5% of all adults age 18 and older have made at least one suicide attempt [27]. While adolescents and young adolescents and young adults have a lower comparative risk (13.2/100,000), suicide is the third leading cause of death in this demographic group. A 2017 Youth Risk Behavior Survey assessment noted that 7.4% of youth in grades 9–12 made at least one suicide attempt in the prior 12 months, with girls attempting suicide twice as often as boys [28].

Suicide is the second leading cause of death among students enrolled in college, trailing only accidents [29]. Alarmingly, suicide rates in the young have climbed gradually over the past 15 years, despite greater awareness and an increased emphasis on prevention [30]. In fact, suicide is one of only three causes of death that are on the rise among the young in the United States [31].

Method of Death from Suicide

In 2015 alone, 500,000 people were hospitalized for suicidal attempts, and data from the CDC suggests that the rate of attempts is increasing [30]. While suicide methods vary by age, gender, and cultural background, lethality of means imparts the biggest risk of successfully completing a suicidal attempt [19]. Nearly half (48.5%) of all people dying from suicide in the United States utilize a firearm. Conversely, suicide is the leading cause of firearm fatality, accounting for two-thirds of firearm fatalities nationally.

Suffocation, typically by hanging, represents the second leading cause of death in the general population, accounting for 28.9% of cases, followed by poisonings and overdose from prescription medication, nonprescription medications, and other chemicals (14.7%). The vast majority of poisonings and overdoses relate to the misuse of prescription medications. Poisoning is the leading means of nonfatal suicidal attempts leading to hospitalization [19].

The Athletic Environment – Risk Factors for Suicide

Athletes at all levels of competition experience stressors that impact their mental health in both common and unique ways. Athletes and nonathletes alike face age-specific risk factors such as a desire for social inclusion, academic achievement, maintaining body image, developing a self-identity, managing family stressors and conflict, and coping with illness. Social media platforms such as Twitter, Instagram, and Facebook, represent new and challenging forums for communication. While these platforms are capable of providing athletes and nonathletes alike with an independent voice and receptive audience, they have also become known as venues for anonymous cyberbullying and cyberhazing [32].

Unlike those who do not compete in sports, athletes routinely possess an identity tied to their participation and success on the playing field. As athletes are identified as pillars of health and wellness, and while this may be the case in some aspects of their lives, they often struggle with mental health in the shadows. Further, the nature of the commitments required to achieve success at the collegiate or professional level leads to an "all-in" mentality, and many athletes consume themselves with their athletic pursuits at the exclusion of developing other facets of their life [33]. Athletes are faced with competing responsibilities to their vocation, their personal lives, and in many cases, to their education or other financial interests. They are faced with the expectations imposed upon them by friends, family, coaches, teammates, and, most importantly, themselves. They may be challenged by the impositions of bullying and hazing upon their identity, social fabric, and well-being. They may contend with the challenges of mental illness, disrupted social and family support, substance and alcohol use, and addiction, as many others do, all the while trying to compete on the playing field often while hiding their struggles in these other arenas of life. Adding to this are factors such as time lost to competition and identity from injury. In recent years, the specter of long-term consequences imparted by brain injury and body injury alike forces many athletes to reconsider their pursuits, and in some cases, their careers for fear of sacrificing their long-term well-being [34].

Adding to the challenge facing athletes is the culture of sport itself, which looks down upon perceived emotional frailty and mental illness. Terms such as "choking," "folding under pressure," "getting the yips" indicate failures in performance related to mental, rather than physical, lapses and have the potential to define the athlete's mental health in unfavorable terms, adding another element of judgment to which an athlete must respond.

As athletes progress toward collegiate and professional competition, the stakes can increase dramatically. For the collegiate or professional athlete, not only is athletic participation at play, but also financial well-being or long-term career prospects. Student-athletes are faced with the challenge of balancing academic performance while trying to excel athletically. The demands of a rigorous practice and competition schedule can weigh heavily on performance in the classroom, and many athletes are forced to prioritize their sports performance over academic achievement [35, 36]. While academic performance can dictate athletic eligibility, successful athletic performance may be necessary for an athlete to maintain his or her athletic scholarship, adding a further twist to the stress and requirements imposed upon scholarship athletes.

Once an athlete has successfully navigated their amateur or collegiate experience and elected to "go pro," additional challenges lie ahead. Many athletes describe an incredible pressure to succeed, having been perceived as "making it" to the professional level. This expectation is countered by the reality that competition at the professional level is stark. For example, the average NFL career lasts 3.3 years, while the typical NBA and MBL career is 5 years [37–39]. In baseball, one in five position players at the major league level has a career that lasts only 1 year. Considering the time and investment placed by so many athletes who hope to play professionally, the harsh reality that the average career only lasts 3–5 years may impart an incredible stress that easily can disturb mental health, even for the most successful athlete [40].

There are a number of suicide risk factors to consider when considering the care of athletes.

1. Gender: Young males, aged 15–24, are 3.5 times as likely as females to die by suicide [41]. Men are more likely to choose firearms as a method for their suicide attempt and thus their suicide attempts are more likely to be fatal [42]. Women are more likely to attempt other means to attempt suicide, including over-the-counter and prescription medications or chemicals [43].
2. Age: While individuals in middle age and the elderly possess the greatest risk of dying by suicide, suicide represents a greater relative risk of death to young people [41]. Suicide remains the second leading cause of death among the young, trailing only accidental death; 8% of individuals aged 15–24% report suicidal thinking. Suicidal ideation appears to be growing in younger people for reasons that are not yet clear [44].
3. Ethnicity and Race: White race is a significant risk factor for suicide [42]. White suicide rates have remained the highest among races (15.2), followed by American Indians and Alaska natives. White males accounted for 7 of every 10 suicide deaths in 2016. Black race imparts a lower risk (6.03/100,000). A number of societal, cultural, and behavioral factors are likely to contribute to these observed differences.
4. Risk taking: Athletes are more likely than their nonathlete peers to consider high-risk activities [45, 46]. Drug and alcohol use and abuse are prevalent in athletic culture and are often tied closely to socialization, bullying, and hazing. Athletes who are depressed and suicidal, exhibit behavior change and may become more vulnerable to substance misuse and inappropriate risk taking, thus positioning then at risk when coupled with their vulnerable state.
5. Bullying and hazing: Bullying and hazing are forms of interpersonal violence in which a power-differential exists or is implied, with resulting consequences. Such behaviors have become increasingly recognized and are commonplace in amateur, collegiate, and professional sports. Prevalence estimates for bullying and hazing vary widely [47, 48]. A study of US high schools reports that 43% of all students are hazed per year, while nearly 80% of NCAA athletes report some level of hazing at the collegiate level [49, 50]. The International Olympic Committee has acknowledged the impact of bullying in Olympic athletic culture and has drafted a document to summarize its impact upon vulnerable populations [51]. Those who suffer from mental illness are more vulnerable to the

negative impacts of such behavior, and by virtue of their emotional frailty, can become the targets of bullying and hazing at moments in which they are most vulnerable.

6. Sexual misconduct. Increasingly recognized in the athletic community is sexual misconduct. Estimates for sexual misconduct and abuse prevalence vary widely by sport and gender, with rates of 19–92% for sexual harassment and 2–49% for sexual abuse [51–53]. A number of studies demonstrate a growing risk of abusive behaviors at the highest levels of sport. Team structures are often hierarchical, and younger athletes are expected to acquiesce to the whims of more established members of the team and coaching staff. Such power dynamics make sexual misconduct challenging to disclose, for fear of reprisal or other consequences. An athlete suffering in the shadows with the distress of being a victim of sexual abuse and assault can be one who sees suicide as a viable option for escape.

7. Financial distress: A number of financial factors can impact the mental health of athletes at all ages. Financial supports may permit or restrict youth athletes interested in playing certain sports that require a pay-to-play model. At the collegiate level, where athletic scholarship support can be revisited annually, athletes are faced with another stress that can impact their mental health [54]. Particularly for those contending with mental illness, performance can suffer, and the added pressure of financial support as dictated by their performance can serve as a difficult challenge to overcome. At the professional level, financial risk factors can be varied, including demand as imposed upon an athlete to maintain lifestyles, support family members and friends, and to attempt to perform to maintain their competitive status [55].

8. Injury. Athletic identity is defined in part by an athlete's ability to participate. When an athlete is injured, they are removed from the field of play, from their social supports, and from the rigorous schedules of their daily lives [56]. Athletes have to recalibrate their routines around their injury, and while many are offered the support of medical staff and the condolences and sympathies of coaches and teammates, the absence of participation can be a substantial stressor for an athlete's mental health [57]. The fear of inability to further participate due to serious injury can be traumatic both physically and emotionally, and an athlete may become suicidal in this context.

9. Concussion: Awareness of concussion and other forms of traumatic brain injury has increased in recent years, and numerous media reports have associated the deaths of prominent athletes from suicide with reports of history of repetitive head trauma and subsequent erratic behavior or cognitive deficit. While preliminary studies reveal an increased likelihood of depression for athletes suffering multiple concussions, there is not sufficient evidence to argue that concussion increases the risk of suicide in athletes [15, 34, 58–60].

10. Performance enhancing drug (PED) use: While the use of performance- enhancing drugs is widely reported through media coverage, studies of PED use among athletes is quite limited, and even more so, potential links to PED use and mental illness or suicide are sparse. A recent study evaluating substance use

among NCAA athletes indicates that only 3.7% of all student-athletes used amphetamines and 0.4% used anabolic steroids within the prior 12 months [61]. In this population, there were no associations drawn between PED use and depression or suicidal behavior, though a recent study of the same population identified higher risk-taking behaviors among those athletes who used PEDs [62]. Recent studies of professional Swedish power sports athletes demonstrate suicide mortality rates 2–4 times higher among former athletes compared to the general population and higher rates of mental health disorders among living athletes who used PEDs, leading the authors to consider widespread PED use in this group as a potential suicide and mental health risk factor [63, 64].

11. Retirement and end of career: Retirement and end of career due to injury or illness represents a life-altering moment in the life of an athlete. Retirement from competitive athletics is not often a choice, as it is in many other aspects of adult life, but is the result of performance decline or injury [55]. Competitive athletes have put in years of effort, time, and energy to their sport and faced with the prospect that their participation is no longer welcomed or permissible. Such moments force them to consider their own identities, prospects, goals, and future employment, and it is not uncommon to struggle in the face of these changes. A recent study of current recently retired former professional soccer athletes identified higher prevalence of anxiety and depression (39%) among retired soccer athletes (39%) compared to current players (26%), with a higher prevalence and greater diversity of psychosocial problems in the recently retired group [13].

The Athletic Environment – Supports

Athletes are routinely offered a number of structural, academic, and social supports that benefit their mental health. The social framework provided by teammates, coaches, and staff provide athletes with structure, friendship, routine, and commitment. An athlete participating on a team is less likely to be socially isolated and more likely to be monitored for performance and behavior. Athletes are more likely to have direct contact with a team medical provider such as a physician, athletic trainer, or physical therapist [65]. With more sets of eyes upon an athlete, dysfunctional or erratic behaviors are more likely to be recognized and addressed.

1. Social structure: Competitive athletes at all levels are granted a unique opportunity to immediately coexist among teammates, who offer friendship, mentorship, and shared competitive vision. Such ready-made social networks offer both pros and cons. Teammates often share similar values, identities, vision, and expectations, and it is common for athletes joining a team to identify immediately with their peers [66].

2. Coaching support: Coaches have a unique investment in the success of their athletes both on and off the playing field. Coaching and team activities provide a structure for social organization, which can provide athletes with a sense of

inclusion and purpose that help to reduce the burden of mental illness. It has been postulated that in the team environment, athletes may be protected, as their behaviors, including maladaptive, risk-taking, and suicidal behaviors, are more likely to be recognized and properly directed to medical care [66].

3. Parental support: Parents are likely to be highly involved in the lives of their children who play competitive sports. The amount of effort required for an athlete to successfully navigate the challenges and logistics of playing on a club, varsity, or professional team necessitates substantial parental effort. In this manner, parents can be more aware of any mental health challenges that their child may be facing and head off suicidal behavior. Prior studies have demonstrated that parental support decreases the risk of depression and suicidal behavior during adolescence, while also conferring reductions in risk taking, substance abuse, and delinquency [67–69]. Whereas depression may erode social supports and peer groups for those suffering from depression, parental support has been demonstrated to be more consistent and immune to more transient forms of social support.

4. Financial gain: For the most competitive and successful of athletes, financial support, in the form of scholarships, sponsorships, and employment provides additional support. Athletes from disadvantaged backgrounds may see athletics and its associated financial rewards as a means of escape. Successfully negotiating a professional contract or college scholarship can have substantial benefits for an athlete's well-being and outlook, while providing opportunities that may not otherwise be accessible.

5. Exercise as treatment: Finally, exercise itself may confer its own protective effect upon suicidal behavior. Exercise has been considered a strategy to manage and mitigate depression, and there is an emerging body of literature to support this claim [70, 71]. More research in non-athletic and athletic populations is needed to clarify associations and the potential for risk reduction of mental illness and suicidality, due to the risk of bias, study design, and other study limitations that currently limit available evidence.

Suicide in High School Athletes

Studies of suicide in athletes are limited in number. Early studies attempting to discern a relationship between participation in high school athletic programs and mental illness suggest that athletes are less depressed and less likely to have suicidal ideation [72]. The most notable research has involved the use of the Youth Risk Behavior Study conducted by the CDC annually [73]. These studies have focused more on suicidal behavior and attempts, as this survey does not track suicide events themselves [74]. Studies of complete suicide in athletes are not currently available, but a study of over 8000 high school student-athletes found that athletes did not differ significantly from nonathletes in reporting suicide attempts [12]. However, both male and female athletes reported lower rates of suicidal ideation and behavior than nonathletes, and female athletes were significantly less likely to consider or plan a suicide than their nonathlete peers. Notably, "highly involved" athletes were significantly less likely to consider suicide than nonathletes (OR 0.58–62, $p < 0.001$).

Suicide in College Athletes

A number of studies have approached suicidality and suicide events in the college athletic population. Initial studies reported that participation of a college sports team reduces the likelihood of considering, planning, or attempting suicide [75]. Male athletes are 2.5 times less likely to be suicidal than their nonathletic peers, while female athletes are 1.7 times less likely. Maron and colleagues reported a suicide and drug -related death rate of 1.3/100,000 over a 10-year retrospective analysis of the US National registry of Sudden Death in Athletes [76]. Rao and colleagues recently performed a 9-year retrospective analysis of an NCAA death registry, identifying 35 cases of suicide among 477 student-athlete deaths spanning greater than 3.7 million individual seasons [11]. They identified an overall college athlete suicide rate of 0.93/100,000, noting suicide to be the fourth leading cause of death among student-athletes, trailing accidents, cardiovascular pathology, and homicide. This same study found that males were 3.7 times more likely than females to die by suicide. Notably, football athletes had a relative risk of 2.2 of dying by suicide as other male college athletes. No specific differences were identified by NCAA division or race. In comparing suicide rates in the general population of college age (11.2/100,000) and published studies of death by suicide in college students (7.5/100,000), college student-athletes appear to be substantially less likely to die by suicide, suggestion that college athlete participation confers a protective benefit against suicide in this population (Fig. 4.1).

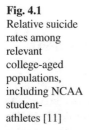

Fig. 4.1
Relative suicide rates among relevant college-aged populations, including NCAA student-athletes [11]

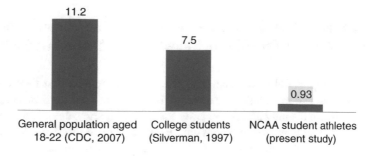

Suicide in Professional Athletes

A number of studies have evaluated suicide in professional athletes. A recent study of 5389 retired professional soccer athletes reported a suicide rate similar to that of the general Italian population [77]. Another study reviewing 214 deaths in current or recently retired soccer athletes from 2017 to 2013 revealed suicide as the third leading cause of death, following disease and accidents, accounting for 11% of all-cause mortality [13]. Due to increased media coverage around suicide in NCAA athletes and the associated debate regarding the potential for mental health consequences to repetitive head trauma and chronic traumatic encephalopathy, a number of studies have evaluated mortality in this population. While one study suggested an attribution of suicide to CTE based on neuropathologic findings of tauopathy on autopsy in a cohort of NFL athletes who died from suicide, a number of other studies suggest that the rates of psychiatric illness and suicide are lower in retired NFL athletes [15, 59, 60, 78]. Baron and colleagues, studying cardiovascular mortality in retired NFL athletes, found substantially lower rates of intentional self-harm in former athletes when compared with men in the general population [14]. Another study led by Lehman reviewing a cohort of 3439 NFL athletes credited with at least four playing seasons between 1959 and 1988 found that suicide rates were significantly less than expected when compared to the general US population (SMR 0.47) [15]. A recent meta-analysis reviewing the potential long-term effects of sports-related concussion notes that multiple concussions appear to be a risk factor for cognitive impairment and mental health problems in some individuals [58]. However, this study concluded that former athletes are not at increased risk of death by suicide.

Many questions regarding the absolute and relative risks of suicide in professional athletes remain. Numerous studies note that the causal relationships and risk factors for suicide in this population remain complicated and multifactorial. The emerging concerns regarding neurodegenerative mortality further complicate both the social and scientific discourse regarding suicide and mental illness in these populations. While most studies show athletic suicide rates to be comparable or less than the suicide in the general population of the same age, some have noted an increase in death rates from suicide in retired athletes from the 1980s forward, suggesting that the demographic and proportional risks may be evolving.

Management Strategies for the Suicidal Athlete (Role of Medical Provider in Suicide Identification and Prevention)

The responsibility for managing the suicidal athlete often falls upon the athlete's affiliated sports medicine care team. Historically, medical providers have lacked the adequate training and preparation for managing the suicidal athlete or dealing with the consequences to a community when an athlete dies from suicide. Prior studies of physicians suggest that while they are comfortable discussing physical health issues, many physicians remain uncomfortable discussing matters of mental health [79]. The goal of this section is to help provide a framework for better managing athletes and communities in mental health crisis.

While some groups have higher suicidal rates, every person is vulnerable to suicide depending on the circumstance and challenges they face. Individuals contemplating suicide are in emotional or physical pain. Previous or current mental health and substance abuse disorders are the greatest risk factors for suicide, and physicians and allied health professions should routinely screen for mental health disorders in their athletes. In some athletic settings, mental health concerns such as substance abuse or risk taking is dismissed or ignored as expected behavior. Further, sports culture does not routinely invite athletes to disclose mental health concerns [17]. In order for members of the medical and coaching communities to overcome their own intrinsic bias, mental health awareness and a willingness to engage in discussions around mental health must increase. Asking an athlete about suicide demonstrates compassion, concern, caring, and a willingness to support when support is most needed.

Medical providers (physicians, ATCs, team allied medical personnel) serve as critical core in the care of their athletes and are perfectly positioned to identify and manage many mental health concerns of their athletes. Two recent studies show that 90–95% of individuals who die by suicide have lived with a mental health disorder, yet only 50% of individuals who die by suicide were seen by a medical provider within a month of their event [80, 81]. Primary care providers are essential to the process of identifying, diagnosing, and following up individuals a risk of suicide. By failing to ask or engage at-risk athletes about their mental health during medical visit, or inviting athletes to discuss their mental health openly and frankly, providers are at risk for missing this important aspect of athlete health.

In order to participate at the high school, collegiate, or professional level, athletes are required to seek pre-participation clearance. These appointments provide opportunities for medical providers to introduce themselves as a resource to athletes for their physical and emotional well-being. By employing a systematic approach to the care of their athletes, members of the athlete's care team can become adept at identifying mental illness, understanding resources in the community, and assisting their athletes with reducing their risk of suicide. A number of widely available strategies for suicide prevention are publicly available for consideration, which can help to guide providers in gaining comfort in managing athletes at risk for suicide. For the sake of simplicity, this chapter summarizes the University of Washington Forefront Suicide Prevention Center's LEARN method, a 3 h online course that teaches point-of-care providers a systematic approach to suicide risk identification and prevention [82]. All physicians in the state of Washington are required complete this course in order to maintain their state medical license. The five steps in the LEARN approach include

- **L**ook for warning signs and risk factors
- **E**mpathize
- **A**sk and assess
- **R**emove dangers and restrict access to lethal means
- Identify **n**ext steps

The steps will be briefly summarized below. However, to secure the full value of this method, sports medicine providers should consider completing this course to prepare to care for suicidal patients, including those in the athletic setting.

Look

The first step of the LEARN method stresses that providers look for warning signs or risk factors that may increase the individual's risk of taking their life. Such signs may include behavior change, social withdrawal, increase in risk-taking activity, substance abuse, worsening symptoms of hopelessness or helplessness, or inappropriate or magnified shame and humiliation. Physicians should consider paying particular attention to patients who have recently suffered the loss of a family member or loved one, the loss of social standing, or financial support. For athletes, a loss of competitive status, through underperformance or injury may be impactful enough to prompt suicidal thoughts. Physicians should review and discuss any substantial behavioral change, such as alternation of sleep pattern, weight change, a change in eating behavior, activities of self-harm such as cutting or irrational risk taking, substance abuse, or giving away prized possessions. Providers should also be aware of patients who have a mental health history, including a prior history of suicide attempts or PTSD, or issues around gender identity or struggles to gain acceptance with their community. Such concerns are not always vocalized, so it is important that physicians and other providers interacting with athletes be aware and ask.

Empathize

Suicidal thoughts are a response to situations in which pain outweighs the capacity of an individual to cope with suffering. Patients can become focused on the task of suicide, developing tunnel vision around their death. As a provider who has identified a patient as suicidal, it is important to show empathy and listen without judgment. Acknowledging one's own inherent biases is an important step that providers must take in pursuing a nonjudgmental approach to the suicidal athlete. Finding empathy in discussions of suicidal behavior or thoughts can be particularly difficult for providers who have not themselves entertained thoughts of suicide or depression or for providers whose own personal experience or cultural makeup frowns upon suicide. Empathetic engagement emphasizes listening without judgment while remaining calm, understanding that the immediate goal does not necessarily involve solving the suicidal patients' dilemmas but rather to show understanding of their situation and to be willing to help.

Ask and Assess

Providers should consider using validated screening tools to look for depression and suicidal thoughts in their athletes. Commonly used tools such as the PHQ-4, PHQ-9, and Beck Depression Inventory include questions concerning a patient's suicidal thoughts. Such tools could feasibly be used as part of a pre-participation evaluation or annual health screen for their patients.

It is an uncomfortable task to ask a patient whether they have considered suicide, but it is necessary for a provider to do so when there is concern. It is important to ask questions directly, using words that do not pass judgment. For example, one can ask "are you thinking about suicide?" Compare this to the question, "Are you thinking of killing yourself?" The latter question implies a judgment around death, while the former asks a direct question without judgment. Similarly, provider should avoid double negative questions such as, "you are not thinking about suicide, are you?", as such questions provide an athlete with a means to evade a truthful answer.

When a patient opens up about suicidal thoughts, reflective listening and repeating the patient's own words to compel them to expand are nonjudgmental ways to express concern. Disclosing suicidal thoughts to another person, particularly a medical provider, can be a difficult experience for the patient. Once an athlete reveals their suicidal thoughts, they often experience relief. The provider should thank the patient for their honesty and their courage to disclose such difficult feelings. This approach permits the provider to ask about the suicidal athlete's plan, access to lethal means, and their timeline.

Remove the Danger

Once a provider has identified a suicidal patient, they should direct their patient to remove or limit access to potential means for suicide. For example, locking away, or limiting access to firearms represent a substantial barrier for those individuals considering taking their lives. The provider should not charge himself or herself with the task of separating a patient from a firearm but should engage that patient's on support network of friends or family to assist. For athletes considering taking their lives by using medications or poisons, similar steps can be taken to remove such substances or make medications available only at nonlethal quantities. Some medications considered to be lethal at high doses include NSAIDs, acetaminophen, hypnotics, opioids, and beta-blockers. Some medications used to treat depression or other mental health disorders, such as SSRIs, and hypnotics are also dangerous to the individual at high doses, and thus care should be taken regarding only insuring that the suicidal patient has access to nonlethal quantities of such medications. Tools such as medication lock blocks may be used to limit medication access. In many instances, even simple barriers to access can have substantial impacts on an individual's ability to carry forward a suicide attempt, as they prolong the time between the decision to attempt suicide and the actual attempt.

Next Steps

Sports medicine providers should encourage a recently identified suicide athlete to seek help through a number of resources and should be clear in providing instructions on how to access those resources. When an athlete is depressed or suicidal, any barrier to seeking care can be monumental, so the provider should be encouraged to follow-up with both the athlete and with referral sources to insure that continuity of care is established and maintained.

In the United States, every suicidal patient should be provided with the National Suicide Prevention Lifeline (1-800-273-8255), a national network of local crisis centers that provides free support to individuals in suicidal ore emotional crisis. This phone number is continuously staffed and free of charge. Patients considering suicide are encouraged to add this phone number to their contact lists, and even to "favorite" this contact for ready access if needed. Those who prefer texting should can "Hello" to 741–741 (Crisis Text Line), which triggers a response typically within 5 min of their text. Finally, patients in crisis may be directed to Crisischat. org, an online chat service of the National Suicide Prevention Lifeline in partnership with CONTACT USA. Please keep in mind that 911 is not an appropriate call unless the athlete is actively suicidal with a plan that they are attempting to enact.

Local resources for suicidal athletes may include, but are not exclusive to, local or campus counseling services, psychologists or psychiatrists who have access and are willing to take on a suicidal patient, staff psychologists for collegiate athletic departments or professional teams, or community mental health partners. Emergency room mental health partners (MHP) are available through most emergency rooms for patients who are actively suicidal with a plan, to consider whether inpatient mental health care is necessary. For athletes who require inpatient hospitalization, a sports medicine provider or affiliated mental health provider should consider an in-office visit, within 1–2 days of hospital discharge.

Summary and Conclusions

Suicide is an emerging concern with athletic communities, with profound and lasting impacts. Athletes struggle with a number of risk factors and personal challenges both common and unique to their experience. While the risk factors and support mechanisms for athletes are complex, athletes at all levels appear to be at lower risk of dying by suicide than comparable members of the general population. Physicians should undergo training to manage athletes identified as suicidal.

References

1. World Health Organization. 2018. http://www.who.int/mental_health/prevention/suicide/suicideprevent/en/. Accessed 21 Dec 2018.
2. Associated Press via CBS sports. 2012. https://www.cbsnews.com/news/junior-seau-found-dead-in-apparent-suicide/. Accessed 21 Dec 2018.
3. Miller L. Losing the will to die just before choosing death. The last days of "Miracle Boy." NY Mag. 2016. http://nymag.com/intelligencer/2016/04/bmx-dave-mirra-last-days.html?gtm=top&gtm=bottom. Accessed 21 Dec 2018.

4. Bishop G. A college QB's suicide. A family's search for answers. Sports Illustrated online. 2018. https://www.si.com/college-football/2018/06/26/tyler-hilinski-suicide-washington-state-qb-cte. Accessed 21 Dec 2018.
5. Fagan K. Honoring the life of Penn student-athlete Madison Holleran and continuing to 'Talk for Maddy'. ESPN. 2017. http://www.espn.com/espnw/voices/article/19859160/honoring-life-penn-student-athlete-madison-holleran-continuing-talk-maddy. Accessed 21 Dec 2018.
6. Hürriyet Daily News. Italian athletes commits suicide in Turkey. 2012. http://www.hurriyetdailynews.com/italian-athlete-commits-suicide-in-turkey%2D%2D21934. Accessed 21 Dec 2018.
7. Associated Press via ESPN. 2012. http://www.espn.com/mlb/story/_/id/8774575/ryan-freel-dies-apparent-suicide. Accessed 21 Dec 2018.
8. NHL.com. Wade Belak found dead in Toronto. 2011. https://www.nhl.com/news/wade-belak-found-dead-in-toronto/c-587564. Accessed 21 Dec 2018.
9. National Federation of State High School Associations. 2018. https://www.nfhs.org/articles/high-school-sports-participation-increases-for-29th-consecutive-year/. Accessed 21 Dec 2018.
10. Bogage J. High school football participation continuesto drop as concerns over cost, injuries pers. The Washington Post. 2018. https://www.washingtonpost.com/news/early-lead/wp/2018/08/28/high-school-football-participation-continues-to-drop-as-concerns-over-cost-injuries-persist/?noredirect=on&utm_term=.06225f9318d6. Accessed 21 Dec 2018.
11. Rao AL, Asif IM, Drezner JA, et al. Suicide in National Collegiate Athletic Association (NCAA) Athletes: a 9-year analysis of the NCAA Resoutions database. Sports Health. 2015;7(5):452–7.
12. Sabo D, Miller KE, Melnick M, et al. High school athletic participation and adolescent suicide: a nationwide U.S> Study. Int Rev Sociol Sport. 2005;40:5–23.
13. Gouttebarge V, Frings-Dresen MHW, Sluiter JK. Mental and psychological health among current and former professional footballers. Occup Med. 2015;65:19–6.
14. Baron SL, Hein MJ, Lehman E, et al. Body mass index, playing position, race, and the cardiovascular mortality of retire professional football players. Am J Cardiol. 2012;109(6):889–96.
15. Lehman EJ, Heln MH, Gersic CM. Suicide Mortality among retired National Football League Players who played 5 of more Seasons. AJSM. 2016;44(10):2486–91.
16. Moreland J, Coxe KA, Yang J. Collegiate athletes' mental health services utilization: a systemic review of conceptualizations, operationalizations, faciliators, and barriers. J Sports Health Sci. 2018;7:58–69.
17. Neal TL, Diamond AB, Goldman S, et al. Inter-association recommendations for developing a plan to recognize and refer student-athletes with psychological concerns at the collegiate level: an executive summary of a consensus statement. J Athl Train. 2013;48:716–20.
18. Centers for Disease Control. Definitions: self-directed violence. 2018. https://www.cdc.gov/violenceprevention/suicide/definitions.html. Accessed 21 Dec 2018.
19. Jack SPD, Petrosky E, et al. Surveillance for violent deaths – National Violent Death Reporting System, 27 states, 2015. MMWR Surveill Summ. 2018;67(11):1–32.
20. Merikangas KR, He JP, Burstein M, et al. Lifetime prevalence of mental disorders in U.S. adolescents: results from the National Comorbidity Survey Replication V Adolescent Supplement (NCS-A). J Am Acad Child Adolesc Psychiatry. 2010;49:980–9.
21. Centers for Disease Control. Preventing suicide. 2018. https://www.cdc.gov/features/preventingsuicide/index.html. Accessed 21 Dec 2018.
22. Centers for Disease Control. Suicide – Facts at a glance. 2015. https://www.cdc.gov/violenceprevention/pdf/suicide-datasheet-a.pdf. Accessed 21 Dec 2018.
23. Gender difference in males in attempt.
24. Gender difference in males in completed.
25. American Foundation for Suicide Prevention. Suicide statistics: https://afsp.org/about-suicide/suicide-statistics/. Accessed 21 Dec 2018.
26. American Foundation for Suicide Prevention. Suicide statistics: https://afsp.org/about-suicide/suicide-statistics/. Accessed 31 July 2018.

27. 2016 National Survey on Drug Use and Health: Detailed Tables. Substance abuse and mental health services administration, Rockville, MD. https://www.samhsa.gov/data/sites/default/files/NSDUH-DetTabs-2016/NSDUH-DetTabs-2016.pdf. Accessed 21 Dec 2018.
28. Centers for Disease Control. Trends in the prevalence of suicide-related behaviors. National YRBS: 1991–2017. https://www.cdc.gov/healthyyouth/data/yrbs/pdf/trends/2017_suicide_trend_yrbs.pdf. Accessed 21 Dec 2018.
29. Silverman MM, Meyer PM, et al. The big ten student suicide study: a 10-year study of suicides on Midwestern University campuses. Suicide Life Threat Behav. 1997;27(3):285–303.
30. Curtin SC, Heron M, Minino AM, et al. Recent increases in injury mortality amoung children and adolescents aged 10–19 years in the United States: 1999–2016. National Vital Stat Rep. 2016;67(4):1–16.
31. Centers for Disease Control. National vital statistic reports. https://www.cdc.gov/nchs/data/nvsr/nvsr67/nvsr67_04.pdf. Accessed 21 Dec 2018.
32. Van Geel M, Vedder P, Tanilon. Relationship between peer victimization, cyberbullying, and suicide in children and adolescents: a meta-analysis. JAMA Pediatr. 2014;168(5):435–42.
33. Bauman NJ. The stigma of mental health in athletes: are mnetal toughness and mental health seen as contradictory in elite sport? Br J Sports Med. 2016;50(30):135–6.
34. Rao AL. Athletic suicide – separating fact from finction and navigating the challenging road ahead. Curr Sports Med Rep. 2018;17(3):83–4.
35. Adler P, Adler PA. From idealism to pragmatic detatchment: the academic performance of college athletes. Sociol Educ. 1985;58(4):241–50.
36. Maloney MT, McCormick RE. An examination of the role that intercollegiate athletic participation plays in academic achievement: athletes' feats in the classrooms. J Hum Resour. 1993;208(3):555–70.
37. Statista Online Statistics Portal. Average playing career length in the National Football League. https://www.statista.com/statistics/240102/average-player-career-length-in-the-national-football-league/. Accessed 21 Dec 2018.
38. https://weaksideawareness.wordpress.com/2011/11/22/average-nba-career-length-for-players-details/. Accessed 21 Dec 2018.
39. Witnauer WD, Rogers RG, Saint Onge JM. Major league baseball career length in the twentieth century. Popul Res Policy Rev. 2007;26(4):371–86.
40. Erpic SC, Wylleman P, Zupancic M. The effect of athletic and non-athletic factors on the sports career termination process. Psychol Sports Exerc. 2004;5(1):45–59.
41. National Institute of Mental Health. Suicide statistics. Suicide. https://www.nimh.nih.gov/health/statistics/suicide.shtml. Accessed 21 Dec 2018.
42. Black SPD, Petrosky E, Lyns BH, et al. Surveillance for violent deaths – National violent death reporting system, 27 states, 2015. MMWR Surveill Summ. 2018;67(11):1–34.
43. Tsirigotis K, Gruszczynski W, Tsirigotis M. Gender differentiation in methods of suicide attemps. Med Sci Monit. 2011;17(8):PH 65–70.
44. Blader JC. Suicidal thoughts and behaviors increased amoung young adults. Why? JAACAP. 2018;57(1):18–9.
45. Nattiv A, Puffer JC, Green GA. Lifestyles and health risks of collegiate athltes: a multi-center study. Clin J Sports Med. 1997;7(4):262–72.
46. Kokotailo PK, Henry BC, et al. Substance abuse and other health risk behaviors in collegiate athletes. Clin J Sports Med. 1996;6(3):183–9.
47. Diamond AB, Callahan ST, et al. Qualitative review of hazing in collegiage and school sports: consequences from a lack of culture, knowledge, and responsiveness. Br J Sports Med. 2016;50(3):149–53.
48. Jeckell AS, Copenhaver EA, Diamond AB. The spectrum of hazing and peer sexual abuse in sports: a current perspective. Sports Health. 2018;10(6):558–64.
49. Hoover NC, Pollard NJ. Initiation rites in American high schools: a national survey. Alfrey, NY: Alfred University; 2000.
50. Hoover NC. National survey: initiation rites and athletics for NCAA teams. Alfred NY: Alfred University; 1999.

51. Montjoy M, Brackenridge C, et al. International Olympic Committee consensus statement: harassment and abuse (non-accidental violence) in sport. Br J Sports Med. 2016;50:1019–29.
52. Vertommen T, Schipper-van Veldhoven NHMJ, et al. Sexual harassment and abuse in sport. The NOC∗NSF helpline. Int Rev Spciol Sport. 2015;50(7):822–39.
53. Timpka T, Jason S, et al. Lifetime history of sexual and physical abuse among competitive athletics (track and field) athletes: cross sectional study of associations with sports and non sports injury. Br J Sports Med. 2019;53:1412–7.
54. Leeds MA, von Allmen P, Matheson VA. The economics of sports. New York: Routledge; 2018.
55. Taylor J, Ogilvie BC. A conceptual model of adaptation to retirement among athletes. J Appl Sports Psych. 1994;6(1):1–20.
56. Putukian M. The psychological response to injury in student athltes: a narrative review with a focus on mental health. Br J Sports Med. 2016;50(3):145–8.
57. Ardern CL, Taylor NF, Fellner JA, Webster KE. A systemic review of the psychological factors associated with returning to sport following injury. Br J Sports Med. 2013;47(17):1120–6.
58. Manley G, Gardner AJ, et al. A systematic review of potential long-term effects of sports-related concussion. Br J Sports Med. 2017;51:969–77.
59. Iverson G. Chronic traumatic encephalopathy and the risk of suicide among former athletes. Br J Sports Med. 2014;48:162–4.
60. Webner D, Iverson GL. Suicide in professional American football players in the past 95 years. Brain Inj. 2016;30(14–14):1718–21.
61. Bracken NM. Substance abuse – National study of substance use trends amound NCAA college student-athletes. Indianapolis, IN: NCAA; 2012.
62. Buckman JF, Farris SG, Yusko DA. A national study of substance use behaviors among NCAA male athletes who used banned performance enhancing substances. Drug Alcohol Depend. 2013;131:50–5.
63. Lindqvist AS, Moberg T, et al. Increased mortality rate and suicide in Swedish former elite male athletes in power sports. Scand J Med Sci Sports. 2014;24:1000–5.
64. Lindqvist AS, Moberg T, et al. A retrospective 30-year follow-up study of former Swedish-elite male athletes in power sports with a past anabolic androgenic steroid use: a focus on mental health. Br J Sports Med. 2013;47:96–9.
65. Dijkstra HP, Pollock N, et al. Managing the health of the elite athlete: a new integrated performance health management and coaching model. Br J Sports Med. 2014;48:523–31.
66. Schroeder PJ. Changing team culture: the perspectives of ten successful head coaches. J Sport Behav. 2010;33(1):63–88.
67. Borowsky IW, Ireland M, Resnick MD. Adolescent suicide attempts; risks and protectors. Pedatrics. 2001;107(3):485–93.
68. Hirsch JK, Barton AL. Positive social support, negative social exchanges, and suicidal behavior in college students. J Am Coll Health. 2011;59(5):393–9.
69. Macalli M, Tournier M, Galera C, et al. Perceived parental support in childhood and adolescence and suicideal ideation in young adults: a cross-sectional analysis of the i-Share study. BMC Psychiatry. 2018;27(18):373.
70. Kvan S, Kleppe CL, Nordhus IH, et al. Exercise as a treatment for depression: a meta-analysis. J Affect Disord. 2016;202:67–86.
71. Schuch FB, Vancampfort D, Richards J, et al. Exercise as a treatment for depression: a meta-analysis adjusting for publication bias. J Psychiatr Res. 2016;77:42–51.
72. Oler MJ, Mainous AG, Martin CA, et al. Depression, suicidal ideation, and substance abuse among adolescents – are atheltes at less risk? Arch Fam Med. 1994;3:781–5.
73. Pate RR, Trost SG, Levin S, et al. Sports participation and health-related behaviors among US youth. JAMA Peds. 2000;154(9):904–11.
74. Taliaferro LA, Rienzo BA, Donovan KA. Relationships between youth sport participation and selected health risk behaviors from 1999 to 2007. J Sch Health. 2010;80(8):399–410.
75. Dr B, Blanton CJ. Physical activity, sports participation, and suicidal behavior among college students. Med Sci Sports Exerc. 2002;34:1087–96.

76. Maron BJ, Haas TS, Murphy CJ, et al. Incidence and causes of sudden death in U.S. college athletes. JACC. 2014;63(16):1636–43.
77. Taioli E. All causes mortality in male professional soccer players. Eur J Public Health. 2007;17(6):600–4.
78. Mez J, Daneshvar DH, Kiernan PT, et al. Clinicopathological evaluation of chronic traumatic enceaphalopathy in platers of American football. JAMA. 2017;318(4):360–70.
79. Mann BJ, Grana WA, Indelicate PA, et al. A survey of sports medicine physicians regarding psychological issues in patient-athletes. Am J Sports Med. 2007;35:2140–7.
80. Ahmedani BK, Simin GE, Steward C, et al. Health care contacts in the year before suicide death. J Gen Intern Med. 2014;29(6):87077.
81. Nock MK, Ramirez F, Rankon O. Advancing our understanding of the who, when, and why of suicide risk. JAMA Psychiat. 2018;
82. University of Washington Forefront Suicide Prevention. All patients safe training for medical professionals. http://www.intheforefront.org/. Accessed 21 Dec 2018.

Chapter 5
Managing Psychiatric Disorders in Athletes

Claudia L. Reardon

Background

Management of psychiatric disorders in athletes is often provided by the sports medicine physician. Thus, a working knowledge of treatments for mental illness, especially with regard to the nuanced ways in which treatment should be undertaken with athletes, is critical. It is helpful if the sports medicine physician has access to consultation with and referrals to a sports psychiatrist as well, but that is not always available.

While treatment for mental illness, including treatment with medications in some cases, is important, there are numerous barriers that can impact an athlete's ability to get this type of needed treatment. The stigma of a mental illness or condition, particularly prominent among athletes, is one such barrier [1], as described earlier in this book. Likewise, athletes are often accustomed to having a team of providers to help them with medical conditions and treatments. Athletes may be less likely to attend psychiatry appointments, pick up psychiatric medication prescriptions, and take psychiatric medication regularly if they receive less support for this type of treatment compared to what they are used to with other physical ailments. For example, an athlete's trainer may accompany them to primary care sports medicine appointments, schedule those appointments for them, and arrange pickup of prescribed medications for medical conditions. That same degree of involvement may not occur with psychiatric treatment, and this may or may not be the preference of the athlete.

There are at least three important, unique considerations when prescribing psychiatric medication to an athlete: (1) potential negative impact on athletic performance; (2) potential performance-enhancing effects; and (3) potential safety risks.

C. L. Reardon (✉)
University of Wisconsin School of Medicine and Public Health, Department of Psychiatry, Madison, WI, USA
e-mail: clreardon@wisc.edu

© Springer Nature Switzerland AG 2020
E. Hong, A. L. Rao (eds.), *Mental Health in the Athlete*,
https://doi.org/10.1007/978-3-030-44754-0_5

Regarding the potential negative impact on performance, prescribers must keep in mind that even "minor" side effects can mean the difference between higher levels of athletic achievement (e.g., with the ability to ascend to the next level of competition or increase income potential) and lower levels of accomplishment. Side effects typically of greatest concern in this regard are sedation, weight gain, cardiac side effects, and tremor [2]. Even an apparently minimal degree of sedation or undesired weight gain, for example, could slow down a track and field sprinter's time by enough to impact their performance in a meaningful way. Similarly, performance-enhancing effects are an important consideration. Many sports governing bodies, e.g., the National Collegiate Athletic Association (NCAA) [3] and the World Anti-Doping Agency (WADA) [4], prohibit medications that have been found to have performance-enhancing effects. Moreover, even if a prescriber is able to obtain a therapeutic use exception (TUE) for a banned medication, there are ethical issues to be considered in terms of whether it is fair to prescribe such a medication for an athlete, particularly those competing at the highest levels. Finally, safety risks that exist with certain psychiatric medications, when taken by athletes exercising at high intensity, are paramount. For example, some medications can reach toxic blood levels in heavily sweating athletes [5]. Medications with any potential cardiac side effects may be of extra concern in heavily exercising athletes as well.

The end result of needing to consider these three variables is that clinicians prescribing psychiatric medication for athletes should tend toward relatively conservative prescribing practices. Thus, a psychiatric prescriber for athletes is well advised not to simultaneously start multiple medications or escalate dosages quickly. Of course, there are always exceptions to these guidelines. In the case of significant mental illness, the athlete's health and well-being must be staunchly prioritized. There is a definite risk of undertreating mental illness in athletes, and care must be taken to avoid that circumstance as well, as certainly ongoing, untreated mental illness is not conducive to high-level sports performance.

There are unique considerations within each category of psychiatric medications when it comes to prescribing for athletes. Unfortunately, there is a paucity of research when it comes to psychiatric medication use in athletes. Studies that attempt to look at the impact of psychiatric medications on athletic performance tend to have several flaws: sample sizes are very small; medications are not used in dosages or time frames that reflect their actual usage in the real world; populations studied are not high-level athletes; very few female athletes are studied; types of performance measures used in studies to determine if a medication has a negative impact on athletic performance may not be representative of real-world performance impact; and study subjects often do not have the psychiatric disorder that the medication is intended to treat [6]. With acknowledgment of the research limitations to date, the remainder of this chapter details what is known about medications prescribed for athletes within numerous major categories of mental illness, and general considerations when it comes to psychiatric prescribing within each of these categories. Non-pharmacologic approaches to management of mental illness in athletes are described elsewhere in this book.

Depression

Medications for depression in athletes have received some research attention. A recent survey of sports psychiatrists noted that bupropion was a top choice of sports psychiatrists for depression, without comorbid anxiety, in athletes [2]. It can be speculated that the relatively energizing effect of this medication and lack of weight gain as a side effect contribute to its top selection. However, this medication must not be prescribed in the presence of an eating disorder, which, depending on the sport and setting, can be a relatively common occurrence in athletes. Use of bupropion in the context of an eating disorder increases the risk of seizure. It is important as well to note that bupropion is currently on WADA's in-competition monitored list, meaning that WADA is monitoring for evidence that this medication may be being used inappropriately, presumably for a performance advantage [7]. Specifically, there is very preliminary evidence suggesting the possibility of performance enhancement for endurance athletes using bupropion as a single, high dose (600 mg) in warm climates [8]. Performance enhancement was not observed when the medication was dosed chronically [9], which is how it would be prescribed in actual clinical practice. A more recent study demonstrated performance enhancement with 300 mg dosing the night before and morning of a cycling time trial in warm climates, but no such enhancement was noted at doses less than 300 mg [10]. The sum of the research on bupropion seems to suggest that it may allow athletes to push themselves to higher core body temperatures and heart rates, thus allowing improved performance, when used at higher doses and in acute rather than chronic dosing time frames [8]. However, such evidence is not to the level that WADA is banning it at this point, and as such, it can be prescribed without restriction or high degrees of concern about safety at this time, especially if athletes are taking it on a daily basis at dosages within approved ranges.

Another very reasonable top choice of antidepressants for athletes is fluoxetine. It has relatively more research than other antidepressants, and specifically more research than any other selective serotonin reuptake inhibitors (SSRIs) have to support that it does not have a negative impact on performance [11, 12]. In an earlier (2000) survey of sports psychiatrists, it had emerged as the top antidepressant choice for athletes [13]. It may be especially reasonable if the depressed athlete has a comorbid eating disorder, as it is FDA-approved for bulimia nervosa.

Serotonin norepinephrine reuptake inhibitors (SNRIs), tricyclic antidepressants (e.g., nortriptyline, amitriptyline), and mirtazapine have not been studied in athletes per se. Tricyclics and mirtazapine may cause sedation and weight gain, which can be problematic for this population. Tricyclics also may have safety concerns in athletes pushing themselves to extremes. Supraventricular and ventricular arrhythmias have been described in young, healthy people taking tricyclics [6]. Additionally, there is a theoretical risk that tricyclic blood levels could become toxic in athletes sweating heavily. One very small study demonstrated mild, temporary increases in tricyclic blood levels in exercising subjects. Though the authors concluded that the increases were unlikely to be dangerous, the subjects were not high-level athletes [5]. In general, tricyclic antidepressants should be avoided in athletes if possible, and if prescribed, blood levels should be monitored [14].

Anxiety

There are important considerations when it comes to prescribing medications for anxiety as well. The mediation that has emerged as sports psychiatrists' top choice for treatment of anxiety in athletes is escitalopram [2]. That said, escitalopram has not been uniquely studied in athletes, and other SSRIs (besides paroxetine, which is unique among the SSRIs in its notable sedation) are often reasonable alternative options. Buspirone may be used as monotherapy or as an add-on to antidepressants (e.g., SSRIs or SNRIs) for anxiety. One small study suggested performance impairment from buspirone, but only a single 45 mg dose of the medication was used, and that is a large dose to be taken at any given time, nonreflective of real-world prescribing [15].

Medications are not generally prescribed to athletes for anxiety that solely presents as performance anxiety and is thus not reflective of a broader anxiety condition such as generalized anxiety disorder. As-needed medications that would be used for situational anxiety such as performance anxiety would have detrimental effects on sports performance. For example, benzodiazepines have been shown to have a negative impact on performance [16, 17]. Such an impact is not surprising given this class's propensity to cause sedation and muscle relaxation. Propranolol and other B-blockers should typically be avoided as well. As blood pressure medications, they may lower blood pressure in athletes who already may have relatively low blood pressure, and may decrease cardiac output. In endurance sports, they can problematically decrease $VO_{2\ max}$ [18]. They are banned in other sports, specifically rifle in the NCAA [3] and archery, automobile, billiards, darts, golf, shooting, some skiing/snowboarding, and some underwater sports at the world level [4] because they improve fine motor control. The B-blocker bans at the world level are in-competition only, except that archery and shooting are also banned out-of-competition [4].

Insomnia

Insomnia may be a symptom of an underlying mental illness, such as depression or anxiety. In such cases, treating the primary psychiatric condition will often result in correction of a sleep disturbance. Consequently, it is often recommended to avoid adding a second medication for sleep, in addition to any medication that is being prescribed for the primary condition, in an effort to avoid polypharmacy in athletes. In addition to optimization of treatment of the primary psychiatric condition, any prescriber should ensure that proper sleep hygiene is being followed. More details are provided in the chapter on sleep within this text, but important and unique issues to consider in athletes, prior to issuing a sedative-hypnotic prescription, include distinguishing insomnia from insufficient allotment of time for sleep in very busy athletes, and the impact of evening workouts and caffeine use.

If a sleep medication is needed, the hope is that it can be a short-term aid in most cases. A major concern with sleeping medications for athletes is potential sedation that carries over into the next morning. Thus, athletes taking any sleep aid should be advised of the importance of allowing a full night of sleep after taking it. Melatonin emerges as the first choice of sports psychiatrists [2], and it is the best-studied sleep medication in athletes [14]. Melatonin has not been shown to have a negative impact on performance [16, 19]. If immediate release melatonin does not have a long-enough duration for a given athlete, extended-release melatonin may be tried, as studies have shown neither formulation to impair performance [14]. A rare side effect of potential concern in athletes taking melatonin is a reduction in blood pressure, as athletes may have relatively low blood pressure at baseline [20]. Importantly, athletes must be advised to obtain melatonin from a reputable company in which it is labeled as the only ingredient. In the United States and Canada, melatonin is an over-the-counter supplement not regulated by the FDA, and thus its purity cannot be guaranteed [14]. If a supplement were to include any prohibited substances, and an athlete ingests those laced substances unknowingly, the athlete will still be held accountable if testing positive for a prohibited agent. Ignorance of the ingredients or improper labeling of supplements is not considered a valid excuse by anti-doping agencies [14].

In the event that melatonin is not sedating enough for an athlete, trazodone has been ranked as a second (off-label) choice among sports psychiatrists [2]. However, it has not been uniquely studied in athletes. Similarly, gabapentin is another off-label option for treating insomnia in athletes, though also not studied in this population [14]. Non-benzodiazepine agonists, for example, zolpidem and zopiclone, are latter options [14]. They have been shown to have less of a next-day sedation effect as compared to benzodiazepines when performance effects have been studied [21–25]. Among the benzodiazepines, agents with longer half-lives have demonstrated more of a detrimental impact on next-day athletic performance compared to shorter-acting agents [17]. The latter finding must be considered alongside the knowledge that benzodiazepine with shorter half-lives are more addictive.

Attention-Deficit/Hyperactivity Disorder

There are critical considerations unique to athletes when prescribing medications for attention-deficit/hyperactivity disorder (ADHD). Stimulants can be problematic in a number of ways. They have been shown to be performance-enhancing in sport via improved strength, acceleration, anaerobic capacity, time to exhaustion, and maximum heart rate [26]. Athletes taking stimulants may be able to exercise to higher core body temperatures without perceiving as much effort or thermal stress as they otherwise would [27]. This raises not only concerns about performance-enhancement, but also about safety, as athletes may be unaware of increasing thermal stress [27]. Stimulants may be used for weight loss as a performance advantage in leanness sports (e.g., lightweight rowing, distance running, diving, gymnastics, figure skating) or in sports with weight classes (e.g., wrestling) and may be inappropriately used by athletes with an eating disorder to aid further weight loss. These medications may also cause side effects, such as insomnia, anxiety, increased heart rate, and an undesired decrease in appetite, all of which may interfere with performance.

The National Collegiate Athletic Association [3] and World Anti-Doping Agency [4] prohibit stimulants. At the level of the NCAA, stimulants are only allowable for ADHD if institutions are able to submit the "NCAA Medical Exception Documentation Report to Support the Diagnosis of Attention Deficit Hyperactivity Disorder (ADHD) and Treatment with Banned Stimulant Medication" and supporting documentation to the NCAA in the event the athlete tests positive for stimulants [28]. This documentation must include: a summary of comprehensive clinical evaluation (referencing Diagnostic and Statistical Manual criteria and including family history, any indication of mood disorders, substance abuse, and previous history of ADHD treatment); blood pressure and pulse readings and comments; notation that alternative non-banned medications (e.g., atomoxetine) have been considered; diagnosis; medication(s) and dosage(s); and follow-up orders [28]. NCAA schools may differ in their internal requirements for validated ADHD testing and documentation. Of note, NCAA schools do not submit information to the NCAA until an athlete is actually tested and found positive for a stimulant medication in their system.

WADA prohibits stimulants at the elite and professional levels [4]. They are only allowable for ADHD with approved Therapeutic Use Exemptions (TUEs) [29]. TUE applications are available at the websites of individual countries' anti-doping organizations (ADOs), for example, the United States Anti-Doping Agency [30]. Completed applications are then submitted to the relevant ADO. Initial TUEs for stimulants are often granted for 12 months, while TUEs for a "well-documented, long-standing" diagnosis of ADHD may be for up to 4 years [29]. Any change of medication or significant adjustment of the dosage should result in a re-submission or advisement to WADA [29].

Given these regulations, medication prescription for ADHD must be undertaken with great care. Behavioral interventions may be tried before prescriptions if symptoms are mild and/or if the athlete is not a student, in which case academic concerns would not be as paramount [31]. Non-stimulants should at least be considered, as articulated in the NCAA exceptions procedures, before stimulants in many cases [28]. Non-stimulant atomoxetine emerges as the number one medication choice for ADHD among sports psychiatrists, presumably owing to the drawbacks of stimulants [2]. Prescribers and athletes should be aware that they need to allow up to 2–3 months to see full benefit from atomoxetine [31]. Non-stimulant bupropion has evidence as an off-label agent for ADHD [32], and as it is an antidepressant, it may be an especially reasonable choice if depression is comorbid.

If stimulants are used, most sports psychiatrists start with long-acting formulations, which are more convenient and less abusable. The top three stimulant choices of sports psychiatrists have been reported to be long-acting agents: lisdexamfetamine (Vyvanse), long-acting methylphenidate (Concerta), and long-acting mixed amphetamine salts (Adderall XR) [2]. However, another potentially reasonable stimulant prescribing strategy involves use of formulations and timing that allow for use during school, study, and work times only and not during practices and competition, thereby decreasing concerns about impact on performance [31]. A final important consideration is that prescribers may wish to advise holding the stimulant medication if the athlete is participating in endurance events in hot temperatures, given the described safety concerns [14].

Eating Disorders

Even more so than with other disorders, psychotropic medication prescribing for eating disorders in athletes should be undertaken only within the context of a multidisciplinary team [33]. Medical evaluation includes laboratory monitoring, physical examination, and consideration of electrocardiography and bone mineral density testing [33], all of which are often undertaken by the sports medicine physician, though sometimes may be conducted or ordered by a psychiatrist. Nutrition and psychotherapy are important aspects of treatment, in addition to any prescriptions for psychiatric medication. There are two medications FDA-approved for eating disorders [33]. Fluoxetine is approved for bulimia nervosa, and, by extension, tends to be a first-line medication used in the presence of any type of eating disorder if depression or anxiety are also present. That said, there is not a significant amount of research supporting its utility in anorexia nervosa alone, apart from any component of depression or anxiety [34].

Lisdexamfetamine is FDA-approved for binge eating disorder (BED), but this is a stimulant and thus is prohibited at collegiate [3] and world [4] levels. As of the time of this publication, the NCAA, USADA, and WADA do not have official, written policies specifically about the potential to apply for a TUE for use of this medication for a diagnosis of BED. However, both the NCAA (oral communication, 2017 April 28) and USADA (written communication, 2018 February 28) report that they would follow a similar protocol as for stimulants to treat ADHD. USADA qualifies that information by noting that it is important to be cognizant of the differences in psychiatric practice in different countries. That is, it is possible that an athlete could receive a TUE from USADA (or any other country) for use of a stimulant to treat BED, but not have it recognized by an International Federation or another country's ADO if it is not yet deemed an accepted practice worldwide. Thus, if an athlete plans to compete internationally, this could be a restricting factor.

Bipolar Disorder

Like anyone else, athletes may suffer from bipolar disorder. However, great care should be taken before making this diagnosis in anyone, definitely including athletes, as the medications can cause significant side effects and safety concerns. With rare exception, medications are necessary to control this disorder. Lamotrigine and lithium tie as the top choice among mood stabilizing medications for athletes with bipolar spectrum disorders [2]. Lamotrigine is an unsurprising choice, given its favorable side effect profile. However, it is unreliable in preventing and treating mania, and rather, has more evidence for preventing and treating depression [2]. Thus, for athletes with full bipolar disorder type I, prescribers must use caution and close monitoring if this is the sole mood stabilizing agent used. Lithium is a full-spectrum mood stabilizer, well established for management of both depression and mania. However, it can be dangerous and life-threatening if an athlete taking it becomes dehydrated (e.g., due to sweating heavily or dehydrating themselves for weigh-ins in certain sports). Thus, its use must occur only with close laboratory and clinical monitoring and insistence on adequate hydration [14]. Most medications for bipolar disorder, apart from lamotrigine, can cause sedation, weight gain, and tremor. These include antipsychotic medications, valproic acid, and lithium [2]. Among the atypical antipsychotics, aripiprazole, lurasidone, and ziprasidone are relatively less likely to cause sedation and weight gain [2]. However, ziprasidone may cause QTc prolongation [35] and thus may not be a first-line choice within this class for athletes. Finally, it is worth noting that within the general population, antipsychotics such as quetiapine are sometimes used off-label for sleep or anxiety, but for the athlete population, in the absence of a bona fide bipolar or psychosis diagnosis, they should generally not be used for these purposes given the side effect burden [14].

Psychotic Disorders

Presumably for the same reasons explained above, aripiprazole emerges as sports psychiatrists' top choice of medications for psychotic disorders in athletes [2]. Typical antipsychotics, for example, haloperidol, appear to be infrequent choices for psychosis in athletes [2]. This is unsurprising, given that class's propensity to cause significant sedation and movement side effects including, but not limited to, tremor, which can interfere with fine motor coordination [36]. Typical antipsychotics also appear more likely than atypical antipsychotics to cause cardiac concerns [35].

Conclusions

It is critical that prescribers of psychiatric medications for athletes be familiar with issues of relevance for athletes, including safety risks, potential positive or negative impact on performance, and competitive regulations surrounding use of certain medications by governing bodies. All treatment team members should be aware of and on the lookout for side effects that may limit performance, especially sedation, weight gain, cardiac side effects, and tremor. Importantly, though, it is a delicate balance between scrutinizing for side effects and not discouraging use of needed medication in mentally ill athletes. Additionally, all treatment team members should be aware of NCAA, WADA, or other prohibited lists and documentation requirements. Athletes should be reminded to always ask their prescribers if a given medication or substance is allowed prior to ingesting it.

Athletes and their treatment teams do well to think of psychiatric medications as one important part of a treatment plan, but rarely should the medication be the only part. An analogy to physical injury is appropriate. With a physical injury, athletes may need medication (e.g., to decrease pain or inflammation), but they may also need to participate in rehabilitation exercises. Similarly, athletes with a psychiatric injury may need medication, but they may also need to participate in rehabilitation exercises in the form of psychotherapy. It is critical that they have the support of all members of their medical treatment team as they undertake any such treatment for mental illness.

References

1. Bauman NJ. The stigma of mental health in athletes: are mental toughness and mental health seen as contradictory in elite sport? Br J Sports Med. 2016;50(3):135–6.
2. Reardon CL, Creado S. Psychiatric medication preferences of sports psychiatrists. Phys Sportsmed. 2016;44(4):397–402.
3. NCAA Sport Science Institute. 2017–2018 NCAA Banned Drugs List [Internet]. Indianapolis, IN: The National Collegiate Athletic Association; 2017. Available from: http://www.ncaa.org/2017-18-ncaa-banned-drugs-list.
4. World Anti-Doping Agency. Prohibited List [Internet]. Quebec, Montreal: World Anti-Doping Agency; 2018. Available from: https://www.wada-ama.org/sites/default/files/prohibited_list_2018_en.pdf
5. de Zwaan M. Exercise and antidepressant serum levels. Biol Psychiatry. 1992;32:210–1.
6. Reardon CL, Factor RM. Sport psychiatry: a systematic review of diagnosis and medical treatment of mental illness in athletes. Sports Med. 2010;40(11):961–80.
7. World Anti-Doping Agency. Monitoring Program [Internet]. Quebec, Montreal: World Anti-Doping Agency; 2018. Available from: https://www.wada-ama.org/en/resources/science-medicine/monitoring-program
8. Watson P, Hasegawa H, Roelands B, Piacentini MF, Looverie R, Meeusen R. Acute dopamine/noradrenaline reuptake inhibition enhances human exercise performance in warm, but not temperate conditions. J Physiol. 2005;565(3):873–83.
9. Roelands B, Hasegawa H, Watson P, Piacentini MF, Buyse L, De Schutter G, et al. Performance and thermoregulatory effects of chronic bupropion administration in the heat. Eur J Appl Physiol. 2009;105(3):493–8.
10. Roelands B, Watson P, Cordery P, Decoster S, Debaste E, Maughan R, et al. A dopamine/noradrenaline reuptake inhibitor improves performance in the heat, but only at the maximum therapeutic dose. Scand J Med Sci Sports. 2012;22(5):e93–8.
11. Parise G, Bosman MJ, Boeeker DR. Selective serotonin reuptake inhibitors: their effect on high-intensity exercise performance. Arch Phys Med Rehabil. 2001;82:867–71.
12. Meeusen R, Piacentini MF, van Den Eynde S, Magnus L, De Meirleir K. Exercise performance is not influenced by a 5-HT reuptake inhibitor. Int J Sports Med. 2001;22:329–36.
13. Baum AL. Psychopharmacology in athletes. In: Begel D, Burton RW, editors. Sport psychiatry. New York, NY: WW Norton & Company; 2000. p. 249–59.

14. Reardon CL. The sports psychiatrist and psychiatric medications. Int Rev Psychiatry. 2016;28(6):606–13.
15. Marvin G, Sharma A, Aston W, Field C, Kendall MJ, Jones DA. The effects of buspirone on perceived exertion and time to fatigue in man. Exp Physiol. 1997;82:1057–60.
16. Paul MA, Gray G, Kenny G, Pigeau RA. Impact of melatonin, zaleplon, zopiclone, and temazepam on psychomotor performance. Aviat Space Environ Med. 2003;74(12): 1263–70.
17. Charles RB, Kirkham AJ, Guyatt AR, Parker SP. Psychomotor, pulmonary and exercise responses to sleep medication. Br J Clin Pharm. 1987;24:191–7.
18. Cowan DA. Drug abuse. In: Harries M, Williams C, Stanish WD, Micheli LJ, editors. Oxford textbook of sports medicine. New York, NY: Oxford University Press; 1994. p. 314–29.
19. Atkinson G, Drust B, Reilly T, Waterhouse J. The relevance of melatonin to sports medicine and science. Sports Med. 2003;33(11):809–31.
20. Herman D, Macknight JM, Stromwall AE, Mistry DJ. The international athlete—advances in management of jet lag and anti-doping policy. Clin Sports Med. 2011;30(3):641–59.
21. Ito SU, Kanbayashi T, Takemura T, Kondo H, Inomata S, Szilagyi G, et al. Acute effects of zolpidem on daytime alertness, psychomotor and physical performance. Neurosci Res. 2007;59:309–13.
22. Grobler LA, Schwellnus MP, Trichard C, Calder S, Noakes TD, Derman WE. Comparative effects of zopiclone and loprazolam on psychomotor and physical performance in active individuals. Clin J Sport Med. 2000;10(2):123–8.
23. Tafti M, Besset A, Billiard M. Effects of zopiclone on subjective evaluation of sleep and daytime alertness and on psychomotor and physical performance tests in athletes. Prog Neuro-Psychopharmacol Biol Psychiatry. 1992;16:55–63.
24. Holmberg G. The effects of anxiolytics on CFF. Pharmacopsychiatry. 1982;15 Suppl: 49–53.
25. Maddock RJ, Casson EJ, Lott LA, Carter CS, Johnson CA. Benzodiazepine effects on flicker sensitivity: role of stimulus frequency and size. Prog Neuro-Psychopharmacol Biol Psychiatry. 1993;17:955–70.
26. Chandler JV, Blair SN. The effect of amphetamines on selected physiological components related to athletic success. Med Sci Sports Exerc. 1980;12(1):65–9.
27. Roelands B, Hasegawa H, Watson P, Piacentini MF, Buyse L, De Schutter G, et al. The effects of acute dopamine reuptake inhibition on performance. Med Sci Sports Exerc. 2008;40(5):879–85.
28. NCAA Sport Science Institute. Drug-testing exceptions procedures [Internet]. Indianapolis, IN: The National Collegiate Athletic Association; 2017. Available from: http://www.ncaa.org/health-and-safety/sport-science-institute/drug-testing-exceptions-procedures
29. World Anti-Doping Agency. Therapeutic use exemptions [Internet]. Quebec, Montreal: World Anti-Doping Agency; 2018. Available from: https://www.wada-ama.org/en/what-we-do/science-medical/therapeutic-use-exemptions
30. U.S. Anti-Doping Agency. Apply for a therapeutic use exemption (TUE) [Internet]. Colorado Springs, CO: U.S. Anti-Doping Agency; 2014. Available from: https://www.usada.org/substances/tue/apply/
31. Reardon CL, Factor RM. Considerations in the use of stimulants in sport. Sports Med. 2016;46(5):611–7.
32. Verbeeck W, Bekkering GE, Van den Noortgate W, Kramers C. Bupropion for attention deficit hyperactivity disorder (ADHD) in adults. Cochrane Database Syst Rev. 2017;
33. Joy E, Kussman A, Nattiv A. 2016 update on eating disorders in athletes: a comprehensive narrative review with a focus on clinical assessment and management. Br J Sports Med. 2016;50:154–62.

34. American Psychiatric Association (APA). Practice guideline for the treatment of patients with eating disorders. 3rd ed. [Internet]. Washington, D.C.: American Psychiatric Association Publishing; 2010. Available from: https://psychiatryonline.org/pb/assets/raw/sitewide/practice_guidelines/guidelines/eatingdisorders.pdf
35. Beach SR, Celano CM, Noseworthy PA, Januzzi JL, Huffman JC. QTc prolongation, torsades de pointes, and psychotropic medications. Psychosomatics. 2013;54(1):1–13.
36. Macleod AD. Sport psychiatry. Aust N Z J Psychiatry. 1998;32:860–6.

Chapter 6
Attention Deficit/Hyperactivity Disorder (ADHD)

Jason M. Matuszak

Introduction/Definition

Attention Deficit/Hyperactivity Disorder is a primarily heritable chronic neurodevelopmental disorder that is the most common neurobehavioral disorder of childhood, but can affect individuals throughout the lifespan. This disorder is typically considered to represent a deficit in behavioral inhibition that results in inattention, hyperactivity, and/or impulsivity. Other features often seen with ADHD include impairment in executive function and self-regulation of behavior [1]. Manifestations of this disorder are usually present in more than one situation (e.g. home, school, work, sports). Children with ADHD may experience adaptation problems because their functional level and behavior may not correspond to their chronological age or expected development [2]. It is unclear what part the role of "relative expected behavior" may have in the diagnosis of ADHD in young people. In one study out of Canada, where the date of birth cutoff for entry to school is December 31, boys were 30% and girls 70% more likely to be diagnosed with ADHD if they were born in December, compared with January [3]. A study from the United States with a September 1 cutoff showed August-born children were 30% more likely to be diagnosed with ADHD than those born in September [4].

ADHD is often apparent early in life, with many cases diagnosed during childhood, while others may become more apparent during adolescence or adulthood. However, since the condition is predominantly diagnosed in younger people, inherent bias by teachers, coaches, or the medical team may prevent college athletes or adults, who have not previously been diagnosed, from being identified.

Individuals with ADHD are at higher risk for injuries, academic underachievement, social difficulties, lower occupational status, substance use, antisocial

J. M. Matuszak (✉)
Excelsior Orthopaedics, Buffalo, NY, USA

University at Buffalo, School of Medicine, Buffalo, NY, USA

© Springer Nature Switzerland AG 2020   69
E. Hong, A. L. Rao (eds.), *Mental Health in the Athlete*,
https://doi.org/10.1007/978-3-030-44754-0_6

behavior, and automobile accidents, and according to the National Institutes of Health "consume a disproportionate share of resources and attention from the health care system, criminal justice system, schools, and other social service agencies" [5].

Pathophysiology

Research suggests there are genetic components altering the synthesis, presynaptic release and reuptake, and postsynaptic reuptake of catecholamines in different regions and networks in the brain. Other possible contributors or risk factors may include brain injury, environmental toxins, premature delivery, or low birth weight. Family studies report a higher incidence of ADHD among first-degree family members and estimates of heritability are as high as 0.76, which places ADHD high among heritable psychiatric conditions [7].

While many of these have anecdotally been implicated, research does not support causation or worsening from eating too much sugar, watching too much television, parenting, poverty, or unstable family situations. [8]

Epidemiology

Approximately 5–6% of children are diagnosed with ADHD, although some estimate that as many as 10% of children suffer from the disorder [9]. It is unclear what affect inherent coping mechanisms some individuals may possess that could result in under-identification, since CDC data shows about 5.5% of children take medication for the treatment of ADHD [9]. More than half of children have symptoms that continue to require treatment in adolescence or young adulthood, with at least 30% having symptoms well into adulthood. Most studies on prevalence have identified the disorder more commonly in boys than in girls [9].

The athlete population appears to closely mirror the general population. Borchers et al. presented data that demonstrated about 5.5% of athletes have ADHD [10]. This suggests that individuals with ADHD can participate successfully in athletic endeavors. One feature of this data that is particularly striking is that there is a 142% rate of participation in contact sports compared with noncontact sports. An association is not clear, but it is a factor that treating providers may have to consider when treating injuries such as concussion.

Diagnosis

Diagnosis of ADHD is made clinically and may be informed by corroborating information from parents or other family members, teachers, coworkers, or other individuals who interface with the patient in different environments. The Diagnostic

Table 6.1 Criteria for Attention Deficity/Hyperactivity Disorder

Attention-Deficit/Hyperactivity Disorder (ADHD)
A. A persistent pattern (>6 months) of inattention and/or hyperactivity-impulsivity that interferes with functioning or development, and is not solely a manifestation of oppositional behavior, defiance, or hostility.
B. Several inattentive or hyperactive-impulsive symptoms were present prior to age 12 years.
C. Several inattentive or hyperactive-impulsive symptoms are present in two or more settings (e.g., at home, school, or work; with friends or relatives; in other activities).
D. There is clear evidence that the symptoms interfere with, or reduce the quality of, social, academic, or occupational functioning.
E. The symptoms do not occur exclusively during the course of schizophrenia or another psychotic disorder and are not better explained by another mental disorder (e.g., mood disorder, anxiety disorder, dissociative disorder, personality disorder, substance intoxication or withdrawal).

Adapted from Diagnostic and Statistical Manual of Mental Disorders, Fifth Edition [6]

and Statistical Manual of Mental Disorders, Fifth Edition (DSM-V) [6] outlines the diagnostic criteria for the disorder (Table 6.1).

In order to be diagnosed historically, ADHD symptoms would have had to be present before the age of 7, DSM-V now suggests that symptoms any time before the age of 12 is sufficient to meet criteria. The three subtypes of ADHD are primarily determined by the predominant symptom pattern and are divided into inattentive type, hyperactive-impulse type, and the combined type [6]. Although a primary diagnosis of ADHD as adult may be made, in order to fulfill the DSM-V criteria, there should be evidence of symptoms during childhood. If history cannot be firmly established, a concurring opinion is often helpful.

There are several tools designed to assist with the diagnosis and monitoring of the disorder. Some of the commonly used tools include the Connors Questionnaire, NICQH Vanderbilt Assessment Tool, the Special Needs Assessment Profile, the SNAP-IV, and the Sawnson, Kotkin, Angler, M-Flynn, and Pelham (SKAMP) Scale [11]. In addition to the reports, a medical exam is usually indicated to evaluate for other possible causes or confounders. This medical evaluation may also include laboratory evaluation. It is important for the clinician evaluating the athlete to consider that adolescents and adults are less likely to exhibit overt hyperactivity and may have developed other coping mechanisms that could affect the clinical diagnosis or alter the perception of other evaluators.

Comorbidities

Depression, bipolar disorder, conduct disorder, oppositional-defiant disorder, and anti-social personality disorder are occasionally comorbid with ADHD, and a number of these diagnoses are more prevalent when ADHD in under- or untreated [2, 12] (Fig. 6.1). Lack of sufficient treatment for ADHD also has been seen to be

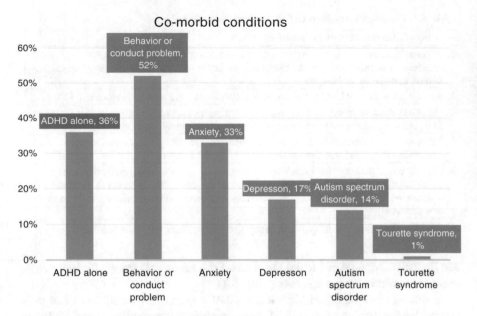

Fig. 6.1 Other conditions often comorbid with ADHD. (Adapted from [2, 12])

associated with learning or language problems and academic underachievement, and increases the risks of substance use, dangerous driving, delinquent behavior, and impulsive sexual activity [13].

Overview in the Athlete

Given the frequency of ADHD in the general and athletic population, any medical provider who is working with athletes will encounter people with the disorder. The Mental Health Team Physician Consensus Statement, published by the collaboration of multiple professional associations concerned about clinical sports medicine issues, suggests that it is essential the team physician recognize the signs and symptoms of ADHD [14]. Further, it is considered desirable the team physician encourage, coordinate, and facilitate referral to the mental health care network; educate or provide resources to the athletic care network about ADHD, the medications used to treat this condition, and potential side effects, including the risk for cardiac and heat-related issues; and understand that with certain medications, documentation may be required for the athlete to meet the conditions for treatment specified by organizing bodies (e.g., NCAA, IOC) [14].

The American Medical Society for Sports Medicine published a position statement on ADHD [15] in the athlete and several governing bodies or sports leagues (e.g., NCAA, IOC, MLB) have published guidelines about the treatment of athletes with ADHD [16, 17].

Treatments

Behavioral/Psychosocial

Behavior therapy represents a broad set of interventions that seek to modify the behavior and are implemented by training parents, teachers, coaches, or peers. These interventions promote positive (as opposed to negative) reinforcement, allow trainees to learn what behaviors can be reduced or eliminated by using planned ignoring, or provide appropriate consequences or punishments for failing to meet goals. These goals or expectations may be increased for each task as they are mastered [18].

Behavioral therapy may be more effective when combined with medications and combined treatment may be more satisfying for parents, teachers, and students [18]. Additionally, the combination of behavioral interventions and medication allowed for the use of lower dosages of stimulants, and possibly reduced risk of adverse effects [18].

Pharmacologic

While behavioral and psychosocial interventions are recommended for everyone with ADHD, the majority of individuals with ADHD will require the use of medication for symptom management [9]. Although not universally accepted as the mainstay of treatment [19], stimulant medications have been reported to be the most effective medication for managing the core symptoms [20]. Other medications have shown to be effective for some patients, but are generally considered second-line treatments (Table 6.2). Sports organizations have their own rules about the use of stimulant versus nonstimulant medication; however, proven failure with a nonstimulant is generally not required for an athlete to be treated with a stimulant medication. Relative contraindications to using stimulants may include hypertension, underlying arrhythmias, or other cardiac conditions.

Since the destabilization of symptom control can lead athletes to demonstrate increase in risk-taking behaviors and conflict situations, and for general treatment

Table 6.2 FDA-approved medications for ADHD

Medication	Class	NCAA exemption needed?	WADA/IOC banned?
Dextroamphetamine	Stimulant	Yes	Yes
Dextroamphetamine/ Amphetamine	Stimulant	Yes	Yes
Lisdexamfetamine	Stimulant	Yes	Yes
Methylphenidate	Stimulant	Yes	Yes
Atomoxetine	Nonstimulant SNRI	No	No

considerations, it is generally considered important to maintain consistent therapeutic dosing of medication through the year, even during competition in most sports. Following the initiation of treatment, monitoring should be performed to assess the effectiveness of the medication until stabilization is reached [15].

Medications sometimes used off-label for ADHD

Armodanfinil	Stimulant	Yes	Yes
Modafinil	Stimulant	Yes	Yes
Buproprion	SSRI	No	No
Imipramine	TCA	No	No
Nortriptyline	TCA	No	No
Amitriptyline	TCA	No	No
Desipramine	TCA	No	No
Clonidine	Alpha-2 adrenergic	No	No
Guanfacine	Alpha-2 adrenergic	No	No

Adapted from White et al. [11] and Stewman et al. [21]

Medical Risks to Athletes as a Result of ADHD or Prescribed Medication

Cardiovascular Considerations

Post-marketing reports of sudden deaths in pediatric patients in the United States prompted the Canadian drug regulatory agency to temporarily suspend the sale of Adderall XR in Canada in 2005, which in turn led the Food and Drug Administration (FDA) to release a "Public Health Advisory for Adderall and Adderall XR" and prompted the addition of a warning to the Adderall labeling to not use in patients with structural heart abnormalities. Because of this, conflicting recommendations were developed about whether or not to obtain a pretreatment electrocardiogram (ECG). The American Heart Association and the American College of Cardiology found it *reasonable* for a physician *to consider* obtaining an electrocardiogram (ECG) [22], whereas the American Academy of Child and Adolescent Psychiatry and the American Academy of Pediatrics, citing both the rareness of sudden cardiac death in patients taking medications for ADHD, (and no higher than that of the general population), and the potential risk for serious implications from untreated ADHD, recommended against obtaining an ECG as part of the pretreatment evaluation of children [23].

Further study by Cooper et al., funded by the FDA and the Agency for Healthcare Research and Quality, in 2011, seeking to clarify the conflicting recommendations, did not find an increased risk of serious cardiovascular events from the use of ADHD medications in more than 1.2 million children and young adults [24]. There does not appear to be an increase in sudden cardiac death risk in healthy athletes without known heart disease who begin stimulant medication use, either. Rates of sudden cardiac death in athletes taking stimulants are substantially lower than the baseline risk of sudden cardiac death in the athlete population as a whole or athletes not taking stimulants.

Studies show a baseline small (estimated at 3–4 mmHg) increase in systolic and diastolic blood pressure and an increase upward of 5 bpm in resting and exertional heart rates [25]; however, there is an absence of evidence to suggest this leads to increased complications. The overall prevalence of hypertensive and pre-hypertensive individuals has been shown to be comparable between groups of children with ADHD on stimulant medications and those with ADHD not on stimulant medications, and children without ADHD [25].

Hyperthermia

A stimulant was implicated in the death of a Danish cyclist in the Olympics in 1960 and of a Tour de France cyclist in 1967. These high-profile deaths helped fuel the advent of the Medical Commission by the International Olympic Committee to help fight doping. The use of stimulants has been shown to increase core temperature directly, possibly by interfering normal thermoregulation in the brain by altering neurotransmitters, but also to allow athletes to push the limits of fatigue, which could elevate core temperature more [26]. It should be noted that the absolute clinical relevance of these changes is unclear and may have been extrapolated from data on toxicity data, cocaine and methamphetamine, supplements such as ephedra, or other labeled or unlabeled medications used as ergogenic aids. Despite large numbers of athletes, and soldiers, who have historically used stimulant medications for medical purposes, there is a paucity of research into the risk of exertional hyperthermia or exertional rhabdomyolysis for athletes with ADHD taking stimulant medication at therapeutic doses and causation remains unproven.

Concussion

Although it is unclear whether individuals with ADHD are any more likely to sustain concussion, neuropsychiatric disorders, such as ADHD, may be important modifiers to consider with concussion. Since ADHD has the potential to affect memory, attention, and concentration, these may have important implications for aspects of the typical concussion evaluation. Further, for athletes who are subject to computerized neurocognitive testing, there may be an effect on both baseline and postinjury test, especially when comorbid with learning disabilities, including differences in verbal and visual memories, processing speed, and reaction time [27], which makes interpretation more challenging, or which may invalidate the results. One study on high school and collegiate athletes found that individuals diagnosed with ADHD reported a greater baseline rate of fatigue, difficulty concentrating, trouble sleeping, difficulty remembering, and balance problems [28].

The presence of ADHD does not appear to affect outcome following concussion [29]; however, mixed data suggests it may alter the recovery trajectory following concussion [29, 30], or may make returning to the classroom more difficult. It is unclear whether this effect could be a result of the injury or differences in interpretation of findings, given the differences in pre- and postinjury symptoms in athletes with ADHD [29]. There does not, however, appear to be a risk of developing new, chronic, or worsened ADHD symptoms following concussion, but it may affect compensatory mechanisms that an individual has developed that keep symptoms below threshold. The effect of this is that a case of newly diagnosed, but not newly developed, ADHD could be seen in the aftermath of the concussive injury.

It is generally recommended that medication treatment plans should be continued for athletes under treatment for ADHD with stimulant medications, although using stimulant medications off-label does not improve recovery or time to return to play.

Monitoring

Monitoring of athletes with ADHD focuses on the effectiveness of treatment by control of symptoms, often using symptom scales, and balances the side effects of the medications, since most people on stimulant medications will report at least one side effect [19]. Common side effects or toxicities for medications used to treat ADHD include, for the stimulants: Insomnia, reduced appetite, headaches, jitteriness, possible decrease in growth velocity (but probably not final height); and for the non-stimulants: somnolence, sexual side effects, possible liver complications [11, 15, 19]. Since untreated ADHD is considered as having detrimental effects on the quality of life and on psychosocial development, during breaks from school, individual clinicians and athletes should weigh the potential risks and benefits of maintenance therapy versus taking a "drug holiday" [15].

Ergogenic Effects

Stimulants have been used in sports for several decades because of real or perceived physical and psychological benefits to sports. Some of the specific cited benefits to athletes include a subjective sense of euphoria, improved concentration, increased aggression, and decreased pain [11, 31]. There is limited data in well-controlled studies to confirm these findings, especially specific to the elite athlete. One older study showed stimulants resulted in increased strength, acceleration, anaerobic capacity, time to exhaustion, and maximum heart rates [32]. Some athletes may use stimulants for their appetite suppression properties, especially those in weight-controlled sports [33].

Doping Considerations

Stimulants may trigger a positive doping test even when taken for a legitimate medical purpose. Another consideration is that a number of over-the-counter supplements may contain unlabeled stimulants [34]. Thus, athletes who consume supplements that are not fully tested, or deemed safe, are at risk of unknowingly taking banned substances. Supplements labeled as "energy-containing or energy-increasing," as well as those touted for appetite suppression or weight loss may be particularly questionable [34].

Sport/Competition-Level Specific Considerations

College Athletes

College athletes participating under national Collegiate Athletic Association (NCAA) governance need to be aware of the NCAA policy enacted in 2009 concerning the use of stimulant medications for treating ADHD. Student-athletes are required to provide "evidence that the student athlete has undergone clinical assessment to diagnose the disorder, is being monitored routinely for use of the stimulant medication and has a current prescription on file."

The minimum requirements to establish the indication for stimulant medication include: (1) a written description of the evaluation process including assessment tools and procedures, (2) a statement of the diagnosis, (3) history of ADHD treatment, (4) a statement that a non-banned ADHD has been *considered*, and (5) a statement regarding follow-up and monitoring visits (Table 6.3).

Table 6.3 National Collegiate Athletic Association Documentation Requirements

Prior to initiation of sport activity:
Athlete has undergone clinical evaluation to diagnose the disorder
Athlete is being monitored routinely for use of stimulant medication
Athlete has a current prescription on file
Yearly, thereafter:
Clinical evaluation and documentation with sports medicine staff and athletic department
Description of the assessment, evaluation tools, or procedures
Statement of diagnosis
History of previous and current ADHD treatment
Statement that a non-banned ADHD alternative medication has been considered
Plan for follow-up and monitoring visits

Adapted from NCAA Handbook

Professional Athletes

Each of the professional leagues/associations has their own rules governing the diagnosis and management of ADHD (Table 6.4). Physicians working with professional athletes of one of the major sports leagues may consider consulting with the league office for specific medical direction. Physicians working with professional athletes who fall under the jurisdiction of a governing body or international federation may consult USADA regarding the pertinent rules. A summary of League/Association rules is presented in the following table.

Olympic/International Federation Athletes

The International Olympic Committee and the World Anti-Doping Agency's current policy, currently in its fifth iteration, permits for the treatment of ADHD even during competition. Athletes may participate and continue medical treatment with prohibited drugs for ADHD, but require the submission of a therapeutic use exemption (TUE) to the Therapeutic Use Exemption Committees detailing the athlete's symptoms, diagnosis, and testing criteria [16].

Athletes undergoing active treatment for ADHD with stimulant medications are subject to annual review by the TUE Committee, although in cases of well-established, stable, and long-standing diagnosis, a TUE can be granted for up to 4 years. [16]

Noncompetitive Athletic Activities

Equestrian-based activities have been shown in one study to help with symptoms of ADHD [35]. Yoga and mindfulness have been advocated; however, studies are plagued by low methodological quality and there are no definitive conclusions [36].

A number of leisure and competitive sports have been anecdotally considered helpful for individuals with ADHD in the lay press or in the public realm, including rock-climbing, surfing, archery and shooting sports, fencing. Data supporting these remain limited or absent.

Pediatric Considerations

While ADHD frequently affects children in a school setting, the effects in an athletic setting are less well understood. It is believed that ADHD may negatively affect balance and coordination and may make some movement patterns more difficult.

Table 6.4 League and Organization specific rules related to Therapeutic Use Exemption or medication treatment of ADHD

League/association	Written policy explicit to stimulants/ADHD?	Stimulants permitted?	Documentation required	Independent examiner required?	Recertify frequency and other documentation
Major League Baseball (MLB)	Yes[1]	With TUE	ACDS Impairment Scale	MLB-Certified Clinician or Review by Expert Panel	Yearly Pharmacy Records
Major League Soccer (MLS)	No	No	N/a		
National Basketball Association (NBA)[2]	No[2]	With TUE	Petition to the Medical Director of the Anti-Drug Program Medical Information and valid prescription		
National Football League (NFL)[3]	Yes[3]	With TUE	History, Physical Exam and Testing: Neurological Evaluation Concussion history (with imaging or neuro-psych testing, if indicated) Evaluation for Mental Health Disorders Laboratory tests Neurocognitive testing Interviews with player and family DSM-V criteria ACDS BFIS Management Plan	NFL-certified psychiatrist	Yearly Must provide documentation of follow-up visits
National Hockey League (NHL)[2]	No[2]	Qualified yes	PES Program Committee can review, consider, and act on a player's application		
Nascar	No	With TUE			

(continued)

Table 6.4 (continued)

League/association	Written policy explicit to stimulants/ADHD?	Stimulants permitted?	Documentation required	Independent examiner required?	Recertify frequency and other documentation
Boxing	Through USADA/VADA/WADA	With TUE	Voluntary program VADA or WADA administered depending on Commission/Competition VADA: Medical History/Exam Labs (if indicated) Imaging (if indicated) WADA: DSM-V criteria Second opinion, if new dx >18 y/o		
Mixed Martial Arts	Through USADA	With TUE	USADA/WADA DSM-V criteria Second opinion, if new dx >18 y/o		

ACDS Adult ADHD Clinician Diagnostic Scale v1.2, *BFIS* Barkley Functional Impairment Scales, *USADA* United States Anti-Doping Association, *VADA* Voluntary Anti-Doping Association, *WADA* World Anti-Doping Association

http://www.mlb.com/pa/pdf/jda.pdf

[2] https://footballplayershealth.harvard.edu/wp-content/uploads/2017/05/08_Ch4_Drugs.pdf

[3] https://nflpaweb.blob.core.windows.net/media/Default/PDFs/ADHD_requirements_2018.pdf

Exercise may benefit pediatric patients since it may decrease inattention or impulsive behavior and improve anxiety and depressive symptoms, although it is unlikely exercise alone can be used as a treatment [15, 19]. There is no evidence that the therapeutic use of stimulants increases aggressive behavior. On the contrary, evidence of lack of control or increased aggression may be the manifestation of undertreatment through subtherapeutic dosing or noncompliance [37]. The risk of developing long-term substance abuse from the therapeutic use of stimulants for the treatment of ADHD is small and may further decrease with long-term use [38]. During the periods of rapid growth during childhood and adolescence, there may be need for frequent dosing changes to maintain symptom control [37].

Adult Considerations

It is generally considered that there is no "adult onset" ADHD; however, in some cases compensatory efforts may push symptoms below threshold for years and symptoms may emerge after compensation efforts are reduced or unavailable [15]. For this reason, in athletes 18 and older, when considering a new diagnosis of ADHD, particular attention should be paid to medical and mental health comorbidities and history of brain injury during the medical evaluation. In some sports organizations, a new diagnosis of ADHD in an adult patient may require a second opinion from an independent specialist medical provider to confirm the diagnosis.

Optimal doses of medications vary substantially across the population; however, it is generally considered preferable to use long-lasting or extended-release formulations, because of their improved adherence to treatment regimens, decreased risk of abuse, avoidance of rebound symptoms, and to provide coverage without multiple dosing [39].

Abuse Considerations

Since stimulant medications are considered ergogenic, there is always the potential for abuse of medication or medication diversion. In a 2008 survey of college students, 5.3% admitted nonmedical misuse of stimulants, which approaches the rate of individuals taking stimulants for legitimate medical indications. This historically may have led treating providers to shift prescribing habits; however, the AMSSM position statement makes clear a position that the fear of potential abuse of stimulants is not justification for withholding pharmacologic treatment of ADHD in the appropriate patient. It is supported that untreated ADHD increases the risk of substance abuse, and it has also been demonstrated that athletes appropriately treated for ADHD actually have a lower risk of substance abuse.

There are numerous anecdotal reports of individuals self-medicating with marijuana for the treatment of ADHD. With the growth of medical and recreational marijuana, this may be a growing area of research and/or concern. One small ($n = 30$) randomized-controlled study by Cooper et al. showed nonstatistically significant trends toward improved symptoms in the treatment group [40].

Other Team Physician Considerations

As a team physician, it is important to recognize that problems with motivation or attitude for athletes, or difficulty following the rules may be a manifestation of ADHD [11]. Other signs may include behavioral issues, being involved in conflict situations, or poor attention during coaching sessions [11, 15].

The team medical provider should understand how an athlete's compliance with their medication regimen may affect symptoms. Some athletes may take medication only during certain times of year or for exams. Some athletes may prefer to participate without being medicated because of the belief it may benefit their spontaneity [41, 42]. Cessation or noncompliance with medication regimens may result in symptom exacerbation or outward signs described above [41]. For the same reasons that younger people are more inconsistent with medication, young athletes may be more inconsistent with their medication regimen than older athletes [41].

The appetite suppression seen with stimulants may be a cause of concern for athletes trying to gain weight, and lead to noncompliance, or alternately, stimulants have the potential for abuse by athletes trying to maintain a lower weight [15, 19, 41].

While exercise may improve ADHD symptomatology, and there is little potential harm in recommending continued physical activity, little evidence suggests exercise alone is an effective treatment of ADHD [15, 19, 43]. Notably, coaching may be more effective when an athlete is therapeutically dosed.

Conclusion

Attention deficit disorders remain a prevalent factor in the mental health of many athletes. Through proper education, treatment, and follow-up, physicians and athletes can navigate the challenges of treatment compliance, potential side effects, consequences of under- and overtreatment, and therapeutic use allowances related to their level of competition. The relative risks of ADHD medications upon the cardiovascular, neurologic, and general health of an individual should be considered in initiating treatment, but these risks appear to be unfounded. Appropriate treatment may promote improved cognitive functioning of affected athletes with this diagnosis.

References

1. Pennington BF, Ozonoff S. Executive functions and developmental psychopathology. J Child Psychol Psychiatry. 1996;37(1):51–87.
2. Pliszka S, Issues AWGoQ. Practice parameter for the assessment and treatment of children and adolescents with attention-deficit/hyperactivity disorder. J Am Acad Child Adolesc Psychiatry. 2007;46(7):894–921.
3. Morrow RL, Garland EJ, Wright JM, Maclure M, Taylor S, Dormuth CR. Influence of relative age on diagnosis and treatment of attention-deficit/hyperactivity disorder in children. CMAJ. 2012;184(7):755–62.
4. Layton TJ, Barnett ML, Hicks TR, Jena AB. Attention deficit-hyperactivity disorder and month of school enrollment. N Engl J Med. 2018;379(22):2122–30.
5. Diagnosis and treatment of attention deficit hyperactivity disorder (ADHD). NIH Consens Statement. 1998;16(2):1–37.
6. Diagnostic and statistical manual of mental disorders: DSM-5. Arlington, VA: American Psychiatric Association; 2013.
7. Faraone SV, Perlis RH, Doyle AE, et al. Molecular genetics of attention-deficit/hyperactivity disorder. Biol Psychiatry. 2005;57(11):1313–23.
8. Cdc. Facts | ADHD | NCBDDD | CDC. 2018.
9. Centers for Disease Control and Prevention. Increasing prevalence of parent-reported attention-deficit/hyperactivity disorder among children – United States, 2003 and 2007. MMWR Morb Mortal Wkly Rep. 2010;59(44):1439–43.
10. Center OSUWM. Athletes with ADHD more likely to choose team sports, could increase injury risk, study finds. 2019.; http://www.sciencedaily.com/releases/2017/05/170511135755.htm. Accessed January 15, 2019.
11. White RD, Harris GD, Gibson ME. Attention deficit hyperactivity disorder and athletes. Sports Health. 2014;6(2):149–56.
12. Larson K, Russ SA, Kahn RS, Halfon N. Patterns of comorbidity, functioning, and service use for US children with ADHD, 2007. Pediatrics. 2011;127(3):462–70.
13. Hamed AM, Kauer AJ, Stevens HE. Why the diagnosis of attention deficit hyperactivity disorder matters. Front Psych. 2015;6:168.
14. Psychological issues related to illness and injury in athletes and the team physician: a consensus statement-2016 update. Med Sci Sports Exerc. 2017;49(5):1043–54.
15. Putukian M, Kreher JB, Coppel DB, Glazer JL, McKeag DB, White RD. Attention deficit hyperactivity disorder and the athlete: an American Medical Society for Sports Medicine position statement. Clin J Sport Med. 2011;21(5):392–401.
16. Agency WA-D. Medical Information to Support the Decisions of TUECS – ADHD. 2017. Located at: Medical Information to Support the Decisions of TUECs.
17. NCAA. NCAA Banned Drugs and Medical Exceptions Policy Guidelines Regarding Medical Reporting for Student-Athletes with Attention Deficit Hyperactivity Disorder (ADHD) Taking Prescribed Stimulants; 2009.
18. Subcommittee on Attention-Deficit/Hyperactivity Disorder, Steering Committee on Quality Improvement and Management, et al. ADHD: clinical practice guideline for the diagnosis, evaluation, and treatment of attention-deficit/hyperactivity disorder in children and adolescents. Pediatrics. 2011;128(5):1007–22.
19. Reardon CL, Factor RM. Considerations in the use of stimulants in sport. Sports Med. 2016;46(5):611–7.
20. Jensen PS, Hinshaw SP, Swanson JM, et al. Findings from the NIMH Multimodal Treatment Study of ADHD (MTA): implications and applications for primary care providers. J Dev Behav Pediatr. 2001;22(1):60–73.
21. Stewman CG, Liebman C, Fink L, Sandella B. Attention deficit hyperactivity disorder: unique considerations in athletes. Sports Health. 2018;10(1):40–6.

22. Vetter VL, Elia J, Erickson C, et al. Cardiovascular monitoring of children and adolescents with heart disease receiving medications for attention deficit/hyperactivity disorder. Circulation. 2008;117(18):2407–23.
23. Perrin JM, Friedman RA, Knilans TK, Black Box Working Group, Section on Cardiology and Cardiac Surgery. Cardiovascular monitoring and stimulant drugs for attention-deficit/hyperactivity disorder. Pediatrics. 2008;122(2):451–3.
24. Cooper WO, Habel LA, Sox CM, et al. ADHD drugs and serious cardiovascular events in children and young adults. N Engl J Med. 2011;365(20):1896–904.
25. Hailpern SM, Egan BM, Lewis KD, et al. Blood pressure, heart rate, and CNS stimulant medication use in children with and without ADHD: analysis of NHANES data. Front Pediatr. 2014;2:100.
26. Roelands B, Hasegawa H, Watson P, et al. The effects of acute dopamine reuptake inhibition on performance. Med Sci Sports Exerc. 2008;40(5):879–85.
27. Elbin RJ, Kontos AP, Kegel N, Johnson E, Burkhart S, Schatz P. Individual and combined effects of LD and ADHD on computerized neurocognitive concussion test performance: evidence for separate norms. Arch Clin Neuropsychol. 2013;28(5):476–84.
28. Nelson LD, Guskiewicz KM, Marshall SW, et al. Multiple self-reported concussions are more prevalent in athletes with ADHD and learning disability. Clin J Sport Med. 2016;26(2):120–7.
29. Iverson GL, Gardner AJ, Terry DP, et al. Predictors of clinical recovery from concussion: a systematic review. Br J Sports Med. 2017;51(12):941–8.
30. Mautner K, Sussman WI, Axtman M, Al-Farsi Y, Al-Adawi S. Relationship of attention deficit hyperactivity disorder and postconcussion recovery in youth athletes. Clin J Sport Med. 2015;25(4):355–60.
31. Bouchard R, Weber AR, Geiger JD. Informed decision-making on sympathomimetic use in sport and health. Clin J Sport Med. 2002;12(4):209–24.
32. Chandler JV, Blair SN. The effect of amphetamines on selected physiological components related to athletic success. Med Sci Sports Exerc. 1980;12(1):65–9.
33. Conant-Norville DO, Tofler IR. Attention deficit/hyperactivity disorder and psychopharmacologic treatments in the athlete. Clin Sports Med. 2005;24(4):829–43, viii.
34. Liddle DG, Connor DJ. Nutritional supplements and ergogenic AIDS. Prim Care. 2013;40(2):487–505.
35. Yoo JH, Oh Y, Jang B, et al. The effects of equine-assisted activities and therapy on resting-state brain function in attention-deficit/hyperactivity disorder: a pilot study. Clin Psychopharmacol Neurosci. 2016;14(4):357–64.
36. Evans S, Ling M, Hill B, Rinehart N, Austin D, Sciberras E. Systematic review of meditation-based interventions for children with ADHD. Eur Child Adolesc Psychiatry. 2018;27(1):9–27.
37. Shier AC, Reichenbacher T, Ghuman HS, Ghuman JK. Pharmacological treatment of attention deficit hyperactivity disorder in children and adolescents: clinical strategies. J Cent Nerv Syst Dis. 2012;5:1–17.
38. Lerner M, Wigal T. Long-term safety of stimulant medications used to treat children with ADHD. Pediatr Ann. 2008;37(1):37–45.
39. Kooij SJ, Bejerot S, Blackwell A, et al. European consensus statement on diagnosis and treatment of adult ADHD: the European Network Adult ADHD. BMC Psychiatry. 2010;10:67.
40. Cooper RE, Williams E, Seegobin S, Tye C, Kuntsi J, Asherson P. Cannabinoids in attention-deficit/hyperactivity disorder: a randomised-controlled trial. Eur Neuropsychopharmacol. 2017;27(8):795–808.
41. Pujalte GGA, Maynard JR, Thurston MJ, Taylor WC 3rd, Chauhan M. Considerations in the care of athletes with attention deficit hyperactivity disorder. Clin J Sport Med. 2019;29(3):245–56.
42. Parr JW. Attention-deficit hyperactivity disorder and the athlete: new advances and understanding. Clin Sports Med. 2011;30(3):591–610.
43. Nazeer A, Mansour M, Gross KA. ADHD and adolescent athletes. Front Public Health. 2014;2:46.

Chapter 7
Risk-Taking Behaviors Among Athletes

Kyle Conley and Ashwin L. Rao

Introduction

There is strong evidence participation in athletics is beneficial for physical, social, and mental health. Individual and team sports offer the benefit of social and organizational schemes that benefit the athlete by providing structure, vision, and a path toward success. Participation in competitive sport requires immense drive and commitment that can have both intended and unintended consequences to athletes. Be it the nature of the sport, a willingness to commit to an activity regardless of risk to their health, or other factors, there is a growing body of evidence to suggest that athletes are at equal or greater risk of exhibiting risk-taking behaviors. Risk-taking behaviors fit into several categories, as defined by the CDC's Youth Risk Behavioral Survey, including (I) behaviors that result in unintentional and intentional injury such as motor vehicle crashes, homicide, and suicide; (II) drug and alcohol use; (III) sexual behaviors that result in sexually transmitted infections (STIs), including human immunodeficiency virus (HIV) infection, or unintended pregnancy; (IV) tobacco use; (V) dietary behaviors that contribute to adult morbidity and mortality; and (VI) physical inactivity [1].

There appears to be a potential paradox in reviewing the healthy and risky behaviors taken by athletes. While many studies suggest that athletes demonstrate healthier lifestyle behaviors, such as diet management and exercise activities, than

K. Conley
University of Washington, Seattle, WA, USA
e-mail: Kylec2@uw.edu

A. L. Rao (✉)
Department of Family Medicine and Section of Sports Medicine, Sports Medicine Fellowship, University of Washington, Seattle, WA, USA

UW Husky Athletics and Seattle Seahawks, Seattle, WA, USA
e-mail: ashwin@uw.edu

© Springer Nature Switzerland AG 2020
E. Hong, A. L. Rao (eds.), *Mental Health in the Athlete*,
https://doi.org/10.1007/978-3-030-44754-0_7

nonathletes, other studies suggest that athletes are likely to participate in high-risk behaviors such as drug use, unsafe sex, and risky driving [2, 3]. This chapter will consider the available research regarding the athlete's risk for high-risk behaviors surrounding seatbelt and helmet omission, riding with an intoxicated driver, driving while intoxicated, carrying a weapon, being involved in physical fighting, gambling, sexual risk-taking, and using tobacco products.

Defining Risk Taking

Risk-taking behaviors include activities that put oneself in immediate danger or confer long-term health detriment. Risk-taking may be consciously or nonconsciously controlled and typically has a perceived uncertainty regarding its outcome, potential benefits and related costs, and its impact on the psychosocial well-being of the risk-taking individual and his or her community.

In the context of sports medicine research, a number of studies have referenced data acquired through the Youth Risk Behavior Surveillance system (YRBSS), a national survey of greater that 16,000 U/S public and private high school students conducted by the U.S. Centers for Disease Control and Prevention (CDC) [1]. This survey includes behaviors that may harbor risks and considers representative samples of adolescents by age, ethnicity, and gender. Data regarding collegiate and professional athletes is available but typically involves smaller study sizes, with more modest research goals or specific clinical questions.

Study Context and Quality

Almost all of the studies reviewed here utilize self-reporting questionnaires to assess behaviors. Such questionnaires have been validated to reliably assess behaviors and are routinely used when assessing behavior prevalence [4–6]. Though the validity of self-reporting has been well-documented, under- or overreporting of behaviors is a reasonable concern in the context of the surveyed populations. Studies involving collegiate athletes, in particular, may be challenged by the athlete's tendency to underreport risk-taking behaviors due to the threat of restriction of their athletic participation status or the stigma attached to disclosure.

Additional factors that could impact risk-taking reporting include sport type, race, ethnicity, gender, and role or leadership status on a team. While it may be simple to clarify an individual as an athlete based on their level of participation and competition, other demographic factors render athlete cohorts as heterogeneous in makeup. Thus, drawing broad conclusions from limited data is not advised. Further, findings should be used in the appropriate context as a means of understanding the risk factor environment of athletic lifestyle [7].

Seatbelt Omission

Seatbelt use reduces motor vehicle crash-related fatalities by up to 50% in the general population and is a frequent target for risk mitigation [8]. In the United States, roughly 10% of adolescents admitted to rarely or never using a seatbelt while riding in a car as a passenger. This behavior is more common among adolescent males [1]. It appears that those high school students who self-identify as athletes are actually less likely to omit seatbelt use than nonathletes, with a greater seatbelt adherence rate among girls than boys [2, 9]. In contrast, several studies have identified that collegiate athletes are less likely to wear seatbelts [10–12]. Among collegiate athletes, males are more likely to exhibit this behavior than females (36% vs. 21%) [13]. Collegiate contact sports athletes in particular report higher levels of seatbelt omission [11].

Riding with an Intoxicated Driver

Riding with an intoxicated driver is a significant health risk to athletes. According to the 2007 YRBSS study, approximately 30% of adolescents reported riding in a vehicle with a driver who had been drinking alcohol in the past month [14]. Male college athletes have consistently been found to ride with an intoxicated driver, more than have female athletes, with differences as high as twofold in some studies [10–12, 15]. In two regional studies of college students, female athletes reported lower rates of riding in car with an intoxicated driver compared to male athletes, while there was no significant difference between female athletes and female non-athletes [12, 15]. One study postulates that this behavior emerges in male athletes at the college level when they and their peers reach the legal drinking age, given the lack of difference seen in adolescent athletes [2]. Contact-sport athletes report higher levels of riding with an intoxicated driver than a noncontact athlete [10, 11]. Data is not yet available to study this behavior in professional or older athletes.

Driving While Intoxicated

The risks and harms imposed by drunk driving are well-documented. Driving while intoxicated typically alludes to the consumption of alcoholic beverages above the legal limit for use or when the sensorium is impaired. Marijuana use is being increasingly considered as a form of intoxication capable of causing impaired driving and has been prosecuted similarly. In most countries, driving while intoxicated represents a criminal offence.

According to the CDC, young individuals who drive impaired have a higher relative risk of motor vehicle accidents. Over 50% of motor vehicle fatalities involve intoxicated young drivers [16]. The 2017 YRBSS identifies at 10% prevalence of adolescent athletes who drive while intoxicated, with a greater relative prevalence in males [1].

Collegiate athletic intoxicated driving rates appear to be higher in males than in females, though rates of intoxicated driving varied by how intoxication was defined [10, 11]. In general, the use of more inclusive definitions of intoxication (i.e., driving under the influence of intoxicating agents, or even simple utilization of use) reveal higher rates of impaired driving among male athletes by as much as twofold (25% vs. 13%) [13]. As is the case with riding with an intoxicated driver, collegiate athletes involved in contact or collision sports appear to be more likely to drive while intoxicated [11].

Among professional sport athletes, data regarding driving while intoxicated or impaired by substances is limited. However, Zhou et al. identified that team sports athletes are more likely to be categorized as hazardous drinkers compared to athletes engaged in individual sports [17]. Further, reported rates of alcohol and substance abuse are reported to be high among current and recently retired professional athletes playing football, soccer, and rugby [18, 19].

Possession and Carriage of a Deadly Weapon

Access, possession, and carriage of a deadly weapon are an important and known risk factor in gun-related violence, including suicide and homicide. Those with access to lethal means such as a firearm are more likely to successfully carryout a suicidal or homicidal act [20–22]. Adolescent males are more likely to possess and carry a weapon and are similarly more likely to die by suicide or homicide [1].

The data regarding the prevalence of weapons carriage among student athletes, compared to nonathletes, is limited. Among adolescent athletes, a number of YRBSS studies show stronger evidence of reduced weapons carriage among adolescent male athletes compared to nonathletes. In contrast, there appears to be no substantial difference in weapon carriage between adolescent female athletes and nonathletes [7, 23, 24].

Among the collegiate athlete population, studies range from showing no difference to showing modest increases in weapon use among contact-sport athletes [2, 11, 25, 26]. Regional and demographic differences cloud the picture of weapon carriage in cited studies. As an example, there may be regional differences in accessibility of guns utilized for hunting purposes that can impact response rates.

Fighting

Engagement in physical fighting puts one at risk for significant bodily harm. YRBSS data from 2017 found males had a higher prevalence of having been in a physical fight [1]. YRBSS data from 1997 to 2007 found that, when analyzed as a whole, adolescent athletes and nonathletes were no different in reporting involvement in physical fights; however, race-specific analyses found non-White males were more likely to have been involved in physical fighting [7, 24]. For female adolescent athletes, only white females were less likely to be involved in a fight at school [24]. Similarly, two studies found adolescent sports participants to be more likely to be involved in fights in the past year [25, 26]. Male and female college athletes as a whole had a higher propensity to be involved in physical fights compared to nonathletes (26% vs. 12%) and contact-sport athletes had a significantly higher risk of fighting than noncontact-sport athletes [11]. Fight-related risk-taking data is lacking for professional athlete populations.

Gambling

A significant literature has accumulated in the field of psychology regarding the relationships between gambling behaviors, impulsivity, and addiction. Some evidence regarding gambling behavior in athletes has emerged over the last 15 years. Among NCAA athletes, males have been found to gamble more often and are up to tenfold as likely to be pathological gamblers as females, potentially due to males gambling for expected financial gain and females for expected fun and enjoyment [27, 28]. In a separate study, 15% of all athletes, demonstrated pathological gambling behavior, while yet another study of Midwest universities found that non-White athletes were most at risk for gambling problems compared to other groups [29].

Gambling behaviors have not been as robustly studied at the high school or professional levels. A study of 316 high school students in Israel found that participation in athletics was positively associated with gambling frequency, and males were more likely to gamble pathologically [30]. While details of the gambling tendencies of athletes in the United States are not available, European professional athletes from various sports were particularly prone to gamble [31]. Nearly 60% of athletes had gambled in the past year and prevalence of pathological gambling was 8.2%. There was also an association between gambling problems with betting on one's own team, betting online, and gambling regularly [31].

There is limited data available that suggests that former athletes are more likely to participate in skill-based forms of gambling (i.e., sports betting, poker), while nonathletes are more likely to participate in games of chance [32].

High-Risk Sexual Behavior

High-risk sexual behaviors include activities that put people at risk for sexually transmitted infections, unplanned pregnancy, or other unintended consequences. Behaviors such as unprotected sex, sexual intercourse with multiple partners, or sex following alcohol consumption represent examples of high-risk sexual behaviors that may bring about unwanted consequences. A substantial body of evidence exists for sexual risk-taking in general with the adolescent or high-school-aged athletes, as well as with specific risky sexual behaviors. A study of 556 Polish high school students in 2015 found sports participation to be a protective factor for females against sexual risk-taking, but a risk factor for males [33]. General sexual risk-taking has not been assessed in large studies, and the evidence is not consistent [34–36]. There is better evidence for specific categories of sexual risk-taking, such as condom use. There is strong evidence of increased rates of condom use in adolescent and high school athletes compared to nonathletes from large, national studies, and these findings have been repeated in a few smaller, regional studies [23, 24, 36, 37]. However, increased condom usage was found only among male athletes when studying a cohort of a few thousand alternative high school students [25]. There is also robust evidence that athlete status for female adolescents is protective against pregnancy and one ever having had a sexually transmitted disease [23, 34–36]. In contrast, a 2018 study of 445 college students evaluating the psychological motifs of goal orientation, sport identities, and risky sexual behavior found that females who reported playing organized sports regularly in high school were more likely than males to engage in risky sexual behavior when in college [38].

Among sexually active NCAA athletes, male athletes reported higher prevalence of unprotected sex (10% vs. 8%) and multiple sex partners (15% vs. 10%) than females [39]. Male athletes appear to engage in riskier sex, have a greater number of sexual partners, higher rates of health-risk outcomes and use less contraceptives compared to nonathletes [11]. When assessing female collegiate students, there has been either no difference or less sexual risk-taking behaviors or health-risk outcomes among female athletes, including condom use and pregnancy [11, 12]. Subgroup analyses from a small study of 168 multiracial female college athletes at two universities in South Florida found Hispanic athletes had more sexual partners in past 3 months compared to Caucasian and African American athlete [40]. When both genders are analyzed together, studies have found more sexual risk-taking in athletes compared to nonathletes, including amongst incoming freshman and college-bound high school graduates [10, 41, 42]. Only one study did not find a difference in athletes' sexual risk-taking [12].

Tobacco Use

The adverse health effects associated with tobacco use are well-known and include malignancy, coronary artery disease, obstructive and inflammatory pulmonary disease, and sudden infant death. In some cases, tobacco use may be seen as recreational and part of the social fabric of certain sports. In other instances, tobacco may be used as a central nerves system stimulant with potential for performance enhancement.

Tobacco use among collegiate student athletes is surprisingly prevalent, in part due to prevalence of smokeless tobacco use. A large study of 991 NCAA Division I, II, and III institutions found that 23% of athletes used smokeless tobacco, with male athletes more likely to use (6–55%) than female athletes (1–22%) [43]. While smokeless tobacco use has been consistently observed, there are some differences between sports. Interestingly, Nattiv et al. found no differences in tobacco usage by college athletes compared to nonathletes, but their analysis excluded baseball athletes, whose culture is known to accept routine tobacco use [11]. In general, college athletes report the less frequent cigarette use but higher frequency of smokeless tobacco utilization.

When considering adolescent athletes, YRBSS data suggests that male athletes are less likely to smoke cigarettes [1]. Amongst the high school and adolescent athlete population, there is robust evidence from several national studies, several regional studies, and even a meta-analysis that athletes of all races/ethnicities, ages and genders are less likely to smoke cigarettes than their nonathlete peers [2, 7, 9, 24, 25, 44–46]. Some studies found a positive correlation with level of athletic involvement, with more high-involved athletes having significantly lower risk than low-involved athletes [5, 47].

Limitations

The studies used above have a number of potential limitations. As previously stated, most included studies rely upon self-reported surveys, which risk athletes misreporting or underreporting risk behaviors. The culture of athletics may dissuade athletes from disclosing their risk-taking behavior, for fear of reprisal. In some instances, their risk-taking may preclude athletic population if known. In other instances, their risk-taking may be considered socially unacceptable. In yet other cases, shame may cloud the athlete's willingness to report.

Many of the studies used focus on specific athlete population. Hence, generalizing assumptions should not be undertaken, as sampling bias may put the provider at risk of making false judgments. Additionally, the studies reviewed cover a 20-year timeframe, during which risk-taking behaviors in athlete populations may have evolved. Finally, a large portion of the data reviewed is retrospective, which limits the value of the information gathered.

Conclusion

Risk-taking remains a large concern among athlete populations, and the range of risk-taking among athletes is broad and may differ by gender, sport, culture, or geographic region. Providers caring for athletes should be aware that athletes are willing to take risks to their own health, and often are unaware of the consequences of their actions. Athletes who appear to be struggling with social integration, successful participation in their sport, or with performance in the classroom should be engaged to assess for risk-taking behaviors.

References

1. Kann L, McManus T, Harris WA, Shanklin SL, Flint KH, Queen B, et al. Youth risk behavior surveillance – United States, 2017. MMWR Surveill Summ. 2018;67(8):1–114.
2. Baumert PJ, Henderson JM, Thompson NJ. Health risk behaviors of adolescent participants in organized sports. J Adolesc Health. 1998;22(6):460–5.
3. Heron M. Deaths: leading causes for 2010. Natl Vital Stat Rep. 2013;62(6):1–96.
4. Bauman KE, Koch GG. Validity of self-reports and descriptive and analytical conclusions: the case of cigarette smoking by adolescents and their mothers. Am J Epidemiol. 1983;118(1):90–8.
5. Dolcini MM, Adler NE, Lee P, Bauman KE. An assessment of the validity of adolescent self-reported smoking using three biological indicators. Nicotine Tob Res. 2003;5(4):473–83.
6. O'Malley PM, Bachman JG, Johnston LD. Reliability and consistency in self-reports of drug use. Int J Addict. 1983;18(6):805–24.
7. Patel DR, Luckstead EF. Sports participation, risk taking, and health risk behaviors. Adolesc Med. 2000;11(1):141–55.
8. Injury prevention: meeting the challenge. The National Committee for Injury Prevention and Control. Am J Prev Med. 1989;5:1–303.
9. Melnick MJ, Miller KE, Sabo DF, et al. Athletic participation and seatbelt omission among U.S. High School students. Health Educ Behav. 2010;37(1):23–36.
10. Nattiv A, Puffer JC. Lifestyles and health risks of collegiate athletes. J Fam Pract. 1991;33(6):585–90.
11. Nattiv A, Puffer JC, Green GA. Lifestyles and health risks of collegiate athletes: a multi-center study. Clin J Sport Med. 1997;7(4):262–72.
12. Kokotailo PK, Henry BC, Koscik RE, Fleming MF, Landry GL. Substance use and other health risk behaviors in collegiate athletes. Clin J Sport Med. 1996;6(3):183–9.
13. Peretti-Watel P, Guagliardo V, Verger P, Pruvost J, Mignon P, Obadia Y. Risky behaviours among young elite-student-athletes: results from a pilot survey in south-eastern France. Int Rev Sociol Sport. 2004;39(2):233–44.
14. Bovard RS. Risk behaviors in high school and college sport. Curr Sports Med Rep. 2008;7(6):359–66.
15. Kokotailo PK, Koscik RE, Henry BC, et al. Health risk taking and human immunodeficiency virus risk in collegiate female athletes. J Am Coll Heal. 1998;46(6):263–8.
16. CDC. Motor vehicle crash deaths: how is the US doing. https://www.cdc.gov/vitalsigns/motor-vehicle-safety/index.html.
17. Zhou J, Heim D, O'Brien K. Alcohol consumption, athlete identity, and happiness among student sportspeople as a function of sport-type. Alcohol Alcohol. 2015;50(5):617–23.
18. Du Preez EJ. Depression, anxiety, and alcohol use in elite rugby league players of a competitive season. Clin J Sport Med. 2017;27(6):530–5.
19. Mez J, Daneshvar DH, Kiernan PT, et al. Clinicopathological evaluation of chronic traumatic encephalopathy in players of American Football. JAMA. 2017;318(4):360–70.
20. Grossman DC, Mueller BA, Dowd RC, et al. Gun storage practice and the risk of youth suicide and unintentional firearm injuries. JAMA. 2005;294(6):707–14.
21. Page RM, Hammermeister J. Weapon-carrying and youth violence. Adoelscence. 1997;32(1278):505–13.
22. Rao AL, Poon S, Drezner JA, et al. Death by homicide in National Collegiate Athletic Association athletes between 2003–2013. Br J Sports Med. 2016;50(3):33–8.
23. Page RM, Hammermeister J, Scanlan A, Gilbert L. Is school sports participation a protective factor against adolescent health risk behaviors? J Health Educ. 1998;29(3):186–92.
24. Taliaferro LA, Rienzo BA, Donovan KA. Relationships between youth sport participation and selected health risk behaviors from 1999-2007. J Sch Health. 2010;80(8):399–410.
25. Johnson KE, McMorris BJ, Kubik MY. Comparison of health-risk behaviors among students attending alternative and traditional high schools in Minnesota. J Sch Nurs. 2013;29(5):343–52.

26. Garry JP, Morrissey SL. Team sports participation and risk-taking behaviors among a biracial middle school population. Clin J Sport Med. 2000;10(3):185–90.
27. Huang J-H, Jacobs DF, Derevensky JL. DSM-based problem gambling: increasing the odds of heavy drinking in a national sample of U.S. college athletes? J Psychiatr Res. 2011;45(3):302–8.
28. St-Pierre RA, Temcheff CE, Gupta R, et al. Predicting gambling problems from gambling outcome expectancies in college student-athletes. J Gambl Stud. 2014;30(1):47–60.
29. Kerber CS. Problem and pathological gambling among college athletes. Ann Clin Psychiatry. 2005;17(4):243–7.
30. Gabriel-Fried B. Attitudes of Jewish Israeli adults towards gambling. Int Gambl Stud. 2015;15(2):196–211.
31. Grall-Bronnec M, Caillon J, Humeau E, Perrot B, Remaud M, Guilleux A, et al. Gambling among European professional athletes. Prevalence and associated factors. J Addict Dis. 2016;35(4):278–90.
32. Weiss SM, Loubier SL. Gambling habits of athletes and nonathletes classified as disordered gamblers. J Psychol. 2010;144(6):507–21.
33. Lipowski M, Lipowska M, Jochimek M, Krokosz D. Resiliency as a factor protecting youths from risky behaviour: moderating effects of gender and sport. Eur J Sport Sci. 2016;16(2):246–55.
34. Sabo DF, Miller KE, Farrell MP, Melnick MJ, Barnes GM. High school athletic participation, sexual behavior and adolescent pregnancy: a regional study. J Adolesc Health. 1999;25(3):207–16.
35. Miller KE, Melnick MJ, Farrell MP, Sabo DF, Barnes GM. Jocks, gender, binge drinking, and adolescent violence. J Interpers Violence. 2006;21(1):105–20.
36. Miller KE, Barnes GM, Melnick MJ, Sabo DF, Farrell MP. Gender and racial/ethnic differences in predicting adolescent sexual risk: athletic participation versus exercise. J Health Soc Behav. 2002;43(4):436–50.
37. Habel MA, Dittus PJ, De Rosa CJ, et al. Daily participation in sports and students' sexual activity. Perspect Sex Reprod Health. 2010;42(4):244–50.
38. Maberry S. Goal orientation, sport identities, and risky sexual behavior. J Study Sports Athl Educ. 2018;12(2):113–32.
39. Huang J-H, Jacobs DF, Derevensky JL. Sexual risk-taking behaviors, gambling, and heavy drinking among U.S. College athletes. Arch Sex Behav. 2010;39(3):706–13.
40. Kuo Y, Perry A, Wang X, et al. Comparison of body composition, eating habits, exercise habits, and high risk behavior in tri-racial female athletes. IJESAB. 2016;8(4):58.
41. Grossbard JR, Lee CM, Neighbors C, et al. Alcohol and risky sex in athletes and nonathletes: what roles do sex motives play? J Stud Alcohol Drugs. 2007;68(4):566–74.
42. Wetherill RR, Fromme K. Alcohol use, sexual activity, and perceived risk in high school athletes and non-athletes. J Adolesc Health. 2007;41(3):294–301.
43. Green GA, Uryasz FD, Petr TA, Bray CD. NCAA study of substance use and abuse habits of college student-athletes. Clin J Sport Med. 2001;11(1):51–6.
44. Diehl K, Thiel A, Zipfel S, Mayer J, Litaker DG, Schneider S. How healthy is the behavior of young athletes? A systematic literature review and meta-analyses. J Sports Sci Med. 2012;11(2):201–20.
45. Older MJ, Mainous AG, Martin CA, et al. Depression, suicidal ideation, and substance abuse among adolescents. Are athletes at less risk? Arch Fam Med. 1994;3(9):781–5.
46. Forman ES, Dekker AH, Javors JR, Davison DT. High-risk behaviors in teenage male athletes. Clin J Sport Med. 1995;5(1):36–42.
47. Davis TC, Arnold C, Nandy I, et al. Tobacco use among male high school athletes. J Adolesc Health. 1997;21(2):97–101.

Chapter 8
The Psychological Response to Injury and Illness

Margot Putukian

Psychological and Sociocultural Risk Factors for Injury

There are several injury risk factors in sport, with psychological and sociocultural factors a subject of consensus statements and systematic review [4, 10, 11, 31]. These are listed in Table 8.1.

Sociocultural risk factors include limited social resources, a lifetime history of physical or sexual abuse [32], social pressures, stress related to negative self-appraisal of academic and athletic performance, stress associated with an athlete's appraisal of the structure and function of their team [33], poor athlete–coach relationship and communication, and the general culture of the team or sport (e.g., a "winning at all costs" mindset) [4, 10, 34, 35]. Psychological risk factors include anxiety/worry, hypervigilance, low self-esteem or poor body image, perfectionism, limited coping resources, life event stress (e.g., major life event stressors such as the death of a family member or starting at a new school), risk-taking behaviors, or low mood state.

The prospective literature regarding most psychological and psychosocial risk factors and injury is sparse, and at times conflicting, with the exception of stress. Life event stress and a high stress response, where there is a negative emotional response to either injury or another stressful event, have (i.e., negative emotional responses after sport injury or other stressful events) been consistently associated with an increased risk of injury [8, 10, 31, 34–39].

Stress can increase muscle tension and impair coordination, and cause inattention, distraction, and increased self-consciousness, all of which can increase the risk

M. Putukian (✉)
Princeton University, Athletic Medicine, University Health Services, Princeton, NJ, USA

Rutgers-Robert Wood Johnson Medical School, University of Medicine and Dentistry of New Jersey, New Brunswick, NJ, USA
e-mail: putukian@princeton.edu

© Springer Nature Switzerland AG 2020
E. Hong, A. L. Rao (eds.), *Mental Health in the Athlete*,
https://doi.org/10.1007/978-3-030-44754-0_8

Table 8.1 Risk factors for injury

Sociocultural	Psychological
Stress	Life event stress
Organizational	Anxiety/worry
Social resources and pressures	Hypervigilance
Athletic/academic roles	Perfectionism
Coaching quality	Body image
Rules of sport	Coping and resources
Culture of sport and team	Risk-taking behaviors
	Mood state
	Self-esteem

Modified from [4]

for injury and impair performance [8, 31, 34–39]. There has also been data to show that when teammates and coaches are sources of life event stress, there is an associated increased risk of both overuse and acute injuries [35]. Involuntary and overly intense emotional reactions (increased emotional reactivity) are also associated with injury and poor on-field performance [6, 40, 41].

Response to Injury and Rehabilitation/Recovery from Illness and Injury

A systematic review identified three factors that are most important in determining outcome of rehabilitation following injury; the cognitive, emotional, and behavioral responses to injury [31]. Though there is little information regarding outcome following illness, it is a reasonable assumption that the same processes occurring after injury, also occur after illness. The cognitive response to injury is how the athlete interprets their illness or injury. Cognitive responses lead to emotional responses, which then can affect an athlete's behavioral response, which can be the athlete's motivation, goal-setting abilities, compliance with treatment, and response to treatment.

The cognitive, emotional, and behavioral responses to injury and illness can be considered either "normal" or "problematic" [4]. When an athlete is injured, one of the first responses is coping with and processing the medical information provided. Cognitive responses to injury include concerns about reinjury, doubts about competency, low self-efficacy, loss of identity, and concerns about competency of the medical staff [4, 42]. Examples of problematic cognitive responses are included in Table 8.2.

Emotional responses to injury or illness may include symptoms of sadness, depression, suicidal ideation, anxiety, isolation, lack of motivation, anger or rage, irritability, frustration, sleep disturbances, changes in appetite, low vigor, disengagement, significant pain, frequent crying or emotional outbursts, and burnout [4, 10, 25]. Whereas emotional responses to injury and illness vary, problematic emotional responses are those that do not resolve, worsen over time, or in which the symptoms seem excessive [4]. Injured athletes report more symptoms of depression and of

Table 8.2 Cognitive responses to injury

Athlete statements	Problematic cognitive response
"I can't do this since it may increase the risk for re-injury"	Concerns about reinjury
"I can't play this sport anymore"	Doubts about competency
"I won't be good enough to play at the elite level anymore"	Low self-efficacy
"Who am I if I'm not an athlete")	Loss of identity
"I'll do twice as much so that I can get better quicker"	Inappropriate strategies
"I don't think my medical staff knows what they are doing"	Concerns about competency of the medical staff

Modified from [4]

generalized anxiety disorder compared to noninjured athletes [24]. Female athletes possibly report symptoms of depression and anxiety, with 48% of female collegiate athletes stating that they felt overwhelming anxiety in the past year, compared to 31% of their male counterparts, and 28% versus 21% of female and male collegiate athletes, respectively, stating that in the past year they had felt so depressed it was difficult to function [43, 44]. Injury (and possibly illness) may trigger or unmask other behavioral responses or underlying mental health disorders, including disordered gambling, disordered eating or eating disorders, and substance use disorders [44–57].

Prevention

A systematic review identified three psychological elements (self-determination theory-autonomy, competence, and relatedness) as the factors most important in positive rehabilitation and return to preinjury level of play [9]. Resiliency and "high mental toughness" are associated with lower injury rates as well as a lower incidence of disruptive emotional disorders including depression, anxiety, stress, and obsessive-compulsive symptoms [45, 57]. How an athlete perceives their injury and recovery, their life outside of sport and their expectations for outcomes both short and long term, and satisfaction with their healthcare providers can all impact their rehabilitation and recovery [9, 58–62]. Individual athlete factors such as pain perception, optimism/self-efficacy, depression, and stress may also impact outcome [9, 58–62]. Athletes that have positive cognitive, emotional, and behavioral responses and lower levels of depression and stress may have improved injury recovery [9, 57–66]. Athletes with more positive cognitive, emotional, and behavioral responses may have improved injury recovery [9, 57–61, 63–66]. Higher levels of optimism and self-efficacy and lower levels of depression and stress are associated with improved recovery from injury. [9, 57–61, 63–65]

Examples of interventions that may improve return to sport include: (a) stress and anxiety reduction strategies using modeling techniques (e.g., watching videos of athletes with similar injuries discussing their stress reduction strategies or pairing athletes in different stages of recovery together), (b) providing athlete education (e.g., increasing athlete autonomy by explaining the purpose of certain exercises, or what to expect with surgical interventions), (c) providing athletes with confidence (e.g., demonstrating their function improvements and setting goals), (d) encouraging social support, and (e) encouraging athletes to stay involved in their sport in some manner (e.g., helping with coaching responsibilities yet avoiding premature return to sport activity) [62, 67].

Role of Team Physicians and Other Healthcare Providers

Healthcare providers are in an ideal situation to recognize when an athlete may be experiencing a problematic response to injury. If the athlete appears to have an unreasonable fear of reinjury, deny the severity of injury, appear to have significant impatience of irritability or emotional outbursts, if they appear withdrawn or express guilt about letting teammates down, or if they have significant complaints that appear unrelated to their original illness or injury, they may benefit from working with a mental health provider [4].

If they have any of the behavioral, physical, or psychological signs and symptoms of stress, they may also benefit from working with a mental health provider [4]. In a cross-sectional study of just over 1200 collegiate athletes, 27% reported using mental skills during injury rehabilitation, including goal setting, positive self-talk/positive thoughts, and imagery, and of these athletes, almost 72% indicated that they felt mental skills helped them rehabilitate faster [68].

The benefits of utilizing mental health providers during recovery from injury include: providing general support for the athlete; providing education to the athlete regarding the response to injury; addressing maladaptive coping strategies and challenges with setting new goals and/or expectations; helping with problem solving; improving resiliency; and exploring fears of reinjury. Team physicians and other healthcare providers play a significant role in communicating with the injured or ill athlete in addressing the psychological response to injury, providing ongoing education, identifying misinformation about the injury identifying and interacting with the support network for the athlete, encouraging the athlete to use specific stress and coping skills, and preparing the athlete, parent, and coaches for the process of recovery. Team physicians and other healthcare providers can also encourage and facilitate referral to a member of the mental health network [4].

References

1. Putukian M. The psychological response to injury in student athletes: a narrative review with a focus on mental health. Br J Sports Med. 2016;50(3):145–8.
2. NCAA Interassociation Consensus Document: understanding and supporting student-athlete mental wellness. Mental health best practices. 2018. Available from http://www.ncaa.org/sites/default/files/SSI_MentalHealthBestPractices_Web_20170921.pdf. Accessed 18 Feb 2018.

3. Putukian M. How being injured affects mental health. In: Brown GT, Hainline B, Kroshus E, et al., editors. Mind, body and sport: understanding and supporting student-athlete mental wellness. Indianapolis: NCAA Press; 2014. p. 72–5.
4. Herring SA, Kibler WB, Putukian M. Psychological issues related to illness and injury in athletes and the team physician: a consensus statement-2016 update. Med Sci Sports Exerc. 2017;49(5):1043–54.
5. Neal TL, Diamond AB, Goldman S, et al. Inter-association recommendations for developing a plan to recognize and refer student-athletes with psychological concerns at the collegiate level: an executive summary of a consensus statement. J Athl Train. 2013;48(5):716–20.
6. Ivarsson A, Johnson U, Podlog L. Psychological predictors of injury occurrence: a prospective investigation of professional Swedish soccer players. J Sport Rehabil. 2013;22(1):19–26.
7. Ivarsson A, Johnson U. Psychological factors as predictors of injuries among senior soccer players. A prospective study. J Sports Sci Med. 2010;9(2):347–52.
8. Ivarsson A, Johnson U, Andersen MB, et al. Psychosocial factors and sport injuries: meta-analyses for prediction and prevention. Sports Med. 2017;47(2):353–65.
9. Ardern CL, Taylor NF, Feller JA, et al. A systematic review of the psychological factors associated with returning to sport following injury. Br J Sports Med. 2013;47(17):1120–6.
10. Wiese-Bjornstal DM. Psychology and socioculture affect injury risk, response, and recovery in high-intensity athletes: a consensus statement. Scand J Med Sci Sports. 2010;20:103–11.
11. Wiese-bjornstal DM, Smith AM, Shaffer SM, et al. An integrated model of response to sport injury: psychological and sociological dynamics. J Appl Sport Psychol. 1998;10(1):46–69.
12. Nippert AH, Smith AM. Psychological stress related to injury and impact on sport performance. Phys Med Rehabil Clin N Am. 2008;19(1):399–418.
13. Glazer JL. Eating disorders among male athletes. Curr Sports Med Rep. 2008;7(6):332–7.
14. DeSouza MJ, Nattiv A, Joy E, et al. 2014 Female Athlete Triad Coalition consensus statement on treatment and return to play of the female athlete triad: 1st International Conference held in San Francisco, CA, May 2012, and 2nd International Conference held in Indianapolis, IN, May 2013. Clin J Sport Med. 2014;24(2):96–119.
15. Nattiv A, Puffer JC, Green GA. Lifestyles and health risks of collegiate athletes: a multi-center study. Clin J Sports Med. 1997;7(4):262–72.
16. Beable S, Fulcher M, Lee AC, et al. SHARPSports mental Health Awareness Research Project: prevalence and risk factors of depressive syptoms and the life stress in elite athletes. J Sci Med Sport. 2017;20(12):1047–52.
17. Drew MK, Raysmith BP, Charlton PC. Injuries impair the chance of successful performance by sportspeople: a systematic review. Br J Sports Med. 2017;51(16):1209–14.
18. Gouttebarge V, Aoki H, Kerkhoffs G. Symptoms of common mental disorders and adverse health behaviours in male professional soccer players. J Hum Kinet. 2015;49(1):277–86.
19. Gouttebarge V, Backx FJ, Aoki H, et al. Symptoms of common mental disorders in professional football (soccer) across five European countries. J Sports Sci Med. 2015;14(4):811.
20. Gouttebarge V, Frings-Dresen M, Sluiter J. Mental and psychosocial health among current and former professional footballers. Occup Med. 2015;65(3):190–6.
21. Gouttebarge V, Jonkers R, Moen M, et al. The prevalence and risk indicators of symptoms of common mental disorders among current and former Dutch elite athletes. J Sports Sci. 2017;35(21):2148–56.
22. Gouttebarge V, Jonkers R, Moen M, et al. A prospective cohort study on symptoms of common mental disorders among Dutch elite athletes. Phys Sportsmed. 2017;45(4):426–32.
23. Gouttebarge V, Hopley P, Kerkhoffs G, et al. A 12-month prospective cohort study of symptoms of common mental disorders among professional rugby players. Eur J Sport Sci. 2018;18(7):1004–12.
24. Gulliver A, Griffiths KM, Mackinnon A, et al. The mental health of Australian elite athletes. J Sci Med Sport. 2015;18(3):255–61.
25. Kilic O, Aoki H, Goedhart E, et al. Severe musculoskeletal time-loss injuries and symptoms of common mental disorders in professional soccer: a longitudinal analysis of 12-month follow-up data. Knee Surg Sports Traumatol Arthrosc. 2018;26(3):946–54.

26. Kilic O, Aoki H, Haagensen R, et al. Symptoms of common mental disorders and related stressors in Danish professional football and handball. Eur J Sport Sci. 2017;17(10):1328–34.
27. Nixdorf I, Frank R, Hautzinger M, et al. Prevalence of depressive symptoms and correlating variables among German elite athletes. J Clin Sport Psychol. 2013;7(4):313–26.
28. Schuring N, Kerkhoffs G, Gray J, et al. The mental wellbeing of current and retired professional cricketers: an observational prospective cohort study. Phys Sportsmed. 2017;45(4):463–9.
29. DiFiori JP, Benjamin HJ, Brenner JS, et al. Overuse injuries and burnout in youth sports: a position statement from the American Medical Society for Sports Medicine. Br J Sports Med. 2014;48(4):287–8.
30. Ivarsson A, Johnson U, Lindwall M, et al. Psychosocial stress as a predictor of injury in elite junior soccer: a latent growth curve analysis. J Sci Med Sport. 2014;17(4):366–70.
31. Forsdyke D, Smith A, Jones M, et al. Psychosocial factors associated with outcomes of sports injury rehabilitation in competitive athletes: a mixed studies systematic review. Br J Sports Med. 2016;50(9):537–44.
32. Timpka T, Janson S, Jacobsson J, et al. Lifetime history of sexual and physical abuse among competitive athletics (track and field) athletes: cross sectional study of associations with sports and non-sports injury. Br J Sports Med. 2019;53(22):1412–7.
33. Fletcher D, Hanton S. Sources of organizational stress in elite sports performers. Sport Psychol. 2003;17(2):175–95.
34. Johnson U, Ivarsson A. Psychological predictors of sport injuries among junior soccer players. Scand J Med Sci Sports. 2011;21(1):129–36. https://doi.org/10.1111/j.1600-0838.2009.01057.x. Published online first: 2011/01/11.
35. Pensgaard AM, Ivarsson A, Nilstad A, et al. Psychosocial stress factors, including the relationship with the coach, and their influence on acute and overuse injury risk in elite female football players. BMJ Open Sport Exerc Med. 2018;4(1):e000317.
36. van der Does HT, Brink MS, Otter RT, et al. Injury risk is increased by changes in perceived recovery of team sport players. Clin J Sport Med. 2017;27(1):46–51.
37. Steffen K, Pensgaard AM, Bahr R. Self-reported psychological characteristics as risk factors for injuries in female youth football. Scand J Med Sci Sports. 2009;19(3):442–51.
38. Kellmann M. Preventing overtraining in athletes in high-intensity sports and stress/recovery monitoring. Scand J Med Sci Sports. 2010;20:95–102.
39. Staufenbiel SM, Penninx BWJH, Spijker AT, et al. Hair cortisol, stress exposure, and mental health in humans: a systematic review. Psychoneuroendocrinology. 2013;38(8):1220–35.
40. Nicholls AR, Levy AR, Grice A, et al. Stress appraisals, coping, and coping effectiveness among international cross-country runners during training and competition. Eur J Sport Sci. 2009;9(5):285–93.
41. Casper D. Psychological predictors of injury among professional soccer players. Sport Sci Rev. 2011;20(5–6):5–36.
42. Hainline B, Turner JA, Caneiro JP, et al. Pain in elite athletes: neurophysiological, biomechanical and psychosocial considerations: a narrative review. Br J Sports Med. 2017;51:1259–64.
43. Culbertson FM. Depression and gender. An international review. Am Psychol. 1997;52(1):25–31.
44. Wolanin A, Hong E, Marks D, et al. Prevalence of clinically elevated depressive symptoms in college athletes and differences by gender and sport. Br J Sports Med. 2016;50(3):167–71.
45. Proctor SL, Boan-Lenzo C. Prevalence of depressive symptoms in male intercollegiate student-athletes and nonathletes. J Clin Sport Psychol. 2010;4(3):204–20.
46. Yang J, Peek-Asa C, Corlette JD, et al. Prevalence of and risk factors associated with symptoms of depression in competitive collegiate student athletes. Clin J Sport Med. 2007;17(6):481–7.
47. Rice SM, Purcell R, De Silva S, et al. The mental health of elite athletes: a narrative systematic review. Sports Med. 2016;46(9):1333–53.
48. Guskiewicz KM, Marshall SW, Bailes J, et al. Recurrent concussion and risk of depression in retired professional football players. Med Sci Sports Exerc. 2007;39(6):903–9.
49. Beals KA, Manore MM. Disorders of the female athlete triad among collegiate athletes. Int J Sport Nutr Exerc Metab. 2002;12(3):281–93.

50. Weigand S, Cohen J, Merenstein D. Susceptibility for depression in current and retired student athletes. Sports Health. 2013;5(3):263–6.
51. Lindqvist AS, Moberg T, Ehrnborg C, et al. Increased mortality rate and suicide in Swedish former elite male athletes in power sports. Scand J Med Sci Sports. 2014;24(6):1000–5.
52. Armstrong S, Oomen-Early J. Social connectedness, self-esteem, and depression symptomatology among collegiate athletes versus nonathletes. J Am Coll Heal. 2009;57(5):521–6.
53. Huang J-H, Jacobs DF, Derevensky JL, et al. Gambling and health risk behaviors among US college student-athletes: findings from a national study. J Adolesc Health. 2007;40(5):390–7.
54. Weinstock J, Whelan JP, Meyers AW, et al. Gambling behavior of student-athletes and a student cohort: what are the odds? J Gambl Stud. 2007;23(1):13–24.
55. Kerr ZY, Marshall SW, Harding HP Jr, et al. Nine-year risk of depression diagnosis increases with increasing self-reported concussions in retired professional football players. Am J Sports Med. 2012;40(10):2206–12.
56. Smith AM, Milliner EK. Injured athletes and the risk of suicide. J Athl Train. 1994;29(4):337.
57. Hammond T, Gialloreto C, Kubas H, et al. The prevalence of failure-based depression among elite athletes. Clin J Sport Med. 2013;23(4):273–7.
58. Ardern CL, Taylor NF, Feller JA, et al. Sports participation 2 years after anterior cruciate ligament reconstruction in athletes who had not returned to sport at 1 year: a prospective follow-up of physical function and psychological factors in 122 athletes. Am J Sports Med. 2015;43(4):848–56.
59. Gignac MAM, Cao X, Ramanathan S, et al. Perceived personal importance of exercise and fears of re-injury: a longitudinal study of psychological factors related to activity after anterior cruciate ligament reconstruction. BMC Sports Sci Med Rehabil. 2015;7(1):4.
60. Flanigan DC, Everhart JS, Glassman AH. Psychological factors affecting rehabilitation and outcomes following elective orthopaedic surgery. J Am Acad Orthop Surg. 2015;23(9):563–70.
61. Podlog L, Banham SM, Wadey R, et al. Psychological readiness to return to competitive sport following injury: a qualitative study. Sport Psychol. 2015;29(1):1–14.
62. Podlog L, Dimmock J, Miller J. A review of return to sport concerns following injury rehabilitation: practitioner strategies for enhancing recovery outcomes. Phys Ther Sport. 2011;12(1):36–42.
63. Everhart JS, Best TM, Flanigan DC. Psychological predictors of anterior cruciate ligament reconstruction outcomes: a systematic review. Knee Surg Sports Traumatol Arthrosc. 2015;23(3):752–62.
64. Czuppon S, Racette BA, Klein SE, et al. Variables associated with return to sport following anterior cruciate ligament reconstruction: a systematic review. Br J Sports Med. 2014;48(5):356–64.
65. Glazer DD. Development and preliminary validation of the injury-psychological readiness to return to sport (I-PRRS) scale. J Athl Train. 2009;44(2):185–9.
66. Tripp DA, Stanish W, Ebel-Lam A, et al. Fear of reinjury, negative affect, and catastrophizing predicting return to sport in recreational athletes with anterior cruciate ligament injuries at 1 year postsurgery. Rehabil Psychol. 2007;52(1):74–81.
67. Hainline B, Derman W, Vernec A, et al. International Olympic Committee consensus statement on pain management in elite athletes. Br J Sports Med. 2017;51:1245–58.
68. Arvinen-Barrow M, Clement D, Hamson-Utley JJ, et al. Athletes' use of mental skills during sport injury rehabilitation. J Sport Rehabil. 2015;24(2):189–97.

Chapter 9
Alcohol and Substance Abuse and Sport

Jason R. Kilmer, Cassandra D. Pasquariello, and Adrian J. Ferrera

Introduction

Substance abuse has long been part of athletic culture. Be it for the purpose of celebration, coping with failure, relaxing, or event preparation, substance use comes in many forms. Substance use by athletes can impair athletic performance, recovery, and overall health and wellbeing by affecting sleep quality, weight gain, anxiety, depressed mood, or other domains. In many instances, athletes may attribute a need for substances as part of their coping strategy, which can represent a powerful barrier to both disclosure and seeking treatment of abusive use patterns. Substance use can be addressed during a clinical encounter regardless of its relation to the athlete's presenting complaint. Utilizing a standardized screening methodology for substance may be helpful at encounters because of the role that substance use can play in causing or exacerbating some of the very issues a person might be seeking help for.

Steps taken to address substance use can be an important part of case conceptualization and care of the athlete. Once conversations related to substance use have commenced, the provider can consider potential contextual impacts and work to elicit personally relevant reasons to change.

J. R. Kilmer (✉)
University of Washington, Psychiatry & Behavioral Sciences, School of Medicine,
Seattle, WA, USA
e-mail: jkilmer@uw.edu

C. D. Pasquariello
University of Wisconsin, Madison, WI, USA
e-mail: cdp@athletics.wisc.edu

A. J. Ferrera
Auburn University, Auburn, AL, USA
e-mail: ajf0044@auburn.edu

© Springer Nature Switzerland AG 2020
E. Hong, A. L. Rao (eds.), *Mental Health in the Athlete*,
https://doi.org/10.1007/978-3-030-44754-0_9

Epidemiology and Pattern of Alcohol and Cannabis Abuse

Alcoholic beverages contain ethanol typically provided by fermentation of grains, fruits, or other sources of sugar. Alcohol plays an important role in many social contexts, including athletic culture. Over 50% of those 12 and older in the United States report drinking alcohol at least once per month, and past-month prevalence rates vary by age group (9.2% of 12–17-year-olds, 57.1% of 18–25-year-olds, 54.6% of those 26 or older) [33]. Among those who consume alcohol, some engage in heavy episodic or "binge drinking." Although the definition of "binge drinking" varies depending on the data source, SUbstance Abuse and Mental Health Services Adminsitration (SAMHSA) considers a "binge" as five or more drinks consumed on the same occasion on at least one of the past 30 days for men and four or more drinks on the same occasion on at least one of the past 30 days for women; "heavy alcohol use" is defined as 5 or more days of binge drinking in the past 30 days. In the United States, of those with past month alcohol use, 47.8% have also had a binge drinking episode, and 11.9% meet criteria for heavy alcohol use. Cannabis use similarly varies based on age group, with 18–25-year-olds being most likely to report past-month marijuana use (20.8%, compared to 6.5% of those 12–17-year-olds and 7.2% of those 26 and older) [33].

Studies of rates of substance use by those involved in athletics are primarily limited to intercollegiate athletes. Approximately 42% of intercollegiate athletes report "binge drinking," with 8% reporting consuming 10 or more drinks in one sitting [24]. Approximately 25% of intercollegiate athletes report marijuana use. Whether or not you see a patient or client involved in competitive athletic, the impact of substance use on athletic performance have relevance to the health, well-being, and participation status of the athlete.

The Social and Legal Context of Alcohol and Other Substance Use

Alcohol purchase and use is legal in many jurisdictions, once an age criteria has been met. While alcohol consumption may be considered appropriate in social contexts, it may be associated with a range of unwanted effects or consequences, including impacts to relationships, health effects, impaired sleep, and factors associated with athletic performance. Marijuana use is associated with decreased cognitive abilities, increased heart rate, impaired driving capacity, and, like with alcohol, impaired athletic performance. A complete review of both substances would be outside the scope of this chapter; however, the opportunity to highlight significant findings potentially relevant to patient or client during a mental health or sports medicine visit will be examined.

First, it is important to consider the context of substance use. Alcohol and other drug (AOD) policies governing substance use for competitive athletes widely range from overarching federal and state law, National Collegiate Athletic Association

(NCAA) policies (and/or conference/league rules), to a specific sport organization/ department. AOD policies vastly differ in content (e.g., specificity, length, AOD testing procedures, safe harbor programs, violations of the policy) across amateur, collegiate, and professional institutions. Many athletic departments set a department-wide policy that is the minimum standard for all student-athletes within the department, but provides discretion to individual sport programs to administer AOD policies that are more restrictive and punitive than the department policy. Certainly, if an athlete is ready to discuss a substance use issue that could impact their ability to maintain eligibility, pointing them in the right direction to confirm what is and is not allowed can be important.

There are potential clinical challenges to addressing AOD use with elite athletes, including demystifying the belief that drinking alcohol has little to no impact on athletic performance, considering their often over-emphasized athletic identity, perfectionism traits, perceived pressure to perform, and loss of star status [17]. These challenges create potential and realistic barriers to working with athletes struggling with substance use. Additional barriers a healthcare provider may face in addressing drug abuse concerns with an elite athlete include: the competitive nature of athletics, the media fishbowl (and what it means for a high-profile athlete to seek assistance in what could be a public office), psychosocial ramifications of injury, athletic identity, hazing traditions among teams, low help-seeking behavior, mandatory drug counseling sessions, league testing policies, and confidentiality.

Substance Abuse Interventions

There are opportunities for brief interventions in the context of consultation or appointments with athletes, and these can have significant impacts on decisions related to alcohol and other substance use. Through motivational interviewing [20], brief interventions can be implemented to alter trajectories and provide early intervention when there are signs of potential risks or existing harms. Motivational interviewing is more impactful for those athletes considering change if it is in line with what motivates an individual, and, if effective, can prompt consideration of change, commitment to change, and initial action. Motivational interviewing is a non-judgmental, non-confrontational clinical approach that emphasizes meeting people where they are in terms of their readiness to change and focuses on eliciting personally relevant reasons to change. One of the key principles of motivational interviewing involves developing discrepancies between an individual's personal values and goals (e.g., "I'm trying to stay in shape") and ways in which the status quo could be in conflict with substance abuse behaviors (e.g., "I'm consuming 4000 calories a week from alcohol").

To date, the use of motivational interviewing and brief interventions is limited. Hingson et al. [14] examined the experiences of a sample of people who had ever consumed alcohol and saw a physician at least once in the past year. Only 14% of those exceeding low-risk drinking guidelines were asked and advised about risky drinking by their provider. Although patients 18–25 years of age were the age group to most often exceed guidelines, they were the ones least often asked about drinking. Clearly, an opportunity for providers to screen exists during any visit with a patient or a client.

Screening for Substance Abuse

The most commonly used screening tool for alcohol abuse is the ten-item Alcohol Use Disorders Identification Test (AUDIT), which is available from the World Health Organization at: http://www.who.int/substance_abuse/publications/audit/en/) [3]. A total score derived from this ten-item measure places the participant into one of four different risk zones for which accompanying recommended actions are provided. For providers desiring a shorter screen, the three-item AUDIT-C is available and focuses on the items related to frequency, quantity, and peak alcohol consumption. For those preferring a single-question screen for alcohol abuse, the National Institute for Alcohol Abuse and Alcoholism (NIAAA) provides a question examining how many times in the past year the person has had 4 or more drinks in a day (for women) or 5 or more drinks in a day (for men), and provides suggestions for possible actions in their manual/guide for providers (available at https://pubs.niaaa.nih.gov/publications/practitioner/PocketGuide/pocket.pdf).

Another point of clarification that must be made prior to moving forward to using any of the aforementioned measures is defining "a standard drink" – if a person is keeping track of containers and not standard drinks, there will be gross underestimates of their actual consumption, and research has even demonstrated estimates changing mid-conversation once it is clarified what "one drink" means [6].

For cannabis/marijuana, targeted questioning, using specific language to encompass different forms of consumption, must be considered. If asked, "have you smoked marijuana," a person who uses edibles (or orally ingests it) can say "no" despite using this substance. Preferably, a provider should ask, "do you use cannabis or marijuana in any form" or "have you used cannabis or marijuana in any form" to capture all forms of use. The Cannabis Use Disorders Identification Test-Revised (CUDIT-R) is modeled after the AUDIT and can help provide a sense of potential harmful or hazardous use [1].

Research Studies Related to Substance Abuse in Athlete Populations

When it comes to identifying potential "hooks" or information that could serve to develop a discrepancy for any given individual, the scientific literature can certainly serve as a basis. The following is a brief summary of studies for possible discussion with clients or patients.

Alcohol and Athletic Performance

Murphy, Snape, Minett, Skein, & Duffield [23] tested the impact of drinking follow-ing a competitive rugby league match among young men (mean age = 19.9 years) in Australia. Participants were randomized to consume drinks containing alcohol or alcohol-free beverages, and counter movement jump test peak (which measures lower-body power) was tested 16 hours post-match. The group that consumed alco-hol improved 2.3% in the 16 hours post-match, while the group that consumed no alcohol improved 10.5%. Additionally, the group that consumed alcohol had reduced decision-making speed and reduced quality of responses to visual stimuli. This led the research team to conclude that alcohol should be avoided within 16 hours of a competition or competitive practice. Barnes, Mündel, & Stannard [4] explored the effects of post-exercise alcohol consumption on concentric, eccentric, and isometric contractions, noticing impairment in recovery measures when alcohol was consumed post-exercise. Differences were dramatic, such that the group that did not drink outperformed the group that drank on every type of muscle contraction (for isometric contractions, the no alcohol group was 12% off peak compared to the alcohol group that were 34% off peak; for concentric contractions, the no alcohol group was 28% off peak, the alcohol group was 40% off peak; for eccentric contrac-tions, the no alcohol group was 19% off peak, the alcohol group was 34% off peak). The authors thus concluded that for any participant in a sport containing intense eccentric muscular work, alcohol should be avoided in the post-event period if opti-mal recovery is the value or goal. For all measures, post-exercise alcohol use magni-fied exercise-induced muscle damage and related decreases in performance. Barnes [5] examined the impact of alcohol use among male athletes and demonstrated that drinking post-competition reduced production of testosterone, which had subse-quent effects on protein synthesis and muscular regeneration. There seems to be fairly clear empirical evidence that for any client or patient for whom competitive edge and/or maximizing performance or recovery is a goal or value, alcohol use could impact these athletic outcomes.

Alcohol and anxiety or daytime sleepiness In the instance of sleep and daytime somnolence, alcohol use can exacerbate or even cause the very concerns that have prompted help-seeking by an individual. For example, if your clients/patients are reporting that they use alcohol as a sleep aid, you can ask them what they've noticed about their sleep (or even be more direct by asking what they notice about their dreaming). They'll likely tell you they don't dream at all; or, if they do, they'll see they dream vividly right before waking up. This is because alcohol can interfere with time spent in rapid eye movement (REM) sleep, and REM deprivation can result in increases in daytime sleepiness, anxiety, irritability, or jumpiness the next day. If the person drinks multiple nights in a row, these effects can be cumulative/additive [30].

Alcohol and weight gain If a person is trying to manage their weight, calculating the caloric impact of their alcohol consumption (and number of calories reduced if they make a change in their drinking) could prompt contemplation of or actual commitment to change alcohol consumption behaviors. Unless there are contraindications related to adding to the anxiety of someone struggling with disordered eating practices, feedback about caloric impact has been identified as a key component of brief interventions in healthcare settings (e.g., Grossberg, et al., [12]).

Alcohol and medication Certainly, it is important to encourage your client or patient to consult with any prescribing provider about contraindications for drinking on a medication. If you are the one prescribing a medication, consider discussing what alcohol use would mean for that person given the presenting issue, performance goals, and the medication in question.

Marijuana and athletic performance Hilderbrand [13] warned that the use of marijuana by athletes prior to competition could result in danger to that individual or those around them as a result of impairment of response and/or decision making. Pesta et al. [29] declared marijuana an ergolytic agent particularly because of decreased exercise performance potentially due to increases in heart rate and blood pressure. Gillman, Hutchison, & Bryan [10] demonstrated that marijuana use decreased physiological work capacity and reduced maximal exercise duration. A review by Kennedy [15] examined 15 published studies exploring the effects of Tetrahydrocannabinol (THC) and exercise and found no evidence of improved aerobic performance, in addition to no evidence of increased strength or endurance. Collectively, the limited literature nevertheless suggests marijuana use can impede progress toward athletic goals and performance.

Marijuana and cardiovascular health Mittleman et al. [21] followed 3882 patients and concluded that in the hour following the use of marijuana, heart attack risk increases 4.8 times. The increased heart rate following marijuana use can also be associated with effects on blood pressure, but certainly for anyone at risk for heart attack, this information can be important.

Marijuana and sleep quality Like with alcohol, people might report using marijuana at night to bring on onset of sleep [7]. However, Angarita et al. [2] demonstrated that "deep sleep" is extended following marijuana use and REM sleep is deprived (like with alcohol). These disruptions to the sleep cycle can impact perceived sleepiness and anxiety on subsequent days.

Separating reported benefits of use from withdrawal symptoms When DSM-5 was released, clear criteria for cannabis withdrawal were included for the first time. Many of the criteria for withdrawal (e.g., anxiety, sleep difficulty, decreased appetite, depressed mood, headaches) are the very reasons or motives for use reported by those who engage in cannabis use. For example, if a patient or client is convinced that marijuana helps their depression, and, as evidence, notes that whenever they abstain for a couple of days, their depression symptoms return, and then promptly go away when use resumes. In effect, resumption of substance abuse is likely to simply be curbing withdrawal symptoms, which mimic depression, anxiety, and other mental health concerns.

Other observations related to mental health Anxiety and depression are highly correlated with substance use among athletes. Some athletes may report using substances as coping mechanisms for symptoms of anxiety and/or depression. For other athletes, the unanticipated side effects of heavy substance use/abuse may be signs and symptoms of anxiety and/or depression. Preliminary findings from Project Rest, an NCAA-funded sleep study on college athletes, suggest that poor sleep quality and insufficient sleep duration are critical risk factors associated with the development of depression, anxiety, and AOD use, in addition to decreased athletic performance [11]. Smith and Milliner [31] interviewed five young American athletes who attempted suicide following a significant injury, and demonstrated the risk factors of strong athletic identity, injury, and prior AOD use, in addition to other factors. There is a dearth of literature noting the relationship between psychosis and college student-athlete AOD use, but anecdotally, in states where marijuana has been legalized, there appears to be a relationship between substance use and prodromal symptoms of psychosis and/or first psychotic break among athletes. This relationship is consistent with non-athlete peers.

Clinical Recommendations

Taken together, substance use is an aspect of health that is implicated in many of the most salient mental and physical outcomes among athletes. Despite this, regulating AOD use, especially as it exacerbates other presenting mental health concerns, represents a potential challenge for the patients and clients we work with. The following is a case example written to demonstrate a common clinical presentation and suggested intervention.

Case Example

Jonathan is a 20-year-old Caucasian male, track and field student-athlete at an NCAA Division I institution. He is currently in his sophomore year and is slowly returning to competition following a stress fracture in his leg he suffered toward the end of his freshman year. Most recently, his team athletic trainer has noticed that Jonathan has been consistently late to his physical therapy appointments and when present, he "goes through the motions" with a seemingly irritated attitude. There have even been days when Jonathan appeared to be "hungover." While he does not have a current prescription for pain medication, in a college environment, Jonathan may have a high likelihood of securing accessibility for non-prescription use of pain medication should he choose to self-medicate. The following evidence-based recommendations can be applied to the case of Jonathan and cases similar to us. It is recommended that all interventions (e.g., individual, team, department wide) designed to address athlete substance use and abuse be both educational in nature and resource driven [8]. Given the complex nature of athletic environments, all staff (e.g., coaches, athletic trainers, support staff) should be trained in recognizing signs and symptoms of behavior change, especially as they relate to substance use [32].

Pre-screening During the required pre-participation examination for college athletes, it is recommended to include instruments such as the AUDIT-C or AUDIT discussed earlier. The screening measures are designed to be reviewed by a team physician and/or mental health professional and may accompany other screens of mental health. Kroshus [16] suggests that athletic departments who have a written plan to identify mental health concerns perform more exhaustive screenings than their peers without a written plan, and roughly half of athletic departments that participated in a study ($N = 365$) screen specifically for alcohol consumption (57.4%), prescription drug abuse (52.2%), and illegal drug use (46.8%).

Role of affiliate medical and team personnel It is likely that athletes may have more daily interactions with an athletic trainer, physical therapist, strength and conditioning coach than they do with a medical physician. These daily interactions lead athletes to trust these individuals and turning to them for advice in times of need. In turn, such daily interactions make it more likely that an appropriately trained athletic trainer or staff member to recognize substance behaviors. While these providers do not need to be experts in mental health and substance use, it is critical for them to be aware of warning signs and symptoms [9, 28]. Additionally, engaging in professional development courses on motivational interviewing [19] and mental health first-aid [18] can allow day-to-day providers to feel better equipped to aid an athlete in crisis. Most importantly, day-to-day providers must be self-reflective and aware of their own comfort and competence level. If at any time a provider believes a situation extends beyond or outside of their competence, it is ethically in the athlete's best interest to refer them to the appropriate resource [9, 26, 27]. On college campuses, it is strongly recommended to partner with the experts on campus who specialize in harm reduction-based psychoeducational 1:1 and group programming [25]. Other recommended approaches include designing and facilitating a psychoeducational support group for injured athletes, in addition to more structured programming [25].

Overcoming barriers Despite increasing attention directed toward mental health concerns in athletic population, specific athletic communities continue to harbor a stigma toward seeking mental health services. Following an analysis of studies focused on mental health services utilization by athletes across an 11-year span, Moreland, Coxe, and Yang [22] found that coaches, parents, teammates, athletic trainers, administrators, and the organizational structure of the athletic department can either facilitate or inhibit athletes from seeking mental health assistance. Furthermore, gender of the athlete or sports provider impacted the utilization or referral of services, with female athletes more willing to seek mental health services, and female coaches and athletic trainers more likely to refer an athlete to mental health services [22].

Once it is decided that an athlete may need mental health assistance, several questions may be raised by the sport staff/provider. Often these important questions serve as barriers to the athlete obtaining proper alcohol and substance use screening. These questions may include: To whom do I refer athlete? How do I know if the provider is qualified? Who else needs to know about this referral? According to the NCAA Mental Health Best Practices [26], athletes with suspected mental health concerns should be referred to a licensed provider who is qualified to provide mental health services (e.g., Clinical or counseling psychologist, psychiatrist, licensed clinical social workers, licensed mental health counselors, team physician comfortable with delivering mental health care). Ideally these providers should have specialized training in working with athletes. Such providers can be found through resources such as the American Psychological Association Society for Sport, Exercise and Performance Psychology and the Association for Applied Sport Psychology [26]. Once a provider is located, Neal and colleagues [27] recommend that a sport medicine provider assist the athlete in making the initial appointment.

Typically, meeting with a mental health professional is confidential. However, depending on the level of competition (youth, collegiate, professional), type of organization (sports medicine clinic, athletic training room, physical therapy clinic), who makes the referral and policies and procedures of the organization, will dictate how much information is shared and with whom (e.g., physician, athletic trainer, coach, parents). Exploring various integrated care models can assist in determining the level of collaboration of providers while minimizing the barriers of mental health treatment for athletes [34]. Regardless of which model is adopted, athletes should be informed of confidentiality and the referral policies and procedures in verbal and written forms.

Conclusion

Substance abuse remains an active concern in most athletic communities. It is imperative for providers and staff that serve or care for athletes, be able to identify signs of substance abuse, and triage their athletes to the appropriate resources that can direct care. A written screening plan must identify whom is responsible, when and how frequent provider visits should take place, and how the follow up plan will executed. Employing screening methods at clinic visit may help to identify substance abuse behaviors. Utilizing motivational interviewing and other similar brief interventions can identify and support athletes prepared to address these behaviors.

References

1. Adamson SJ, Kay-Lambkin FJ, Baker AL, Lewin TJ, Thornton L, Kelly BJ, Sellman JD. An improved brief measure of Cannabis misuse: the Cannabis Use Disorders Identification Test – Revised (CUDIT-R). Drug Alcohol Depend. 2010;110:137–43.
2. Angarita GA, Emadi N, Hodges S, Morgan PT. Sleep abnormalities associated with alcohol, cannabis, cocaine, and opiate use: a comprehensive review. Addict Sci Clin Pract. 2016;11:9.

3. Babor T, Higgins-Biddle JC, Saunders JB, Monteiro MG. The alcohol use disorders identification test: guidelines for primary care. 2nd ed. Geneva, Switzerland: World Health Organization: Department of Mental Health and Substance Dependence; 2001.
4. Barnes MJ, Mündel T, Stannard SR. Acute alcohol consumption aggravates the decline in muscle performance following strenuous eccentric exercise. J Sci Med Sport. 2010;13:189–93.
5. Barnes MJ. Alcohol: impact on sports performance and recovery in male athletes. Sports Med. 2014;44:909–19.
6. Bergen-Cico D, Kilmer J. Reported changes in students' alcohol consumption following a brief education of a standard drink. J Alcohol Drug Educ. 2010;15:72–84.
7. Conroy DA, Kurth ME, Strong DR, Brower KJ, Stein MD. Marijuana use patterns and sleep among community-based adults. J Addict Dis. 2016;35:135–43.
8. Cox CE, Ross-Stewart L, Foltz BD. Investigating the prevalence and risk factors of depression symptoms among NCAA division I college athletes. J Sports Sci. 2017;5:14–28.
9. Etzel EF. Understanding and promoting college student-athlete health: essential issues for student affairs professionals. NASPA J. 2006;43(3):518–46.
10. Gillman AS, Hutchison KE, Bryan AD. Cannabis and exercise science: a commentary on existing studies and suggestions for future directions. Sports Med. 2015;45:1357–63.
11. Grandner MA. Sleep and health in student-athletes. 2017. Retrieved from https://www.ncaa.org/sites/default/files/2017RES_InnoGrant_Grandner_FinalReport_20170206.pdf.
12. Grossberg PM, Halperin A, MacKenzie S, Gisslow M, Brown D, Fleming MF. Inside the physician's black bag: critical ingredients of brief alcohol interventions. Subst Abus. 2010;31:240–50.
13. Hilderbrand RL. High-performance sport, marijuana, and cannabimimetics. J Anal Toxicol. 2011;35:624–37.
14. Hingson RW, Heeren T, Edwards EM, Saitz R. Young adults at risk for excess alcohol consumption are often not asked or counseled about drinking alcohol. J Gen Intern Med. 2012;27:179–84.
15. Kennedy MC. Cannabis: exercise performance and sport. A systematic review. J Sci Med Sport. 2017;20:825–9.
16. Kroshus E. Variability in institutional screening practices related to collegiate student-athlete mental health. J Athl Train. 2016;51(5):389–97.
17. Lisha NE, Sussman S. Relationship of high school and colleges sports participation with alcohol, tobacco, and illicit drug use: a review. Addict Behav. 2010;35:399–407.
18. Lucksted A, Mendenhall AN, Frauenholtz SI, Aakre JM. Experiences of graduates of the Mental Health First Aid-USA course. Int J Ment Health Promot. 2015;17:169–83.
19. Martens MP, Kilmer JR, Beck NC. Alcohol and drug use among college athletes. In: Etzel EF, editor. Counseling and psychological services for college student-athletes. West Virginia: Fitness Information Technology; 2009. p. 451–75.
20. Miller WR, Rollnick S. Motivational interviewing: helping people change. 3rd ed. New York: Guilford Press; 2013.
21. Mittleman MA, Lewis RA, Maclure M, Sherwood JB, Muller JE. Triggering myocardial infarction by marijuana. Circulation. 2001;103:2805–9.
22. Moreland JJ, Coxe KA, Yang J. Collegiate athletes' mental health services utilization: a systematic review of conceptualizations, operationalizations, facilitators, and barriers. J Sport Health Sci. 2018;7:58–69.
23. Murphy AP, Snape AE, Minett GM, Skein M, Duffield R. The effects of post-match alcohol ingestion on recovery from competitive rugby league matches. J Strength Cond Res. 2014;27:1304–12.
24. National Collegiate Athletic Association. NCAA National study on substance use habits of college student athletes. NCAA. 2018. Retrieved from http://www.ncaa.org/sites/default/files/2017RES_Substance_Use_Executive_Summary_FINAL_20180611.pdf.
25. NCAA. Mind, body, and sport. Understanding and supporting student-athlete wellness. 2014. Retrieved from http://www.NCAAPublications.com.

26. NCAA. Interassociation consensus document: understanding and supporting student-athlete mental wellness. Mental health best practices. 2016. Retrieved from http://www.NCAAPublications.com.
27. Neal TL, Diamond AB, Goldman S, Klossner D, Morse ED, Pajak DE, Putukian M, Quandt EF, Sullivan JP, Wallack C, Welzant V. Inter-association recommendations for developing a plan to recognize and refer student-athletes with psychological concerns at the collegiate level: an executive summary of a consensus statement. J Athl Train. 2013;48(5):716–20.
28. Neal TL, Diamond AB, Goldman S, Liedtka KD, Mathis K, Morse ED, Putukian M, Quandt EF, Ritter SJ, Sullivan JP, Welzant V. Inter-association recommendations for developing a plan to recognize and refer student-athletes with psychological concerns at the secondary school level: a consensus statement. J Athl Train. 2015;50(3):231–49.
29. Pesta DH, Angadi SS, Burtscher M, Roberts CK. The effects of caffeine, nicotine, ethanol, and tetrahydrocannabinol on exercise performance. Nutr Metabol. 2013;10:71.
30. Roehrs T, Roth T. Sleep, sleepiness, and alcohol use. Alcohol Res Health. 2001;25:101–9.
31. Smith AM, Milliner EK. Injured athletes and the risk of suicide. J Athl Train. 1994;29(4):337–41.
32. Strohle A. Sports psychiatry: mental health and mental disorders in athletes and exercise treatment of mental disorders. Eur Arch Psychiatry Clin Neurosci. 2017; https://doi.org/10.1007/s00406-018-0891-5.
33. Substance Abuse and Mental Health Services Administration. Key substance use and mental health indicators in the United States: results from the 2016 National Survey on Drug Use and Health (HHS Publication No. SMA 17–5044, NSDUH Series H-52). Rockville, MD: Center for Behavioral Health Statistics and Quality, Substance Abuse and Mental Health Services Administration; 2017. Retrieved from https://www.samhsa.gov/data/.
34. Sudano LE, Collins G, Miles CM. Reducing barriers to mental health care for student-athletes: an integrated Care Model. Fam Syst Health. 2017;35(1):77–84.

Chapter 10
Coping with Doping: Performance-Enhancing Drugs in the Athletic Culture

David M. Siebert

Introduction

In 1981, bodybuilder Daniel Duchaine self-published and began independent distribution of his work entitled *Underground Steroid Handbook for Men and Women*. The handbook highlighted a number of different compounds, from anabolic steroids to diuretics and others, as potential performance-enhancing drugs (PEDs) for the athlete. Duchaine's publication is considered one of the first works to widely publicize the use of off-label or illicit substances to the general athlete population. Duchaine himself was later arrested in 1987 for involvement in a steroid distribution ring [1].

By 1984, "Goldman's dilemma" gained infamy as a representation of the lengths to which elite athletes would be willing to go to attain a competitive advantage. Goldman reports that when offered a theoretical drug that would ensure Olympic success at the cost of certain death 5 years later, over 50% of athletes would make the choice of taking the drug. This figure reportedly held steady year after year, though he did not clarify the methodology that lead to these results [2]. Recent research has suggested that Goldman's 50% figure is potentially sensationalized and not reproducible with more rigorous study designs or in contemporary culture [3, 4]. While the modern applicability of the lore of Goldman's dilemma has been called into question, performance-enhancing drug (PED) use and abuse remain a significant problem in the competitive and recreational athletic communities for athletes seeking a performance advantage. For example, as many as 5% of high school athletes [5] and 24% of community gym members [6] have reported abusing human growth hormone (HGH). In the same gym population, 70% reported

D. M. Siebert (✉)
Department of Family Medicine, Sports Medicine Section,
Seattle, WA, USA
e-mail: siebert@uw.edu

© Springer Nature Switzerland AG 2020
E. Hong, A. L. Rao (eds.), *Mental Health in the Athlete*,
https://doi.org/10.1007/978-3-030-44754-0_10

anabolic-androgenic steroid (AAS) use [6]. Furthermore, PED polypharmacy may be as high as 100% in select populations [7].

Precise figures are not as readily available at the elite athlete level, likely due to the inherent secrecy behind illicit use and the potential punishments that may be levied. Nevertheless, former Senator George Mitchell's 2007 report on PED abuse in Major League Baseball revealed dozens of professional athletes connected to various compounds [8], and league suspensions or other athlete punishments continue to surface in the media annually.

Given the documented and ongoing problem of PED abuse in the sporting world, the Sports Medicine clinician may find him or herself face to face with an abusing or at-risk athlete. Pre-conceived strategies to address PED use and abuse, as well as any co-existing psychiatric symptoms or disorders, will help improve the health of an athlete and foster a productive clinician-patient relationship.

PED Prohibition and Testing

The World Anti-Doping Agency (WADA) maintains a list of banned substances, such as AAS and HGH, as well as prohibited performance-enhancing techniques, such as blood doping (Table 10.1) [9]. The use of certain classes of substances is prohibited at all times, while others are prohibited during seasons or competition only.

Major professional and collegiate athletic leagues and associations in the United States have enacted similar lists of prohibited substances [10, 11]. Athlete testing procedures and punishments vary from league to league (Table 10.2) [12–16].

Adverse Systemic Effects of PEDs

Rules prohibiting the use of various substances are grounded in ensuring fair play while also protecting the health and safety of competing athletes. A number of adverse effects may occur with PED use and abuse, and the precise potential effects depend on the substance in question. For example, AAS abuse has been linked to diseases of the cardiovascular system such as dyslipidemia [17], hypertension [18], left ventricular dysfunction, and accelerated coronary artery atherosclerosis [19]. AAS use can also lead to hepatotoxicity [20], endocrine abnormalities, psychiatric disorders, and neurologic consequences [21]. HGH excess is linked to acromegaly [22], which is characterized by bony overgrowth and may precipitate other cardiovascular, neurological, and possibly neoplastic diseases [23, 24]. Finally, erythropoietin abuse has been linked to heart failure and thromboembolic events [25].

Table 10.1 Classes of substances and performance-enhancing methods prohibited by the WADA [9]

Class of substance	Example compounds	Time of prohibition
Non-approved substances	Experimental drugs, designer drugs, veterinary compounds	All times
Anabolic agents	Testosterone, oxandrolone, clenbuterol	All times
Peptide hormones, growth factors, related substances, and mimetics	Human growth hormone, insulin-like growth factor 1, erythropoietin	All times
Beta-2 agonists	Formoterol, salmeterol	All times
Hormone and metabolic modulators	Anastrozole, tamoxifen, clomiphene	All times
Diuretics and masking agents	Acetazolamide, furosemide	All times
Stimulants	Amphetamine, methylphenidate, modafinil	During competition
Narcotics	Morphine, oxycodone	During competition
Cannabinoids	Natural and synthetic cannabinoids	During competition
Glucocorticoids	Prednisone, dexamethasone, triamcinolone	During competition
Beta-blockers	Propranolol, metoprolol	In certain sports, such as archery, billiards, and shooting
Type of methodology	*Example method*	*Time of prohibition*
Manipulation of blood and blood components	Autologous, homologous, or heterologous blood or blood product infusion	All times
Chemical and physical manipulation	Testing sample tampering, urine substitution	All times
Gene doping	Gene editing agents	All times

Table 10.2 Punishments for positive PED tests by league

League	Punishment (1st positive test)	2nd positive test	3rd positive test
NFL [12]	4-game suspension	8-game suspension	2-season suspension; must apply for reinstatement
MLB [13]	80-game suspension	162-game suspension	Lifetime ban; may apply for reinstatement after 2 years
NBA [14]	20-game suspension	45-game suspension	Lifetime ban; may apply for reinstatement after 2 years
NHL [15]	20-game suspension	60-game suspension	Lifetime ban; may apply for reinstatement after 2 years
NCAA [16]	1-year suspension, 1-year loss of eligibility	Lifetime suspension, loss of remaining eligibility	–

NFL National Football League, *MLB* Major League Baseball, *NBA* National Basketball Association, *NHL* National Hockey League, *NCAA* National Collegiate Athletic Association

PED Use, Abuse, and Dependence

The *Diagnostic and Statistical Manual of Mental Disorders, Fifth Edition (DSM V)* does not explicitly define AAS- or HGH-use disorders, though stimulant use, intoxication, and withdrawal syndromes are outlined. However, the *DSM V* does describe diagnostic criteria for "other substance" use, intoxication, and withdrawal disorders, into which PEDs could potentially fit [26]. AAS dependence was described as early as 1988 [27]. In 2009, the disorder was highlighted as likely quite prevalent by Kanayama et al. [28] of Dr. Harrison Pope Jr.'s leading research group, who also proposed a model to define explicit *DSM V* AAS dependence criteria [29]. These criteria were ultimately not included in the *DSM V*, as substance "dependence" diagnosis criteria were eliminated entirely and merged into broader "substance use disorders" in the transition from the *DSM IV* [30] to *DSM V* [26]. Regardless, Kanayama et al. provide a framework from which to assess for AAS dependence, which may develop in as many as 30% of illicit AAS users [29, 31–36]. With a proposed AAS lifetime-use prevalence of 2.9–4.0 million in the United States [37] alone, 1 million of whom may exhibit signs of dependence [37], Sports Medicine clinicians and mental health providers would benefit from understanding the AAS dependence model [29].

AAS and Co-morbid Psychiatric Disorders

The relationship between AAS use and other co-morbid psychiatric disorders is, by far, the most rigorously investigated in comparison to other PED use. A 2014 Endocrine Society statement details adverse health consequences of PED use, and a correlational relationship between AAS use and psychopathology is well documented [21]. Importantly, the degree of a causal relationship remains uncertain [21].

In a systematic review, Piacentino et al. identified 37 manuscripts focusing on the overlap between AAS use and abuse and athlete mental health [38]. While documenting numerous sources of evidence linking AAS to psychiatric disorders, the authors highlight the complexity of such a relationship and suggest that the link between AAS use and psychopathology is in large part correlational or possibly a self-fulfilling or circular cycle [38].

The range of psychiatric disorders tied to AAS use and abuse is large and includes mood disorders in male [36, 39] and female [40] athletes, symptoms of psychosis [39], anxiety disorders [41, 42], somatoform, and eating disorders [38]. Higher rates of mood symptoms during periods of AAS use compared to non-use have been reported, suggesting some degree of a causal link [36]. Furthermore, dependent AAS users reported an anxiety disorder twice as often as non-dependent users [41].

The risk of suicide as it relates to AAS use has been theorized by case reports and retrospective studies [21, 38]. Past studies have postulated a link of violent or psychotic behavior to AAS [38, 39]. One study demonstrated a higher rate of violent deaths in AAS users compared to users of other illicit drugs [43]. A causal link between testosterone levels and risk of suicidality has not been definitively established, and polypharmacy with other PEDs or illicit substances may be a contributing factor [38]. As with other co-morbid psychiatric conditions, one prevailing theory is that those who use AAS may already be predisposed to developing behavioral disorders and symptoms such as suicidality [44].

Long-term mental health effects of AAS use are also an important consideration. A retrospective 30-year review of AAS users showed an increased lifetime prevalence of seeking mental health care compared to non-users [45]. This concern, along with the concern of long-term neurotoxic effects, was reiterated by Dr. Pope's group in 2018 [46, 48]. They suggest that the problem may only grow in scope due to the relatively recent development of the AAS abuse epidemic. As the original AAS generation enters the middle and later stages of life, they may begin to exhibit more frequent and severe mental and physical health problems [46, 48].

Psychological and Psychiatric Effects of Other PEDs

Data and studies on the psychiatric aspects and effects of other PEDs with relation to athletes are relatively lacking. HGH excess in the form of acromegaly has been linked to neuropsychiatric effects [22, 47], but investigations on the psychiatric effects of exogenous HGH are few. Stimulant use disorders are explicitly defined in the *DSM V* [26], and neuropsychological symptoms such as restlessness and agitation are among potential adverse effects [48]. Stimulants are also well known to be addictive substances in general, and substance use as a whole is a widely accepted risk factor for, and potential cause of, co-morbid psychiatric conditions [26].

PEDs and Risk-Taking Behavior

Previous works have suggested that college athletes are at higher risk of maladaptive lifestyle behaviors [49, 50]. Included in those behaviors is a greater risk of AAS use compared to non-athletes [50], and a potential correlation between PED or AAS use and risk-taking behavior has been demonstrated [51]. Polysubstance abuse is a prime example, such as combining AAS with opioid pain relievers to counteract the perceived effects of AAS use [51]. Risky AAS injection practices [52, 53] and higher rates of multiple sexual partners have also been described among AAS-using subjects, with one group postulating that AAS users exhibit an inherent risk-taking trait [52].

Legal Issues and PED Sources

AASs were not included within the original text of the 1970 Controlled Substances Act due to lack of widespread use at that time [54]. The Anabolic Steroids Control Act of 1990 amended the 1970 law, established AAS as a schedule III drug, and outlined punishments for illegal possession and distribution [55]. A first possession federal offense carries a maximum one-year prison sentence and minimum $1000 fine. Distribution may carry a maximum prison sentence of 5 years and a fine of $250,000 [56].

Also addressed in the Anabolic Steroids Control Act was the criminalization of the distribution of HGH. Though not a controlled substance, "the distribution and possession, with the intent to distribute" of HGH "for any use...other than the treatment of disease or other recognized medical condition [...] pursuant to the order of a physician" may lead to a five-year prison sentence [57]. Amphetamines and several other stimulants are currently listed as schedule II substances, as well [58].

The Drug Enforcement Administration (DEA) has found that the bulk of illicit AAS supply arises from smuggling from other countries where the compounds can be purchased over the counter. The inappropriate prescribing or theft of steroids is also a contributing source, as is the illicit synthesis and distribution from laboratories [56].

Illicit HGH distribution stems from off-label prescribing, the black market, smuggling, or theft. Off-label or inappropriate HGH prescribing often originates from so-called anti-aging websites or pharmacies that are "often partnered with a physician willing to write prescriptions for a fee without a physical examination" [57].

For the motivated athlete, obtaining PEDs appears to be remarkably simple. An internet search of the phrase "buy steroids" returns a lengthy list of websites, forums, and even instructional videos posted by users. Low-quality black market websites offer steroids for purchase similar to other internet shopping websites, and online steroid forums are inundated with pharmaceutical marketing. HGH is similarly marketed, and sources can be easily identified online.

PED Subculture and the At-Risk or Using Athlete

While not mainstream until years later, AAS use dates back as far as the 1950s. Dr. John Ziegler, then team physician for the United States weightlifting team, was one of the first to experiment with AAS on his athletes. He was also perhaps one of the first to watch the competitive athlete mindset take over and cause harm. After some athletes consumed 20 times his recommended dose and developed liver pathology, he developed a distaste for the use of the compounds and ceased experimentation [59, 60].

Decades later, anecdotal evidence suggests that such a "more is better" mindset persists in select communities. A cursory overview of online AAS forums is revealing. Some users publish online use diaries in order to promote their expertise and experience with particular PED regimens. Others may post requests for advice from others on how to convince a physician to prescribe a higher dose of testosterone. Others bemoan the reluctance of most physicians to monitor or manage PED use, making statements that "good" doctors are ones that are willing to work with them to support PED use, while "bad" doctors simply disparage use.

A "cycle" is a period of using testosterone, often for a few to several weeks, to gain the desired effect. A steroid "cycle" is a colloquial term in the PED community that refers to a period of time of using testosterone, often a few to several weeks, to gain the desired effect. Exogenous testosterone or analogs may suppress endogenous production, and users may attempt to harness this fact to carefully time laboratory testing in order to reveal an artificially low serum testosterone level. According to one user, this can serve as a potential catalyst for a clinician to prescribe higher doses of intramuscular testosterone.

Whereas the deterrence of PED seeking and use is a priority, it is easy to envision a scenario where a Sports Medicine practitioner is asked to prescribe, manage, or discuss non-indicated "treatment" with PEDs. Clearly, a clinician should not prescribe controlled substances or PEDs for performance enhancement reasons. Rather, counseling regarding the adverse health effects of PEDs and discouraging their use should instead be focuses of such an office visit. Education regarding over-the-counter dietary supplements, their components, and their potential negative health effects are also important topics to consider.

As anecdotal steroid forum evidence suggests, engaging in a respectful conversation about the above issues is paramount, as a patient may be inclined to simply seek care from another provider should he or she feel judgment or conflict. Athletes may present in the pre-contemplative state of the transtheoretical model of change [61]. While no consensus exists regarding the optimal method of counseling, motivational interviewing has been proposed as a potentially effective method [62, 63]. Motivational interviewing is a type of counseling strategy that aims to reduce ambivalence and facilitates the development of readiness for change within a patient [64]. Providers who incorporate a motivational interviewing style should resist the urge to directly counsel in favor of eliciting information and perspective from the patient.

Components of a motivational interviewing session may include attempting to understand a patient's reasons behind substance use or abuse, discussing the risks and benefits of continuing to use a given substance, and identifying the risks and benefits of decreasing or ceasing use. During the conversation, the clinician assesses the patient's readiness for change and helps identify alternative routes down which to proceed but does not insist on one path over another. Instead, the patient's unique beliefs, values, behaviors, and goals for their health take priority, and the clinician aims to facilitate the formulation of a treatment plan with these in mind [62–64].

Motivational interviewing has been used previously and successfully in substance use disorders [65], thus strengthening its potential role in counseling an athlete abusing PEDs. It may be necessary to start this conversation at a follow-up appointment in order to attain a more longitudinal relationship before engaging in the discussion. While counseling, a clinician must also remember that his or her role is not to "catch" a patient in the act but rather help him or her maintain a healthy lifestyle and meet fitness and athletic goals in a safe manner. Providers may also wish to consult with a sports dietician, sports psychologist, psychiatrist, or addiction medicine specialist when appropriate.

Education is an important PED abuse preventative measure [66]. At the high-school athlete levels, peer-led programs can effectively deter substance abuse. ATLAS (Adolescents Training and Learning to Avoid Steroids) for male athletes [67] and ATHENA (Athletes Targeting Healthy Exercise and Nutrition Alternatives) for female athletes [68] have set the standard. Run by coaches and athletes themselves, these programs do not require substantial preparation time and can be carried out during a competition season [69, 70].

Potential Fallout from a Positive PED Test

A large body of literature focuses on symptoms of psychiatric disorders in athletes, exacerbating factors, and treatment guidelines. Estimates of the prevalence of depression symptoms in collegiate athletes are as high as 21–23.7% [71, 72]. Injury has been described as a stressor that may precipitate psychological and psychiatric symptoms or distress in certain cases [73]. Given that positive PED tests often result in lengthy bans from competition, it is reasonable to assume that similar challenges to the athlete's mental health could be provoked by a positive test.

The fact that peer and public perception of an athlete may change substantially following a positive PED test can only complicate matters. Barry Bonds, MLB's all-time home-run leader with substantial ties to PED use and legal issues, has not been elected to baseball's Hall of Fame on numerous consecutive ballots [74]. Hall of Fame Vice Chairman Joe Morgan reiterated his concerns in 2017 with a mass email to voters, pleading for them refrain from electing those linked to steroids, other PEDs, or the Mitchell Report [75].

When an athlete is removed from competition for any reason, in addition to being removed from a major component of his or her life, he or she often loses at least some degree of access to a major social circle and support network. A Sports Medicine clinician must have a keen eye to identify signs of a problematic response that could be a harbinger of future struggles [74]. Given the co-morbid psychiatric disorders that often coincide with PED use – polysubstance abuse, mood disorders, and others – suspended athletes may represent a unique population at particularly high risk of developing serious mental health symptomatology. Further research is needed to elucidate the extent and severity of these increased risks, if present.

Conclusions

Previously relegated to select populations, the use and abuse of PEDs, especially AAS, has grown significantly in recent years. The pediatric population is among those increasingly affected. The WADA and other United States and international sports leagues and associations maintain lists of prohibited substances as well as punishments levied for positive tests. The adverse health consequences of PEDs are well documented, including the emergence of an AAS dependence syndrome that may develop in as many as 30% of users. Furthermore, the body of literature linking psychiatric symptoms and disorders to AAS use is established. The relationship between mental health and AAS use, abuse, and dependence is complex and likely resembles a correlative and bi-directional relationship rather than a purely causative one, though the bulk of evidence does suggest at least some degree of causation. Future research is needed to further elucidate the intricacies of the relationship between AAS abuse and mental health. The psychiatric aspects and consequences of the use and abuse of other PEDs are less well studied.

PED use and distribution carries with it significant legal and other risks, including fines and imprisonment, and it has been suggested that PED abuse may represent a manifestation of previously existing risk-taking tendencies. The "more is better" mindset, first seen in the 1950s with regard to AAS, persists to this day. An abundance of lay online steroid and PED forums guides users, potentially dangerously. These forums provide a unique look into the veritably existing PED subculture. When confronted with a patient using or at risk, a clinician must keep this subculture in mind when deciding how to best approach the situation, and motivational interviewing has been described as one potentially effective strategy. Preventative education measures are paramount, and programs like ATLAS and ATHENA are two examples of success stories.

Competitive and elite athletes may be confronted with unique mental health challenges when faced with a prolonged absence from competition, such a suspension following a positive PED test. Literature regarding the psychiatric risk profile of these athletes is lacking, but it is reasonable to assume that the period of time following suspension may represent a particularly vulnerable time for certain athletes.

References

1. Schachter J. Ex-Olympian arrested in steroid crackdown. LA Times. 1987. http://articles.latimes.com/1987-05-22/local/me-1093_1_steroid-crackdown. Accessed 29 Jul 2018.
2. Goldman B, Bush PJ, Klatz R. Death in the locker room. South Bend: Icarus Press; 1984.
3. Connor J, Woolf J, Mazanov J. Would they dope? Revisiting the Goldman dilemma. Br J Sports Med. 2013;47:697–700.
4. González JM, Johnson FR, Fedoruk M, Posner J, Bowers L. Trading health risks for glory: a reformulation of the Goldman Dilemma. Sports Med. 2018;48:1963–9.
5. Rickert VI, Pawlak-Morello C, Sheppard V, Jay MS. Human growth hormone: a new substance of abuse among adolescents? Clin Pediatr (Phila). 1992;31:723–6.
6. Baker JS, Graham MR, Davies B. Steroid and prescription medicine abuse in the health and fitness community: a regional study. Eur J Intern Med. 2006;17:479–84.
7. Brennan BP, Kanayama G, Hudson JI, Pope HG Jr. Human growth hormone abuse in male weightlifters. Am J Addict. 2011;20:9–13.
8. Michell GJ. Report to the commissioner of baseball of an independent investigation into the illegal use of steroids and other performance enhancing substances by players in Major League Baseball. 2007. http://files.mlb.com/mitchrpt.pdf. Accessed 29 Jul 2018.
9. World Anti-Doping Agency. 2018 list of prohibited substances and methods. 2018. https://www.wada-ama.org/en/content/what-is-prohibited. Accessed 26 Jul 2018.
10. MLB. Prohibited substances list. 2015. http://mlb.mlb.com/pa/pdf/prohibited-substances.pdf. Accessed 26 Jul 2018.
11. NCAA. 2018-19 NCAA banned drugs list. 2018. http://www.ncaa.org/2018-19-ncaa-banned-drugs-list. Accessed 26 Jul 2018.
12. NFLPA. Drug program resources. https://www.nflpa.com/active-players/drug-policies. Accessed 26 Jul 2018.
13. MLB. Major League Baseball's Joint Drug Prevention and Treatment Program. http://mlb.mlb.com/pa/pdf/jda.pdf. Accessed 26 Jul 2018.
14. NBA. NBA, NBPA to add HGH testing into anti-drug program. 2015. http://www.nba.com/2015/news/04/16/nba-and-nbpa-to-introduce-hgh-blood-testing/. Accessed 26 Jul 2018.

15. NHL. NHL, NHLPA team up against performance-enhancing substances. 2005. http://www.nhl.com/ice/page.htm?id=26397. Accessed 26 Jul 2018.
16. NCAA. Frequently asked questions about drug testing. http://www.ncaa.org/sport-science-institute/topics/frequently-asked-questions-about-drug-testing. Accessed 26 Jul 2018.
17. Palatini P, Giada F, Garavelli G, Sinisi F, Mario L, Michieletto M, Baldo-Enzi G. Cardiovascular effects of anabolic steroids in weight-trained subjects. J Clin Pharmacol. 1996;36:1132–40.
18. Achar S, Rostamian A, Narayan SM. Cardiac and metabolic effects of anabolic-androgenic steroid abuse on lipids, blood pressure, left ventricular dimensions, and rhythm. Am J Cardiol. 2010;106:893–901.
19. Baggish AL, Weiner RB, Kanayama G, Hudson JI, Lu MT, Hoffmann U, Pope HG Jr. Cardiovascular toxicity of illicit anabolic-androgenic steroid use. Circulation. 2017;135:1991–2002.
20. Søe KL, Søe M, Gluud C. Liver pathology associated with the use of anabolic-androgenic steroids. Liver. 1992;12:73–9.
21. Pope HG Jr, Wood RI, Rogol A, Nyberg F, Bowels L, Bhasin S. Adverse health consequences of performance-enhancing drugs: an Endocrine Society scientific statement. Endocr Rev. 2014;35:341–75.
22. Katznelson L, Laws ER Jr, Melmed S, Molitch ME, Murad MH, Utz A, Wass JA, Endocrine Society. Acromegaly: an endocrine society clinical practice guideline. J Clin Endocrinol Metab. 2014;99:3933–51.
23. Rokkas T, Pistiolas D, Sechopoulos P, Margantinis G, Koukoulis G. Risk of colorectal neoplasm in patients with acromegaly: a meta-analysis. World J Gastroenterol. 2008;14:3484–9.
24. Wolinski K, Czarnywojtek A, Ruchala M. Risk of thyroid nodular disease and thyroid cancer in patients with acromegaly--meta-analysis and systematic review. PLoS One. 2014;9:e88787.
25. La Gerche A, Brosnan MJ. Cardiovascular effects of performance-enhancing drugs. Circulation. 2017;135:89–99.
26. American Psychiatric Association. Diagnostic and statistical manual of mental disorders. 5th ed. Washington, DC: American Psychiatric Publishing; 2013.
27. Tennant F, Black DL, Voy RO. Anabolic steroid dependence with opioid-type features. N Engl J Med. 1988;319:578.
28. Kanayama G, Brower KJ, Wood RI, Hudson JI, Pope HG Jr. Anabolic-androgenic steroid dependence: an emerging disorder. Addiction. 2009;104:1966–78.
29. Kanayama G, Brower KJ, Wood RI, Hudson JI, Pope HG Jr. Issues for DSM-V: clarifying the diagnostic criteria for anabolic-androgenic steroid dependence. Am J Psychiatry. 2009;166:642–5.
30. American Psychiatric Association. Diagnostic and statistical manual of mental disorders. 4th ed. Washington, DC: American Psychiatric Publishing; 2000.
31. Brower KJ, Blow FC, Young JP, Hill EM. Symptoms and correlates of anabolic-androgenic steroid dependence. Br J Addict. 1991;86:759–68.
32. Copeland J, Peters R, Dillon P. Anabolic-androgenic steroid use disorders among a sample of Australian competitive and recreational users. Drug Alcohol Depend. 2000;60:91–6.
33. Midgley SJ, Heather N, Davies JB. Dependence-producing potential of anabolic-androgenic steroids. Addict Res. 1999;7:539–50.
34. Perry PJ, Lund BC, Deninger MJ, Kutscher EC, Schneider J. Anabolic steroid use in weightlifters and bodybuilders: an internet survey or drug utilization. Clin J Sport Med. 2005;15:326–30.
35. Malone DA Jr, Dimeff RJ, Lombardo JA, Sample RH. Psychiatric effects and psychoactive substance use in anabolic-androgenic steroid users. Clin J Sport Med. 1995;5:25–31.
36. Pope HG Jr, Katz DL. Psychiatric and medical effects of anabolic-androgenic steroid use. A controlled study of 160 athletes. Arch Gen Psychiatry. 1994;51:375–82.
37. Pope HG Jr, Kanayama G, Athey A, Ryan E, Hudson JI, Baggish A. The lifetime prevalence of anabolic-androgenic steroid use and dependence in Americans: current best estimates. Am J Addict. 2014;23:371–7.

38. Piacentino D, Kotzalidis GD, Del Casale A, Aromatario MR, Pomara C, Girardi P, Sani G. Anabolic-androgenic steroid use and psychopathology in athletes. A systematic review. Curr Neuropharmacol. 2015;13:101–21.
39. Pope HG Jr, Katz DL. Affective and psychotic symptoms associated with anabolic steroid use. Am J Psychiatry. 1988;145:487–90.
40. Gruber AJ, Pope HG Jr. Psychiatric and medical effects of anabolic-androgenic steroid use in women. Psychother Psychosom. 2000;69:19–26.
41. Ip EJ, Lu DH, Barnett MJ, Tenerowicz MJ, Vo JC, Perry PJ. Psychological and physical impact of anabolic-androgenic steroid dependence. Pharmacotherapy. 2012;32:910–9.
42. Ip EJ, Trinh K, Tenerowicz MJ, Pal J, Lindfelt TA, Perry PJ. Characteristics and behaviors of older male anabolic steroid users. J Pharm Pract. 2015;28:450–6.
43. Lindqvist AS, Moberg T, Eriksson BO, Ehrnborg C, Rosén T, Fahlke C. A retrospective 30-year follow-up study of former Swedish-elite male athletes in power sports with a past anabolic androgenic steroids use: a focus on mental health. Br J Sports Med. 2013;47:965–9.
44. Thiblin I, Runeson B, Rajs J. Anabolic androgenic steroids and suicide. Ann Clin Psychiatry. 1999;11:223–31.
45. Petersson A, Garle M, Holmgren P, Druid H, Krantz P, Thiblin I. Toxicological findings and manner of death in autopsied users of anabolic androgenic steroids. Drug Alcohol Depend. 2006;81:241–9.
46. Kanayama G, Kaufman MJ, Pope HG Jr. Public health impact of androgens. Curr Opin Endocrinol Diabetes Obes. 2018;25:218–23.
47. Siebert DM, Rao AL. The use and abuse of human growth hormone in sports. Sports Health. 2018; https://doi.org/10.1177/1941738118782688. [Epub ahead of print].
48. Momaya A, Fawal M, Estes R. Performance-enhancing substances in sports: a review of the literature. Sports Med. 2015;45:517–31.
49. Nattiv A, Puffer JC. Lifestyles and health risks of collegiate athletes. J Fam Pract. 1991;33:585–90.
50. Nattiv, Puffer JC, Green GA. Lifestyles and health risks of collegiate athletes: a multi-center study. Clin J Sport Med. 1997;7:262–72.
51. Arvary D, Pope HG Jr. Anabolic-androgenic steroids as a gateway to opioid dependence. N Engl J Med. 2000;342:1532.
52. Midgley SJ, Heather N, Best D, Henderson D, McCarthy S, Davies JB. Risk behaviours for HIV and hepatitis infection among anabolic-androgenic steroid users. AIDS Care. 2000;12:163–70.
53. Larance B, Degenhardt L, Copeland J, Dillon P. Injecting risk behavior and related harm among men who use performance- and image-enhancing drugs. Drug Alcohol Rev. 2008;27:679–86.
54. United States Department of Justice, Drug Enforcement Administration. Title 21 United States Code (USC) Controlled Substances Act. https://www.deadiversion.usdoj.gov/21cfr/21usc/. Accessed 29 Jul 2018.
55. 101st Congress. H.R. 4658 – Anabolic Steroids Control Act of 1990. 1990. https://www.congress.gov/bill/101st-congress/house-bill/4658. Accessed 29 Jul 2018.
56. Drug Enforcement Administration. Anabolic steroids. 2004. https://www.deadiversion.usdoj.gov/pubs/brochures/steroids/public/. Accessed 29 Jul 2018.
57. Drug Enforcement Administration. Human growth hormone. 2013. https://www.deadiversion.usdoj.gov/drug_chem_info/hgh.pdf. Accessed 29 Jul 2018.
58. Drug Enforcement Administration. Controlled substance schedules. https://www.deadiversion.usdoj.gov/schedules/. Accessed 29 Jul 2018.
59. Wade N. Anabolic steroids: doctors denounce them, but athletes aren't listening. Science. 1972;176:1399–403.
60. Bowers LD, Clark RV, Shackleton CH. A half-century of anabolic steroids in sport. Steroids. 2009;74:285–7.
61. Prochaska JO, Velicer WF. The transtheoretical model of health behavior change. Am J Health Promot. 1997;12:38–48.

62. Creado S, Reardon C. The sports psychiatrist and performance-enhancing drugs. Int Rev Psychiatry. 2016;28:564–71.
63. Johnson MC, Sacks DN, Edmonds WA. Counseling athletes who use performance-enhancing drugs: a new conceptual framework linked to clinical practice. J Soc Behav Health Sci. 2010;4:1–29.
64. Miller WR, Rollnick S. Motivational interviewing: preparing people to change addictive behaviour. London: Guilford Press; 1991.
65. Hettema J, Steele J, Miller WR. Motivational interviewing. Annu Rev Clin Psychol. 2005;1:91–111.
66. Reardon CL, Creado S. Drug abuse in athletes. Subst Abus Rehabil. 2014;5:95–105.
67. Goldberg L, Elliot DL, Clarke GN, MacKinnon DP, Zoref L, Moe E, Green C, Wolf SL. The Adolescents Training and Learning to Avoid Steroids (ATLAS) prevention program. Background and results of a model intervention. Arch Pediatr Adolesc Med. 1996;150:713–21.
68. Elliot DL, Goldberg L, Moe EL, Defrancesco CA, Durham MB, McGinnis W, Lockwood C. Long-term outcomes of the ATHENA (Athletes Targeting Healthy Exercise & Nutrition Alternatives) program for female high school athletes. J Alcohol Drug Educ. 2008;52:73–92.
69. Oregon Health and Science University, School of Medicine, Health Promotion and Sports Medicine. ATLAS. https://www.ohsu.edu/xd/education/schools/school-of-medicine/depart-ments/clinical-departments/medicine/divisions/hpsm/research/atlas.cfm. Accessed 29 Jul 2018.
70. Oregon Health and Science University, School of Medicine, Health Promotion and Sports Medicine. ATHENA. https://www.ohsu.edu/xd/education/schools/school-of-medicine/depart-ments/clinical-departments/medicine/divisions/hpsm/research/athena.cfm. Accessed 29 Jul 2018.
71. Yang J, Peek-Asa C, Corlette JD, Cheng G, Foster DT, Albright J. Prevalence of and risk factors associated with symptoms of depression in competitive collegiate student athletes. Clin J Sport Med. 2007;17:481–7.
72. Wolanin A, Hong E, Marks D, Panchoo K, Gross M. Prevalence of clinically elevated depressive symptoms in college athletes and differences by gender and sport. Br J Sports Med. 2016;50:167–71.
73. Putukian M. The psychological response to injury in student athletes: a narrative review with a focus on mental health. Br J Sports Med. 2016;50:145–8.
74. Jaffe J. Despite hall of fame's wishes, Barry Bonds is trending toward induction. Sports Illustrated. 2017. https://www.si.com/mlb/2017/12/12/barry-bonds-hall-fame-ballot-2018. Accessed 29 Jul 2018.
75. Jaffe J. Joe Morgan's Plea to Ban steroid users from the hall of fame is simplistic and reactionary. Sports Illustrated. 2017 https://www.si.com/mlb/2017/11/21/joe-morgan-hall-of-fame-letter-steroid-users. Accessed 29 Jul 2018.

Chapter 11
The Female Athlete Triad

Andrea Kussman and Aurelia Nattiv

Introduction

The female athlete triad (Triad) is comprised of three interrelated conditions: low energy availability (with or without disordered eating), menstrual dysfunction, and low bone mineral density. Low energy availability contributes to both menstrual dysfunction and low bone mineral density, and menstrual dysfunction also contributes to low bone mineral density. As illustrated in Fig. 11.1, these three conditions occur on a spectrum ranging from optimal health (adequate energy availability, eumenorrhea, and normal bone mineral density) to the end-stage that includes eating disorder, amenorrhea, and osteoporosis. Athletes with the female athlete triad can present with these three conditions in different stages at different periods of time, and diagnosis of the Triad does not require simultaneous clinical manifestations of all three conditions [1, 2].

It is crucial that sports medicine physicians are comfortable diagnosing and treating the female athlete triad. If untreated, the consequences of the Triad can be devastating, and include compromised reproductive health, increased rates of bone stress injuries, and other soft tissue musculoskeletal injuries, osteoporosis, and eating disorders. Early recognition and prompt treatment may help patients avoid the end-stage outcomes of the Triad.

A. Kussman (✉)
Stanford University, Department of Orthopaedics, Stanford, CA, USA

A. Nattiv
UCLA Department of Family Medicine, Division of Sports Medicine, UCLA Department of Orthopaedics, Los Angeles, CA, USA
e-mail: anattiv@mednet.ucla.edu

© Springer Nature Switzerland AG 2020
E. Hong, A. L. Rao (eds.), *Mental Health in the Athlete*,
https://doi.org/10.1007/978-3-030-44754-0_11

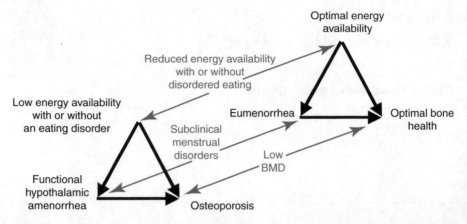

Fig. 11.1 The spectrum of the female athlete triad. The three inter-related components of the Triad are energy availability, menstrual status, and bone health. Energy availability affects menstrual status, and both energy availability and menstrual status affect bone health. (Reprinted with permission from Wolters Kluwer: Medicine & Science in Sport & Exercise [1])

Terminology

In 1992 the American College of Sports Medicine (ACSM) convened a panel of experts, which resulted in the initial description of the Triad [3] and subsequently in the 1997 ACSM Position Stand on the Female Athlete Triad [4]. They defined the Triad as a syndrome affecting active girls and women, comprised of the interrelated conditions of disordered eating, amenorrhea, and osteoporosis. Since this time, there has been a significant body of research dedicated to understanding the female athlete triad, its diagnosis, its management, and its consequences. This has resulted in two major updates. In 2007, the ACSM published an updated Position Stand on the Female Athlete Triad, re-defining the Triad as low energy availability, menstrual dysfunction, and decreased bone mineral density (BMD) [1]. An important feature of this update was the recognition that each component of the Triad may exist on a spectrum ranging from healthy, to subclinical or mild disturbances, to end-stage consequences including eating disorders, amenorrhea, and osteoporosis. The 2007 Position Stand illustrated the Triad as a prism (see Fig. 11.1), where athletes could move along the different axes of the prism at different rates, highlighting the importance of early recognition and treatment. In 2014, The Female Athlete Triad Coalition Consensus Statement on Treatment and Return to Play of the Female Athlete Triad was published to provide further guidance on clinical management of the Triad and return to play decision making [2]. As our understanding of the female athlete triad expands, we have also observed the existence of a similar condition in males [5, 6] – most recently termed the male athlete triad [7]. This is comprised of low energy availability, hypogonadism, and low bone mineral density. The male athlete triad remains a promising area for future research and is further detailed below in section "Return-to-Play Guidelines."

In 2014, the International Olympic Committee (IOC) published a paper on Relative Energy Deficiency in Sport (RED-S) [5], which was followed by an update in 2018 [8]. These papers are based upon research on the female athlete triad, and are similar in that they describe the impacts of low energy availability (EA) on athlete well-being. The RED-S model depicts low EA as the "hub" at the center of a wheel. Each "spoke" of the wheel illustrates the downstream effects of low EA on multiple organ systems, including those involved in the Triad (menstrual function and bone health), as well as several others (immunologic, cardiovascular, etc.). Although research does agree that low EA is the causative mechanism behind the menstrual dysfunction and impaired bone health seen in the Triad, there is not yet sufficient scientific evidence to directly link low EA to each of the other "spokes" of the RED-S model. As such, we will continue to use the more researched term "the female athlete triad." Ongoing research on the health and performance effects of low EA is welcomed and encouraged.

Epidemiology

Unfortunately, the female athlete triad is very common. Because individual athletes may present at different points on each of the three spectra (low EA, menstrual dysfunction, and low BMD), it may be easier to quantify the prevalence of each of the individual components of the Triad. In one study of 425 female collegiate athletes at seven US universities, 3.3% reported a diagnosis of anorexia and 2.3% reported a diagnosis of bulimia nervosa; however, the Eating Attitudes Test (EAT-26) identified "at-risk" behaviors in 15.2% of athletes, and the Eating Disorder Inventory Body Dissatisfaction Subscale (EDI-BD) identified 32.4% of athletes as having "at risk" behaviors for eating disorders [9]. Eating disorders are also more common in athletes than in the general population. In one large study of 1620 athletes and 1696 controls, 20% of female athletes met criteria for an eating disorder compared to 9% of controls [10]. Even in the absence of a formal eating disorder, athletes also demonstrate a high frequency of disordered eating behaviors [11, 12]. Studies have shown that in weight class sports, as many as 70% of athletes may rely on dieting and disordered eating behaviors to make weight [13].

Menstrual irregularities have been reported in 31% of athletes not using oral contraceptives [9]. Other studies have found that the prevalence of secondary amenorrhea may be as high as 65% in elite distance runners [14], and 79% in elite dancers [15]. A Croatian study found rates of secondary amenorrhea were three times higher in athletes when compared to a non-athlete control group [14].

Prevalence of low bone mass ranges from 22% to 50%, and prevalence of osteoporosis ranges from 0% to 13% in athletes [16]. However, it should be noted that the World Health Organization definitions of low bone mass (osteopenia) and osteoporosis in postmenopausal women were used at the time of this study, instead of the current definitions for premenopausal women. Therefore T-scores were used in young women instead of Z-scores. One review found that while 16–60% of athletes had at least one component of the Triad, 2.7–27% had two components, and 0–15.9% of athletes exhibited all three components of the Triad [17].

The incidence of the Triad remains highest in "lean sports" which include aesthetic sports (synchronized swimming, figure skating), sports with weight classes (wrestling, lightweight rowing), and endurance sports (distance running, cycling). In a population of high school athletes, the prevalence of both disordered eating and menstrual irregularity was 15.4% in aesthetic sports, 10.1% in endurance sports, and 7.6% in team/anaerobic sports [18]. A Norwegian study found similar trends – the prevalence of eating disorders in aesthetic sports was 42%, in endurance sports it was 24%, in technical sports it was 17%, and in ballgame sports it was 16% [10]. In a similar study on elite German athletes, the prevalence of eating disorder was 17% in aesthetic sports, 2% in ball sports, and 2% in non-athletes [19].

Although the Triad can occur in all races, the majority of research to date has been performed in Caucasian populations, and further research is needed on the influence of race on the Triad.

Low Energy Availability

Low energy availability (EA) occurs when an individual's nutritional intake is not sufficient to meet their body's energy expenditure, including the energy expended during exercise. This is defined as: energy intake (kcal) minus energy expenditure (kcal) divided by the kg of fat free mass. Research has suggested that optimal physiologic function occurs at an energy availability of 45 kcal/kg FFM. Energy availabilities of 30 kcal/kg FFM and less have been associated with abnormal metabolic markers and Triad symptoms in female athletes.

Low EA affects GnRH, which decreases LH pulsatility and estrogen levels [20]. The hypoestrogenic state contributes to menstrual dysfunction and decreases in BMD. In addition, low EA can also decrease resting energy expenditure, decrease total T3, increase Ghrelin, increase PYY, decrease leptin, decrease insulin-like growth factor (ILGF-1), and increase cortisol [21, 20]. Even in athletes who have adequate EA when averaged overall, periods of low EA throughout the day can contribute to some of the above hormonal changes [20].

Although low EA is easily defined, it can be challenging to calculate in clinical settings. Energy intake can be assessed via a food log or food frequency questionnaire. Energy expenditure can be estimated via metabolic equivalents of a task, heart rate monitoring, or accelerometer. Lastly, fat free mass can be calculated via dual-energy x-ray absorptiometry (DXA), air displacement plethysmography, bioelectrical impedance, or skin fold caliper measurement [22]. Many clinicians will use low body mass index (BMI) as an indicator of low energy availability. BMI is defined as a patient's weight (in kg) divided by their height (in meters) squared. Although normal ranges for BMI can vary considerably due to differences in body composition and varying sport demands, a BMI of less than 18.5 is generally regarded as low. Caution should be used when relying solely on BMI as an indicator of energy availability however, since evidence suggests that the body responds to chronic low EA by decreasing the resting metabolic rate [20]. Although not a direct measurement of EA, screening for restrictive eating patterns may identify red flags which suggest low EA. These behaviors might include highly restrictive diets, avoiding certain food groups completely, or skipping meals. In some patients who have developed an eating disorder, physical exam findings may be present, such as lanugo, Russell's sign (callus on finger from self-induced emesis), dental erosion, or large parotid glands. Given the challenges of identifying low energy availability in the clinical setting, it is very helpful to work with a sports dietitian whenever possible.

It is also important to note that low energy availability may be intentional or unintentional. Unintentional low energy availability usually results from a lack of awareness about the body's nutritional needs, or from a recent increase in training volume without a compensatory increase in dietary intake. A classic example can be seen in the freshman collegiate athlete who transitions to a more intense training schedule without making the necessary dietary changes their body needs in order to compensate for their higher level of training.

Intentional low energy availability may occur due to disordered eating (DE) behaviors, or if more severe, may meet criteria for an eating disorder (ED). According to the DSM-V criteria, anorexia nervosa is defined as persistent restriction of energy intake leading to significantly low body weight ("less than minimally normal in adults or less than expected weight in children and adolescents"), fear of gaining weight or persistent behavior that interferes with weight gain despite being at a low weight, and a disturbance in the way one's body weight/shape is experienced or a persistent lack of awareness of the seriousness of the low body weight [23]. Changes from the DSM-IV include removing the diagnostic criteria of having amenorrhea, and also adding that clinicians may infer fear of gaining weight or of body image disturbance from patient behaviors, even if the patient does not admit to these thoughts. Bulimia nervosa is defined as binge episodes and compensatory behaviors which occur on average at least once per week for 3 months [23]. This DSM-V diagnosis is also a change from the prior edition, as it reduces the minimum frequency of binging episodes required to meet diagnostic criteria. Research demonstrates that eating disorders are more common in athletes than in non-athletes [24]. Unfortunately eating disorders have one of the highest mortality rates of all mental health conditions, and also have a wide range of severe of health complications which can affect nearly every organ system in the body [24]. For this reason, it is important to diagnose eating disorders as soon as possible in order to facilitate prompt access to treatment.

Many athletes exhibit concerning behaviors or thought patterns around food, without meeting full diagnostic criteria for one of the above eating disorders. There are numerous disordered eating behaviors which fall into this category, including over-exercising, making meals contingent on exercise, purging behaviors (such as self-induced vomiting, or the use of laxatives and diuretics), avoiding certain food groups completely, intentionally restricting intake, etc. Because patients with eating disorders often deny or try to hide their condition, and eating disorders are associated with such significant health consequences, clinicians who identify disordered eating behaviors should screen athletes for eating disorders, and should have a low threshold to refer them for further work-up or treatment as indicated.

DE and ED tend to be more common in "lean sports," and part of this may be propagated by the belief that a lower body weight will improve athletic success. However, one large study which relied on self-report via online questionnaire found that athletes with low EA were more likely to report decreased training response, decreased coordination, decreased concentration, impaired judgment, irritability, depression, and decreased endurance performance [25]. Another study on ten elite junior swimmers found decreased performance results associated with ovarian suppression due to low EA [26]. A population of elite level rowers who increased their training volume without increasing their energy intake demonstrated reductions in body mass and fat mass but also showed decreased performance in timed 5K racing [27]. Similarly, in a study on elite endurance athletes, Tornberg et al. found decreased neuromuscular performance in amenorrheic athletes when compared to eumenorrheic athletes [28].

As will be detailed below, low EA predisposes athletes to bony injuries such as stress fractures, which further impair training and performance. However, evidence also suggests that high school athletes who reported some disordered eating were twice as likely to sustain a musculoskeletal injury in general [18]. In addition, low EA is often associated with low iron levels, which can further reduce endurance performance [29, 22].

Menstrual Dysfunction

Athletes should be regularly screened for menstrual dysfunction, because this is associated with significant short-term and long-term consequences for bone health. Menstrual dysfunction may take several different forms, including delayed menarche, oligomenorrhea, or amenorrhea. Delayed menarche is generally defined as starting one's period at age 15 or older. Oligomenorrhea refers to menstrual cycles of 35 days or longer, or less than 9 menses per year. Secondary amenorrhea is diagnosed when it has been greater than 3 months since a patient's last menstrual cycle. Primary amenorrhea refers to a patient who has not yet undergone menarche. All of these forms of menstrual dysfunction have been associated with increased incidence of bone stress injuries (BSI) and low BMD [30]. Furthermore, athletes who reported menstrual irregularities (oligomenorrhea/amenorrhea) may be up to three times as likely to sustain a musculoskeletal injury [31]. Even in patients who do have regular menstrual cycles, there may be subclinical menstrual disturbances such as luteal phase defects and anovulatory cycles, which may only be appreciated on detailed hormonal panels [20]. One study in recreational runners found the prevalence of luteal phase defects to be as high as 79% over a 3-month period [32].

Patients with functional hypothalamic amenorrhea resulting from low EA demonstrate decreased LH pulsatility, decreased FSH, decreased estrogen, and decreased progesterone [20]. Estrogen plays a key role in balancing bone formation and bone resorption and also inhibits bone turnover.

Table 11.1 Suggested studies for the work-up of patients with secondary amenorrhea

Suggested studies for the work-up of secondary amenorrhea
Luteinizing hormone (LH)
Follicle stimulating hormone (FSH)
Estradiol
Thyroid stimulating hormone (TSH)
Free T4
Total T3
Dehydroepiandrosterone (DHEA)
Testosterone (free and total)
Pregnancy test
Prolactin

All female athletes should be screened for menstrual dysfunction at their preparticipation physical exams, and more frequently as clinically indicated. When screening for menstrual irregularities, it is important to inquire about any form of contraception that the athlete is using, as hormonal forms of contraception may mask or artificially induce menses. For example, an athlete with a history of amenorrhea may have regular periods if taking an oral contraceptive pill; however, this does not mean that she would be cycling regularly on her own, or that her bone mineral density is adequate.

If amenorrhea is identified, then further work-up is indicated in order to identify the cause of amenorrhea. While one of the most common causes of amenorrhea in the athlete is functional hypothalamic amenorrhea due to low EA, it is important to rule out other potential causes of amenorrhea including polycystic ovarian syndrome (PCOS), thyroid disease, prolactinemia, premature ovarian failure, or pregnancy. A suggested list of initial diagnostic studies for the work-up of secondary amenorrhea can be found in Table 11.1 and may need to be modified based on individual clinical presentations. Young female athletes with primary amenorrhea may require additional work-up including imaging to rule out structural abnormalities [2].

Low Bone Mineral Density

Low EA has been associated with low BMD (defined by low Z-scores) and also with abnormal bone turnover markers [20]. Triad-related effects on bone health are primarily due to two mechanisms: estrogen-dependent and estrogen-independent. In the estrogen-dependent mechanism, hypoestrogenism associated with amenorrhea causes upregulation of bone resorption and promotes bone loss by inducing osteoclastogenesis. The estrogen-independent mechanism is energy-dependent and involves metabolic hormone adaptations to low EA such as IGF-1, leptin, and T3. IGF-1 usually stimulates osteoblastogenesis and bone formation but is impaired in low EA states. Similarly, leptin is also impaired in low EA states, and it normally plays a role in osteoblast proliferation. T3 (also low in low EA states) normally stimulates osteoblast proliferation and differentiation and promotes bone formation [20].

Estrogen acts on osteoblasts and osteoclasts via a direct receptor-mediated fashion and has indirect effects on calcitonin, parathyroid hormone, cytokines, and growth factors [33].

Low bone mineral density (BMD) is very concerning in athletes and is associated with an increased incidence of bone stress injuries. Even excluding BSI, high school athletes with a BMD Z-score < −1.0 were 3.6 times more likely to incur a musculoskeletal injury [31]. Furthermore, low BMD predisposes athletes to BSIs in more high-risk areas, including those in trabecular bone, which are associated with prolonged recovery and complications such as non-union. A study in collegiate runners found that lower BMD was associated with prolonged return-to-play times for athletes with a BSI and also that athletes with multiple triad risk factors were more likely to have a BSI in a high-risk location like the sacrum or femoral neck [34]. Similarly, Barrack et al. found that patients with multiple Triad risk factors had increasing incidence of BSIs [35].

In addition to decreased BMD, newer modalities such as HR-pQCT suggest that menstrual status affects the microstructure of bone. Ackerman et al. found greater strength parameters (greater stiffness and failure load) at the tibia in eumenorrheic athletes, but amenorrheic athletes lost this effect when compared to non-athletes. Furthermore, the bone strength parameters seen in the amenorrheic athletes at non-weight-bearing sites such as the distal radius were even lower than those seen in non-athletes [36].

Adequate BMD is also of great concern because many patients with the Triad present during periods of peak bone accrual. If an individual is expected to reach their maximal BMD by age 30, then compromised bone health in one's 20s may significantly increase the risk of osteoporosis. Osteoporosis is an important health concern in the United states, where 52% of adults over age 50 have low bone mass at the femoral neck or lumbar spine and 1.5 million people sustain an osteoporotic fracture each year [33].

In order to identify athletes with low BMD, it may be helpful to obtain a DXA scan. DXA scans should be obtained on any athlete with one or more "high-risk" Triad risk factors, as defined by the 2014 Triad Consensus Statement: history of an eating disorder; BMI < 17.5, <85% of estimated weight, or weight loss >10% in 1 month; menarche at age 16 or older; current or history of less than 6 menses within 12 months; two prior BSI, one high risk BSI, or a low-energy non-traumatic fracture; or prior Z-score < −2.0. In addition, athletes with two or more "moderate-risk" Triad risk factors should also have a DXA. "Moderate-risk" factors include current or history of disordered eating for >6 months; BMI between 17.5 and 18.5, <90% estimated weight, or recent weight loss of 5–10% in 1 month; menarche between age 15–16; current or history of 6–8 menses over 12 months; one prior BSI; and prior Z-score between −1.0 and −2.0. In addition, clinicians should consider screening athletes with one or more traumatic fractures in the setting of other Triad risk factors, or athletes on medications which may affect bone health (such as Depo-Provera or oral prednisone). In athletes found to have low BMD, DXA scans should be repeated every 1–2 years to monitor response to treatment. For premenopausal women, Z-scores should be used, as these reflect a comparison to age-matched controls [2]. The American College of Sports Medicine (ACSM) defines low BMD or BMC to be a Z-score of <-1.0 in females engaged in weight-bearing sports [1].

Screening

All athletes should be screened for the Triad during their preparticipation physical examination (PPE). Screening questions for the Triad are included in the PPE Monograph [37], and additional questions are suggested in the 2014 Female Athlete Triad Consensus Statement [2]. Furthermore, the menstrual cycle can be used as a vital sign at the PPE, in order to help identify athletes with the Triad [38]. If screening identifies any one component of the Triad, thorough screening for the other two components is strongly recommended [20]. The 2014 Female Athlete Triad Consensus Statement also provided a cumulative risk assessment (CRA) tool intended to help physicians quantify a female athlete's risk level for bone stress injury and poor bone health (see Fig. 11.2) [2]. This is discussed further in section "Follow Up." The CRA may be used at the time of the PPE, or when making return-to-play decisions [39, 40].

Risk factors	Magnitude of risk		
	Low risk = 0 points each	Moderate risk = 1 pont each	High risk = 2 points each
Low EA with or without DE/ED	☐ No dietary restriction	☐ Some dietary restriction‡; current/past history of DE;	☐ Meets DSM-V criteria for ED*
Low BMI	☐ BMI ≥ 18.5 or ≥ 90% EW** or weight stable	☐ BMI 17.5 < 18.5 or < 90% EW or 5 to < 10% weight loss/month	☐ BMI ≤17.5 or < 85% EW or ≥ 10% weight loss/month
Delayed menarche	☐ Menarche < 15 years	☐ Menarche 15 to < 16 years	☐ Menarche ≥16 years
Oligomenorrhea and/or Amenorrhea	☐ > 9 menses in 12 months*	☐ 6-9 menses in 12 months*	☐ < 6 menses in 12 months*
Low BMD	☐ Z-score ≥ -1.0	☐ Z-score-1.0*** < -2.0	☐ Z-score ≤ -2.0
Stress reaction/fracture	☐ None	☐ 1	☐ ≥ 2; ≥ 1 high risk or of trabecular bone sites†
Cumulative Risk (total each column, then add for total score)	_____ points +	_____ points +	_____ points = _____Total Score

Fig. 11.2 The female athlete triad cumulative risk assessment tool. The cumulative risk assessment provides an objective method of determining an athlete's risk using risk stratification and evidence-based risk factors for the Female Athlete Triad. This assessment is then used to determine an athlete's clearance for sport participation (see Fig. 11.3). ‡Some dietary restriction as evidenced by self-report or low/inadequate energy intake on diet logs; *current or past history; ** ≥90% EW; absolute BMI cut-offs should not be used for adolescents. ***Weight-bearing sport; † high-risk skeletal sites associated with low BMD and delay in return to play in athletes with one or more components of the Triad include stress reaction/fracture of trabecular sites (femoral neck, sacrum, pelvis). BMD bone mineral density, BMI body mass index, DE disordered eating, EA energy availability, EW expected weight, ED eating disorder. (Reprinted with permission from BJSM [2])

For many athletes with the Triad, their initial presenting symptom is a bone stress injury, so all athletes with stress reactions and stress fractures should also be thoroughly screened for the Triad.

Treatment

Treatment of the female athlete triad is best accomplished with a multidisciplinary team that includes the physician, sports dietitian, athletic trainer, and mental health provider (as indicated), and otherwise as available resources may dictate. In many cases, patients may require additional consultants based on their individual presentations and complications. Good communication between members of the treatment team is essential to success. In cases involving disordered eating or eating disorders, the athlete often exhibits reluctance to "buy in" to the treatment plan. In such situations, a medical contract may be very helpful. This serves to clarify expectations for the athlete and to describe the conditions necessary for ongoing sport participation. The use of contracts is highly individual and must be tailored to the unique circumstances of each patient. An example contract is provided in the 2014 Female Athlete Triad Consensus Statement [2].

Since the Triad is the result of low EA, treatment of low EA is crucial to success. This is accomplished either through an increase in nutritional intake, a decrease in training volume, or a combination of both. As mentioned above, this is best done with the assistance of a registered sports dietitian, who can provide tailored guidance to the athlete, and also continue to provide an assessment of energy availability. There is robust evidence that restoration or normalization of body weight is associated with resumption of menses and improvements in BMD [2]. Some athletes may need to increase caloric intake, but other athletes may benefit from adjusting the timing of meals and snacks, or altering the content of meals rather than the volume. If an athlete has been diagnosed with an eating disorder, their treatment team should include a mental health provider, as this is essential to treatment. For patients with eating disorders, providing nutritional advice in isolation is not likely to result in any clinical improvement. Most athletes with disordered eating behaviors would also benefit from seeing a mental health provider, in order to help treat dysfunctional attitudes towards food and body image concerns.

For patients with menstrual dysfunction, the treatment goal is to regain normal menses. As mentioned above, all patients with amenorrhea should undergo work-up to rule out alternative causes of amenorrhea (such as thyroid dysfunction), which would require different treatment approaches. For patients who have a laboratory work-up consistent with functional hypothalamic amenorrhea, the first-line treatment is to improve energy availability (see above). Although oral contraceptive pills may be indicated for patients who require protection against pregnancy, they are not indicated to treat menstrual dysfunction. Taking oral contraceptive pills may result in resumption of menses, but this does not correlate with the return of spontaneous menses or improvements in BMD, and may provide a false sense of reassurance

[41]. The lack of benefit on BMD has been associated with first-pass effects of hepatic metabolism on IGF-1 [2]. In cases of hypothalamic amenorrhea, which persists for more than 1 year, despite non-pharmacologic treatment, treatment with transdermal estrogen (which bypasses hepatic metabolism) and cyclic oral progesterone may be considered [2, 33]. It is important to note, however, that transdermal estrogen and cyclic progesterone have not been proven to prevent pregnancy, so patients should be counseled that this is not adequate for contraception.

The treatment of low BMD should also focus on improving EA. Monitoring for the spontaneous return of regular menses can serve as a positive clinical indication that factors which influence bone health are improving.

If low BMD is identified, patients should optimize their intake of calcium and vitamin D in order to provide the important building blocks for bone formation and remodeling. One study of female navy recruits found that the incidence of BSI was reduced by as much as 20% with calcium and vitamin D supplementation [42]. Another study found that higher intakes of calcium, skim milk, and dairy products were all associated with lower rates of stress fractures in active women. For every additional cup of skim milk consumed per day, there was a 62% reduction in stress fracture incidence [43]. Kelsey et al. also found that stress fractures were more common in female runners with low dietary calcium intake [44]. Per Institute of Medicine (IOM) guidelines, the Recommended Dietary Allowance (RDA) of calcium ranges from 1000 mg to 1300 mg per day for adults, with higher values recommended for adolescents and the elderly [45]. It is recommended that whenever possible, the majority of a patient's calcium intake should be from their diet, rather than supplements. This is particularly important since some studies have suggested increased incidence of kidney stones and cardiovascular disease in patients with high doses of oral calcium supplementation [46, 47].

Per IOM guidelines, the RDA for vitamin D is 600 international units (IU) per day for adolescents, pregnant or lactating women, and adults up to age 70. Adults older than age 70 have an RDA of 800 IU per day [45]. In patients who have low BMD or a strong history of bone stress injuries, it is recommended to check a vitamin D-25(OH) level. If vitamin D deficiency or insufficiency is identified, then patients may require higher levels of vitamin D supplementation. One study of professional football players found increased incidence of fractures in patients with vitamin D deficiency, and possibly decreased performance [48]. Another study in competitive distance runners found that even among runners with normal vitamin D levels, a higher vitamin D level in those with a history of bone stress injury was associated with less time off from running [49]. However, it is worth noting that at very high levels of vitamin D (such as may result from taking daily doses of 10,000 to 50,000 IU for extended periods of time), vitamin D intoxication may be seen [45]. Vitamin D intoxication may include hypercalcemia, hypercalciuria, vascular and tissue calcifications, renal complications, and heart arrhythmias [45]. One study examined the effects of a single annual high dose of vitamin D (500,000 IU) and actually found increased rates of falls and fractures in the elderly [50].

The specific sport played also affects BMD. Sports with multi-directional loading and higher impact, such as basketball, volleyball, or soccer, have been associated with improved bone health. One study demonstrated that runners who played a ball sport in their childhood had a 50% lower risk of stress fracture [51]. In another study, athletes in high-impact sports had a 3–22% higher BMD compared to athletes in low-impact and moderate-impact sports [52]. Some low-impact sports, such as swimming or cycling, may result in decreased BMD, while running (repetitive impact but without multidirectional loading) seems to have a relatively neutral effect on BMD. This evidence supports the health benefits of being a multisport athlete, and demonstrates some of the potential dangers of early sports specialization.

Pharmacologic measures should be considered as a second-line option only when there is a lack of response to non-pharmacologic treatment for at least a year, and if new fractures occur during non-pharmacologic management [2]. As mentioned above, pharmacologic treatment may include transdermal estrogen with cyclic oral progesterone. Bisphosphonates may be considered in unique cases in consultation with an endocrinologist, but are not currently FDA-approved for treatment in premenopausal women. Furthermore, they are known to be teratogenic, which is particularly concerning in reproductive age women, given the long half-life of bisphosphonates. Specific criteria for the use of pharmacologic measures can be found in the 2014 Female Athlete Triad Consensus Statement [2].

Follow-up

When treating low BMD, it is advantageous to obtain follow-up DXA scans at 1–2 year intervals to monitor for improvements in bone health over time. Time to restoration of menses is highly variable, but in some cases, it may take longer than a year of non-pharmacologic treatment [53]. Furthermore, one study found that resumption of menses took longer in athletes who had amenorrhea for >8 months, compared to those who had amenorrhea <8 months [54]. It is also concerning that although restoration of adequate EA and resumption of menses results in improvements in BMD, it is not clear whether patients can return to normal BMD compared to healthy controls [55, 56]. This highlights the importance of early recognition and prompt treatment of the Triad to minimize long-term health consequences.

Return-to-Play Guidelines

The 2014 Female Athlete Triad Consensus Statement provided a cumulative risk assessment (CRA) tool to help clinicians quantify an athlete's Triad risk factors (Fig. 11.2) [2]. This tool may be implemented at the time of an athlete's annual PPE, in order to quantify their risk level and connect the athlete with resources to improve their bone health and reduce their risk of injury. In addition, it may also be used when an athlete has been diagnosed with a BSI or with the Triad, as a tool to help

	Cumulative risk score*	Low risk	Moderate risk	High risk
Full clearance	0 – 1 point	☐		
Provisional/limited clearance	2 – 5 points		☐ Provisional clearance ☐ Limited clearance	
Restricted from training and competition	≥ 6 points			☐ Restricted from training/competition-provisional ☐ Disqualified

Fig. 11.3 The female athlete triad clearance and return-to-play guidelines based on risk assessment score. The cumulative risk score is calculated using evidence-based risk factors displayed in Fig. 11.2. Athletes have differing clearance recommendations based on their risk assessment scores. *Cumulative Risk Score determined by summing the score of each risk factor (low, moderate, high risk) from the Cumulative Risk Assessment (Fig. 11.2). Clearance status for athletes who are moderate-to-high risk for the Triad: provisional clearance—clearance determined from risk stratification at time of evaluation (with possibility for status to change over time depending on athlete's clinical progress); limited clearance—clearance granted, but with modification in training as specified by physician (with possibility for status to change depending on clinical progress and new information gathered); restricted from training/competition (provisional)—athlete not cleared at present time, with clearance status re-evaluated by physician and multidisciplinary team with clinical progress; disqualified—not safe to participate at present time, clearance status to be determined at future date depending on clinical progress, if appropriate. It is the recommendation of the Consensus Panel that athletes diagnosed with anorexia nervosa who have a body mass index (BMI) <16 kg/m^2 or with moderate-to-severe bulimia nervosa (purging >4 times/week) should be categorically restricted from training and competition. Future participation is dependent on treatment of their eating disorder, including ascertainment of BMI >18.5 kg/m^2, cessation of bingeing and purging and close interval follow-up with the multidisciplinary team. (Reprinted with permission from BJSM [2])

guide their safe return to participation. Based on the athlete's risk score, different clearance recommendations are suggested – full clearance, restricted/provisional clearance, and restriction from training and competition (Fig. 11.3). Studies have demonstrated that an athlete's risk score does correlate with future risk of BSI [39, 40]. Since the Triad occurs on a spectrum of severity and represents a complex relationship between the three conditions which comprise the Triad, return-to-play decisions for patients with the Triad must always be individualized. For example, several of the points gained in the CRA tool are for non-modifiable risk factors. An athlete with a history of delayed menarche will always carry risk points for this, even if she has improved her overall energy availability. Other non-modifiable risk factors include a prior history of an eating disorder and history of past BSI. Clinician judgment is necessary for situations such as these. It has been suggested that a modified weighted risk assessment tool may be useful for follow-up assessments. In addition, physicians should utilize their individual judgment regarding consideration of other

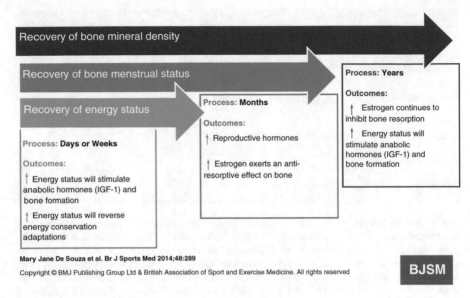

Mary Jane De Souza et al. Br J Sports Med 2014;48:289

Copyright © BMJ Publishing Group Ltd & British Association of Sport and Exercise Medicine. All rights reserved

BJSM

Fig. 11.4 Recovery from the female athlete triad. The three components of the Triad recover at different rates, and full recovery may be a long process lasting months to years. The three components of the Triad recover at different rates with the appropriate treatment. Recovery of energy status is typically observed after days or weeks of increased energy intake and/or decreased energy expenditure. Recovery of menstrual status is typically observed after months of increased energy intake and/or decreased energy expenditure, which improves energy status. Recovery of bone mineral density may not be observed until years after recovery of energy status and menstrual status has been achieved. IGF-1, insulin-like growth factor-1. (Reprinted with permission from BJSM [2])

known risk factors which are not included in the CRA, such as family history of osteoporosis, vitamin D deficiency, low dietary calcium intake, or malabsorptive disorders such as celiac disease [30]. The IOC has proposed a return-to-play model based on red light (high risk), yellow light (moderate risk), and green light (low risk) groups [5] (Fig. 11.4).

Because safe return-to-play is often contingent on specific criteria (such as the athlete continuing to meet regularly with members of their care team), the use of contracts may be helpful. These are documents which specify all of the necessary conditions for ongoing safe participation, such as keeping appointments, adhering to an exercise or meal plan, or achieving certain minimum weight or body composition. In addition, a contract may specify the consequences of failure to follow the care plan, such as restricted participation, decreased training mileage, or even removal from team training. The contract should be reviewed and agreed upon by all members of the care team, and then reviewed with the athlete as well. The goal of the medical contract is to establish the plan for safe return-to-play which prioritizes an athlete's health and wellbeing, and does not expose them to undue risk during their return to sport. An example of a contract can be found in the 2014 Female Athlete Triad Consensus Statement [2].

The Male Athlete Triad

Although historically most of the research on the Triad has been done in female athletes, male athletes have also been found to have low EA and increased risks of BSI. This has led to a description of the Male Athlete Triad, which mirrors the female athlete triad, and consists of low energy availability, hypogonadism, and decreased BMD [6, 7]. As in female athletes, low energy availability can be intentional or unintentional. Although eating disorders are more common in female athletes than in male athletes, male athletes have a higher prevalence of eating disorders than male non-athletes. In one study, 20% of female athletes and 8% of male athletes met criteria for an eating disorder, compared to 9% of female controls and 0.5% of male controls [10]. As in female athletes, eating disorders are particularly common in male athletes who participate in lean sports. One study found rates of eating disorders to be 22% in antigravitational sports, 9% in endurance sports, and 5% in ball sports [10]. Another study found the prevalence of eating disorders to be 42% in antigravitational sports, 17% in weight class sports, and 10% in endurance sports [57]. As was noted in female athletes, male athletes also demonstrate high levels of disordered eating behaviors even in the absence of a formal eating disorder diagnosis [58, 12, 59, 60, 61].

Evidence suggests that the EA cut-off for observing physiologic effects (impact on reproductive and metabolic hormones) may be lower in male athletes than in female athletes [62, 63]. One study found that a period of low EA reduced leptin and insulin levels in men (similar to changes seen in women) but did not observe changes in ghrelin, T3, testosterone, and IGF-1 [63]. More research is needed to better understand the physiologic effects of low EA in male athletes [5, 6, 8].

Male athletes do not have menstrual periods that provide an easily observed indicator of hypothalamic function; however, studies suggest that male athletes with high training volumes or low EA may have decreased testosterone levels or sperm counts, or may see changes in the hypothalamic-pituitary-gonadal axis [6]. As in females, low EA and hypogonadism have important consequences for bone health. One study found that either low estrogen (in females) or low testosterone (in males) was associated with 4.5-fold increased risk of BSI [64]. A study in male adolescent runners found that risk factors for low BMD were cumulative and included weight less than 85% of expected, average weekly mileage greater than 30, prior history of stress fracture, and less than one serving of calcium per day [65]. Furthermore, adolescent male runners had lower weight, lower BMI, and lower spine BMD Z-scores when compared with adolescent male athletes who were not runners. It is therefore important to screen not only our female athletes but also our male athletes for the Triad.

The Triad in Para-Athletes

Similar to the general athlete population, para-athletes may also present with the Triad [5]; however, para-athletes may have unique differences in their energy demands, bone health, and menstrual function [66, 8]. Energy availability may vary for para-athletes – athletes in wheelchairs may have lower energy demands, but some athletes with prosthetics, or with involuntary movements such as dyskinesis or athetosis, may have increased metabolic demands. Central nervous system injuries that disrupt the hypothalamic-pituitary axis may also affected menstrual function. Para-athletes may also be predisposed to disuse osteopenia or osteoporosis from altered skeletal loading patterns, which can further compound the effects of the Triad. Para-athletes should also be screened for the Triad, and clinicians should be mindful of factors which may affect a para-athlete's presentation with the Triad. Although awareness of Triad risk factors in para-athletes is increasing, more research is needed in this area.

Prevention

As we have detailed earlier in this chapter, the potential long-term health consequences of the Triad are significant. The sports medicine community should seek to increase awareness of the Triad as much as possible. Increased awareness among athletes, parents, coaches, athletic trainers, and physicians may help prevent the Triad and may also assist in identifying athletes with the Triad as early as possible in order to facilitate prompt treatment.

Unfortunately, studies have demonstrated that knowledge of the Triad is low in several of these groups. In a study on US High School nurses, only 19% were able to identify the three components of the Triad and only 25% reported working proactively with coaches to help prevent health issues in their female athletes. However, more than 95% expressed interest in learning more about the Triad [67]. In a survey of multi-specialty physicians, only 37% had heard of the Triad, and of these respondents, they named an average of 2.1 components of the Triad correctly [68]. In one small study, 30% of coaches had heard of the Triad, but only 10% could name the three components of the triad. Furthermore, 30% of the coaches thought that menstrual irregularities were normal in athletes. When asked to list consequences of low energy or disordered eating, 70% of the coaches listed impaired performance, but only 30% listed menstrual dysfunction, and 20% listed injury [69]. NCAA Division I collegiate coaches faired slightly better, in that 43% were able to correctly identify the components of the Triad; however, this still leaves significant room for improvement [70]. In one study on Australian women who exercised regularly, only 10% of respondents could name all three components of the Triad, and 45% did not think amenorrhea could affect bone health. Athletes in lean sports, or with a history of amenorrhea or stress fracture, were all significantly less likely to take action about amenorrhea [71]. When athletic trainers at NCAA institutions were surveyed, almost all (98%) had heard of the triad, but on average respondents could only identify two of the three components [72]. Given these numbers, it is not surprising that many young women feel it is "normal" for a competitive athlete to have irregular periods. Beliefs like these are important to address, in order to avoid the long-term health consequences of the Triad.

In addition to raising awareness of the Triad, it is also important to create a healthy approach to exercise and nutrition at home and at school. Several promising evidence-based educational programs have been used in high school or college populations. One study in female college athletes found that two behavioral modification programs were effective at reducing end-points associated with eating disorders at 6 weeks and at 1 year. Furthermore, after the programs, several athletes came forward to seek medical care for the Triad [73]. Another study demonstrated short- and long-term improvement in disordered eating behaviors and body image among high school students who went through the ATHENA program (Athletes Targeting Healthy Exercise and Nutrition Alternatives), which is a sport team-based harm reduction and health promotion program [74]. Research has also shown that in female college students, both clinician-led and peer-led dissonance-based eating disorder prevention programs were effective in reducing eating disorder risk factors and eating disorder onset, and both were more effective than an online program [75].

Conclusion

In conclusion, the Female Athlete Triad is comprised of the three interrelated conditions: low energy availability, menstrual dysfunction, and decreased BMD. Each of these three conditions can occur along a spectrum, and patients may move along each portion of the spectrum at different rates. There are serious potential long-term consequences of the Triad, and early recognition is key in order to facilitate prompt treatment and reduce the risk of long-term complications. Clinicians should be comfortable identifying and treating each of the three primary components of the Triad. Working with a multidisciplinary team is key to successful treatment, and the team should include a mental health professional whenever disordered eating or eating disorders are present. The first-line treatment for the Triad is increasing EA either by reducing energy expenditure, increasing energy intake, or both. If menstrual dysfunction is identified, alternative causes of amenorrhea or oligomenorrhea should be ruled out. In addition, clinicians should optimize bone health as much as possible, including dietary intake of calcium and vitamin D. Return-to-play decisions in athletes with the Triad are complex, and clinicians should rely on the risk assessment tool provided in the 2014 Female Athlete Triad Consensus Statement as well as their own clinical judgment. There is increasing evidence for the Male Athlete Triad, and male athletes should also be screened for low EA, hypogonadism, and decreased BMD. Due to the potential serious health consequences of the Triad, preventative efforts are of the utmost importance. Evidence suggests the need for increased awareness of the Triad. Educational programs about body image and healthy eating demonstrate long-term efficacy and may help to promote healthy attitudes towards exercise and nutrition.

References

1. Nattiv A, Loucks AB, Manore MM, Sanborn CF, Sundgot-Borgen J, Warren MP, et al. American College of Sports Medicine position stand. The female athlete triad. Med Sci Sports Exerc. 2007;39(10):1867–82.
2. De Souza MJ, Nattiv A, Joy E, Misra M, Williams NI, Mallinson RJ, et al. 2014 Female Athlete Triad coalition consensus statement on treatment and return to play of the female athlete triad: 1st international conference held in San Francisco, California, May 2012 and 2nd international conference held in Indianapolis, Indiana, May 2013. Br J Sports Med. 2014;48(4):289.
3. Yeager KK, Agostini R, Nattiv A, Drinkwater B. The female athlete triad: disordered eating, amenorrhea, osteoporosis. Med Sci Sports Exerc. 1993;25(7):775–7.
4. Otis CL, Drinkwater B, Johnson M, Loucks A, Wilmore J. American College of Sports Medicine position stand. The female athlete triad. Med Sci Sports Exerc. 1997;29(5):i–ix.
5. Mountjoy M, Sundgot-Borgen J, Burke L, Carter S, Constantini N, Lebrun C, et al. The IOC consensus statement: beyond the Female Athlete Triad--Relative Energy Deficiency in Sport (RED-S). Br J Sports Med. 2014;48(7):491–7.
6. Tenforde AS, Barrack MT, Nattiv A, Fredericson M. Parallels with the female athlete triad in male athletes. Sports Med. 2016;46(2):171–82.
7. Fredericson M, Nattiv A. ACSM symposium – the male athlete triad: updates and parallels with the female athlete, ACSM 65th annual meeting proceedings, Abstract A-18. 2018: p. 6.
8. Mountjoy M, Sundgot-Borgen JK, Burke LM, Ackerman KE, Blauwet C, Constantini N, et al. IOC consensus statement on relative energy deficiency in sport (RED-S): 2018 update. Br J Sports Med. 2018;52(11):687–97.
9. Beals KA, Manore MM. Disorders of the female athlete triad among collegiate athletes. Int J Sport Nutr Exerc Metab. 2002;12(3):281–93.
10. Sundgot-Borgen J, Torstveit MK. Prevalence of eating disorders in elite athletes is higher than in the general population. Clin J Sport Med. 2004;14(1):25–32.
11. Reinking MF, Alexander LE. Prevalence of disordered-eating behaviors in undergraduate female collegiate athletes and nonathletes. J Athl Train. 2005;40(1):47–51.
12. Glazer JL. Eating disorders among male athletes. Curr Sports Med Rep. 2008;7(6):332–7.
13. Sundgot-Borgen J, Torstveit MK. Aspects of disordered eating continuum in elite high-intensity sports. Scand J Med Sci Sports. 2010;20(Suppl 2):112–21.
14. Dusek T. Influence of high intensity training on menstrual cycle disorders in athletes. Croat Med J. 2001;42(1):79–82.
15. Abraham SF, Beumont PJ, Fraser IS, Llewellyn-Jones D. Body weight, exercise and menstrual status among ballet dancers in training. Br J Obstet Gynaecol. 1982;89(7):507–10.
16. Khan KM, Liu-Ambrose T, Sran MM, Ashe MC, Donaldson MG, Wark JD. New criteria for female athlete triad syndrome? As osteoporosis is rare, should osteopenia be among the criteria for defining the female athlete triad syndrome? Br J Sports Med. 2002;36(1):10–3.
17. Gibbs JC, Williams NI, De Souza MJ. Prevalence of individual and combined components of the female athlete triad. Med Sci Sports Exerc. 2013;45(5):985–96.
18. Thein-Nissenbaum JM, Rauh MJ, Carr KE, Loud KJ, McGuine TA. Associations between disordered eating, menstrual dysfunction, and musculoskeletal injury among high school athletes. J Orthop Sports Phys Ther. 2011;41(2):60–9.
19. Thiemann P, Legenbauer T, Vocks S, Platen P, Auyeung B, Herpertz S. Eating disorders and their putative risk factors among female German professional athletes. Eur Eat Disord Rev. 2015;23(4):269–76.
20. De Souza MJ, Koltun KJ, Etter CV, Southmayd EA. Current status of the female athlete triad: update and future directions. Curr Osteoporos Rep. 2017;15(6):577–87.
21. Brown KA, Dewoolkar AV, Baker N, Dodich C. The female athlete triad: special considerations for adolescent female athletes. Transl Pediatr. 2017;6(3):144–9.
22. Kim BY, Nattiv A. Health considerations in female runners. Phys Med Rehabil Clin N Am. 2016;27(1):151–78.

23. American Psychiatric Association. Diagnostic and statistical manual of mental disorders. 5th ed. Arlington: American Psychiatric Association; 2013.
24. Joy E, Kussman A, Nattiv A. 2016 update on eating disorders in athletes: a comprehensive narrative review with a focus on clinical assessment and management. Br J Sports Med. 2016;50(3):154–62.
25. Ackerman KE, Holtzman B, Cooper KM, Flynn EF, Bruinvels G, Tenforde AS, et al. Low energy availability surrogates correlate with health and performance consequences of relative energy deficiency in sport. Br J Sports Med. 2018;53(10):bjsports-2017-098958.
26. Vanheest JL, Rodgers CD, Mahoney CE, De Souza MJ. Ovarian suppression impairs sport performance in junior elite female swimmers. Med Sci Sports Exerc. 2014;46(1):156–66.
27. Woods AL, Garvican-Lewis LA, Lundy B, Rice AJ, Thompson KG. New approaches to determine fatigue in elite athletes during intensified training: resting metabolic rate and pacing profile. PLoS One. 2017;12(3):e0173807.
28. Tornberg Å, Melin A, Koivula FM, Johansson A, Skouby S, Faber J, et al. Reduced neuromuscular performance in amenorrheic elite endurance athletes. Med Sci Sports Exerc. 2017;49(12):2478–85.
29. Petkus DL, Murray-Kolb LE, De Souza MJ. The unexplored crossroads of the female athlete triad and iron deficiency: a narrative review. Sports Med. 2017;47(9):1721–37.
30. Joy EA, Nattiv A. Clearance and return to play for the female athlete triad: clinical guidelines, clinical judgment, and evolving evidence. Curr Sports Med Rep. 2017;16(6):382–5.
31. Rauh MJ, Nichols JF, Barrack MT. Relationships among injury and disordered eating, menstrual dysfunction, and low bone mineral density in high school athletes: a prospective study. J Athl Train. 2010;45(3):243–52.
32. De Souza MJ, Miller BE, Loucks AB, Luciano AA, Pescatello LS, Campbell CG, et al. High frequency of luteal phase deficiency and anovulation in recreational women runners: blunted elevation in follicle-stimulating hormone observed during luteal-follicular transition. J Clin Endocrinol Metab. 1998;83(12):4220–32.
33. Goolsby MA, Boniquit N. Bone health in athletes. Sports Health. 2017;9(2):108–17.
34. Nattiv A, Kennedy G, Barrack MT, Abdelkerim A, Goolsby MA, Arends JC, et al. Correlation of MRI grading of bone stress injuries with clinical risk factors and return to play: a 5-year prospective study in collegiate track and field athletes. Am J Sports Med. 2013;41(8):1930–41.
35. Barrack MT, Gibbs JC, De Souza MJ, Williams NI, Nichols JF, Rauh MJ, et al. Higher incidence of bone stress injuries with increasing female athlete triad-related risk factors: a prospective multisite study of exercising girls and women. Am J Sports Med. 2014;42(4):949–58.
36. Ackerman KE, Putman M, Guereca G, Taylor AP, Pierce L, Herzog DB, et al. Cortical microstructure and estimated bone strength in young amenorrheic athletes, eumenorrheic athletes and non-athletes. Bone. 2012;51(4):680–7.
37. Bernhardt DT, Roberts WO, American Academy of Family Physicians, American Academy of Pediatrics. PPE: preparticipation physical evaluation. Elk Grove Village: American Academy of Pediatrics; 2010.
38. American College of Gynecologists. Committee opinion 702: female athlete triad. Obstet Gynecol. 2017;129(6):e160–7.
39. Tenforde AS, Carlson JL, Chang A, Sainani KL, Shultz R, Kim JH, et al. Association of the female athlete triad risk assessment stratification to the development of bone stress injuries in collegiate athletes. Am J Sports Med. 2017;45(2):302–10.
40. Kussman A, Fredericson M, Kraus E, Singh S, Deakins-Roche M, Miller E, Kim BY, Tenforde A, Barrack M, Sainani K, Nattiv A. The female athlete triad cumulative risk assessment score implemented at the preparticipation physical exam correlates with risk of bone stress injury in collegiate distance runners: a 4-year prospective study. Abstract published in Clin J Sport Med. 2018;28(2):247.
41. Cobb KL, Bachrach LK, Sowers M, Nieves J, Greendale GA, Kent KK, et al. The effect of oral contraceptives on bone mass and stress fractures in female runners. Med Sci Sports Exerc. 2007;39(9):1464–73.

42. Lappe J, Cullen D, Haynatzki G, Recker R, Ahlf R, Thompson K. Calcium and vitamin d supplementation decreases incidence of stress fractures in female navy recruits. J Bone Miner Res. 2008;23(5):741–9.
43. Nieves JW, Melsop K, Curtis M, Kelsey JL, Bachrach LK, Greendale G, et al. Nutritional factors that influence change in bone density and stress fracture risk among young female cross-country runners. PM R. 2010;2(8):740–50; quiz 94.
44. Kelsey JL, Bachrach LK, Procter-Gray E, Nieves J, Greendale GA, Sowers M, et al. Risk factors for stress fracture among young female cross-country runners. Med Sci Sports Exerc. 2007;39(9):1457–63.
45. Institute of Medicine. Dietary reference intakes for calcium and vitamin D. Washington DC: National Academies Press; 2011. 1132 p.
46. Bolland MJ, Avenell A, Baron JA, Grey A, MacLennan GS, Gamble GD, Reid IR. Effect of calcium supplements on risk of myocardial infarction and cardiovascular events: meta-analysis. BMJ. 2010;341:c3691.
47. Curhan GC, Willett WC, Speizer FE, Spiegelman D, Stampfer MJ. Comparison of dietary calcium with supplemental calcium and other nutrients as factors affecting the risk for kidney stones in women. Ann Intern Med. 1997;126(7):497–504.
48. Maroon JC, Mathyssek CM, Bost JW, Amos A, Winkelman R, Yates AP, et al. Vitamin D profile in National Football League players. Am J Sports Med. 2015;43(5):1241–5.
49. Kim BY, Kraus E, Fredericson M, Tenforde A, Singh S, Kussman A, Barrack M, Deakins-Roche M, Nattiv A. Serum vitamin D levels are inversely associated with time lost to bone stress injury in a cohort of NCAA Division I distance runners. Abstract published in Clin J Sport Med. 2016;26(2):e58–68.
50. Sanders KM, Stuart AL, Williamson EJ, Simpson JA, Kotowicz MA, Young D, et al. Annual high-dose oral vitamin D and falls and fractures in older women: a randomized controlled trial. JAMA. 2010;303(18):1815–22.
51. Fredericson M, Ngo J, Cobb K. Effects of ball sports on future risk of stress fracture in runners. Clin J Sport Med. 2005;15(3):136–41.
52. Torstveit MK, Sundgot-Borgen J. Low bone mineral density is two to three times more prevalent in non-athletic premenopausal women than in elite athletes: a comprehensive controlled study. Br J Sports Med. 2005;39(5):282–7; discussion -7.
53. Arends JC, Cheung MY, Barrack MT, Nattiv A. Restoration of menses with nonpharmacologic therapy in college athletes with menstrual disturbances: a 5-year retrospective study. Int J Sport Nutr Exerc Metab. 2012;22(2):98–108.
54. Cialdella-Kam L, Guebels CP, Maddalozzo GF, Manore MM. Dietary intervention restored menses in female athletes with exercise-associated menstrual dysfunction with limited impact on bone and muscle health. Nutrients. 2014;6(8):3018–39.
55. Jonnavithula S, Warren MP, Fox RP, Lazaro MI. Bone density is compromised in amenorrheic women despite return of menses: a 2-year study. Obstet Gynecol. 1993;81(5 (Pt 1)):669–74.
56. Keen AD, Drinkwater BL. Irreversible bone loss in former amenorrheic athletes. Osteoporos Int. 1997;7(4):311–5.
57. Rosendahl J, Bormann B, Aschenbrenner K, Aschenbrenner F, Strauss B. Dieting and disordered eating in German high school athletes and non-athletes. Scand J Med Sci Sports. 2009;19(5):731–9.
58. Thiel A, Gottfried H, Hesse FW. Subclinical eating disorders in male athletes. A study of the low weight category in rowers and wrestlers. Acta Psychiatr Scand. 1993;88(4):259–65.
59. Chatterton JM, Petrie TA. Prevalence of disordered eating and pathogenic weight control behaviors among male collegiate athletes. Eat Disord. 2013;21(4):328–41.
60. Steen SN, Brownell KD. Patterns of weight loss and regain in wrestlers: has the tradition changed? Med Sci Sports Exerc. 1990;22(6):762–8.
61. Riebl SK, Subudhi AW, Broker JP, Schenck K, Berning JR. The prevalence of subclinical eating disorders among male cyclists. J Am Diet Assoc. 2007;107(7):1214–7.

62. Fagerberg P. Negative consequences of low energy availability in natural male bodybuilding: a review. Int J Sport Nutr Exerc Metab. 2018;28(4):385–402.
63. Koehler K, Hoerner NR, Gibbs JC, Zinner C, Braun H, De Souza MJ, et al. Low energy availability in exercising men is associated with reduced leptin and insulin but not with changes in other metabolic hormones. J Sports Sci. 2016;34(20):1921–9.
64. Heikura IA, Uusitalo ALT, Stellingwerff T, Bergland D, Mero AA, Burke LM. Low energy availability is difficult to assess but outcomes have large impact on bone injury rates in elite distance athletes. Int J Sport Nutr Exerc Metab. 2018;28(4):403–11.
65. Barrack MT, Fredericson M, Tenforde AS, Nattiv A. Evidence of a cumulative effect for risk factors predicting low bone mass among male adolescent athletes. Br J Sports Med. 2017;51(3):200–5.
66. Blauwet CA, Brook EM, Tenforde AS, Broad E, Hu CH, Abdu-Glass E, et al. Low energy availability, menstrual dysfunction, and low bone mineral density in individuals with a disability: implications for the para athlete population. Sports Med. 2017;47(9):1697–708.
67. Kroshus E, Fischer AN, Nichols JF. Assessing the awareness and behaviors of U.S. High School nurses with respect to the female athlete triad. J Sch Nurs. 2015;31(4):272–9.
68. Curry EJ, Logan C, Ackerman K, McInnis KC, Matzkin EG. Female athlete triad awareness among multispecialty physicians. Sports Med Open. 2015;1(1):38.
69. Brown KN, Wengreen HJ, Beals KA. Knowledge of the female athlete triad, and prevalence of triad risk factors among female high school athletes and their coaches. J Pediatr Adolesc Gynecol. 2014;27(5):278–82.
70. Pantano KJ. Current knowledge, perceptions, and interventions used by collegiate coaches in the U.S. regarding the prevention and treatment of the female athlete triad. N Am J Sports Phys Ther. 2006;1(4):195–207.
71. Miller SM, Kukuljan S, Turner AI, van der Pligt P, Ducher G. Energy deficiency, menstrual disturbances, and low bone mass: what do exercising Australian women know about the female athlete triad? Int J Sport Nutr Exerc Metab. 2012;22(2):131–8.
72. Kroshus E, DeFreese JD, Kerr ZY. Collegiate athletic trainers' knowledge of the female athlete triad and relative energy deficiency in sport. J Athl Train. 2018;53(1):51–9.
73. Becker CB, McDaniel L, Bull S, Powell M, McIntyre K. Can we reduce eating disorder risk factors in female college athletes? A randomized exploratory investigation of two peer-led interventions. Body Image. 2012;9(1):31–42.
74. Elliot DL, Goldberg L, Moe EL, Defrancesco CA, Durham MB, McGinnis W, et al. Long-term outcomes of the ATHENA (Athletes Targeting Healthy Exercise & Nutrition Alternatives) program for female high school athletes. J Alcohol Drug Educ. 2008;52(2):73–92.
75. Stice E, Rohde P, Shaw H, Gau JM. Clinician-led, peer-led, and internet-delivered dissonance-based eating disorder prevention programs: acute effectiveness of these delivery modalities. J Consult Clin Psychol. 2017;85(9):883–95.

Chapter 12
Mental Health Manifestations of Concussion

Anthony P. Kontos, Raymond Pan, and Kouros Emami

Introduction

Nearly 30% of athletes report one or more mental health-related symptoms following concussion [1]. If we extrapolate this number to the 1.8–3.6 million sport-related concussions (SRC) that are estimated to occur in the US annually [2], approximately 522,000 to 1,044,000 athletes may experience these symptoms. Among the mental health-related symptoms that are reported by athletes following a concussion are sadness, anxiety or nervousness, irritability, changes in personality, behavioral changes, and sleep disruptions to name a few. However, the most commonly reported and studied mental health-related issues are depressed mood, anxiety, and post-traumatic stress (PTS).

The purpose of the current chapter is to review key mental health issues that athletes may face following concussion, including anxiety, mood, and other less common, but more substantial issues such as functional neurological and somatic symptom disorders, malingering, and suicide. We will also explore the etiology of these mental health issues and analyze how mental health issues often overlap with other concussion profiles or subtypes, including migraine, vestibular, and cognitive. In so doing we will discuss some issues that may be driving some of the anxiety and fear associated with this injury including neurodegeneration (i.e., chronic traumatic

A. P. Kontos (✉)
University of Pittsburgh, Department of Orthopaedic Surgery, Pittsburgh, PA, USA

UPMC Sports Medicine Concussion Program, Pittsburgh, PA, USA
e-mail: akontos@pitt.edu

R. Pan
University of Pittsburgh, Department of Psychiatry, Pittsburgh, PA, USA
e-mail: panrj@upmc.edu

K. Emami
UPMC Sports Medicine Concussion Program, Pittsburgh, PA, USA

© Springer Nature Switzerland AG 2020 149
E. Hong, A. L. Rao (eds.), *Mental Health in the Athlete*,
https://doi.org/10.1007/978-3-030-44754-0_12

encephalopathy [CTE]). Finally, we will synthesize the information from the chapter using a case illustration to demonstrate what these concepts look like in clinical practice. However, we will begin with a brief discussion of a new conceptual framework from which to better understand mental health issues following concussion and how they may relate to other symptoms and impairment associated with this injury.

Clinical Profiles and Mental Health Issues Following Concussion

There is support in the literature for distinct concussion subtypes or clinical profiles involving specific clusters of these mental health-related symptoms and associated clinical findings [1, 3, 4]. Among these profiles of concussion are cognitive, migraine, ocular, vestibular, and, most relevant to our discussion here, anxiety/mood. In addition, other issues or modifiers such as cervical injury or sleep disturbance may accompany each concussion clinical profiles. It is also important to note that concussion clinical profiles may overlap or co-occur, resulting in complex presentation that can be difficult to distinguish and subsequently treat [4]. For example, one athlete may experience migraine, vestibular, and anxiety/mood profiles following a single concussion, whereas another athlete may only experience a cognitive profile. Another challenge in determining clinical profiles following concussion is prioritizing which profile(s) is primary, secondary, and so on. This "triaging" of profiles allows clinicians to more effectively target treatment strategies. Among the more challenging clinical profiles to assess and treat following concussion is anxiety/mood.

The anxiety/mood clinical profiles, which are described in depth by Sandel and colleagues [5], are characterized by two sets of symptoms that may overlap or occur in isolation. The anxiety symptoms include cognitive anxiety symptoms such as nervousness and worry/fear and somatic anxiety symptoms including nausea, sweating, dizziness, and nausea [5, 6]. The mood symptoms include primarily emotional symptoms involving loss of interest or energy, feelings of hopelessness, sadness, and anger/irritability [5, 6]. Behaviorally, athletes with this clinical profile may constantly think about their injury, be hyper-aware and fixate on their symptoms, and/or isolate themselves from others [4]. Many factors may influence why certain athletes develop the anxiety/mood clinical profile following a concussion including a personal or family history of psychiatric issues, premorbid or comorbid migraine, current stressors, and poor sleep hygiene [4].

The mental health-related symptoms associated with the anxiety/mood clinical profile may be unfamiliar to many athletes who, in a way, are preselected for mental wellness within the psychologically stressful world of competitive sports. As such, athletes who experience mental health-related symptoms following concussion may be unprepared for these symptoms and struggle to cope with them in the absence of familiarity and experience. Moreover, athletes are unlikely to discuss mental health and coping strategies with each other and as a result may struggle to cope with their symptoms in isolation. While athletes may be able to cope successfully with ortho- pedic injuries, they may be less familiar and effective in coping with concussion and its associated mental health symptoms. In fact, researchers have reported that concussed athletes engage in less coping overall than their orthopedically injured counterparts [7]. Consequently, following a concussion, athletes may not openly cope with or even discuss their concussion, choosing instead to deal with it on their own. If athletes are experiencing mental health-related symptoms following their concussion, they may be even less likely to discuss their injury given the stigma and perceived weakness associated with mental health in sport. This internalizing approach can set the stage for athletes to exacerbate many of the symptoms dis- cussed previously. However, not all athletes respond in this manner following a concussion.

In our experience, concussion can often serve as a "door opener" for athletes to discuss or address other mental health conditions under the guise of concussion treatment. Concussion carries with it less stigma and negativity than does a mental health disorder such as depression or anxiety. For example, an athlete with a concus- sion may reveal symptoms of depression that were preexisting or concurrent to their injury, but do so under the cover of their injury. In so doing, the athlete avoids the perceived negative perceptions from coaches, teammates, and family members for seeking mental health care, as the symptoms and treatment occurred in the context of their concussion care. This phenomenon highlights the challenge to sports medi- cine professionals working with concussed athletes who report symptoms associ- ated with mental health conditions following concussion, namely, determining the etiology of their symptoms.

Etiology of Mental Health Symptoms Following Concussion

Extricating mental health symptoms from concussion symptoms in athletes is prob- lematic, as many symptoms may overlap [4]. In addition, the etiology or underlying cause of mental health issues that might accompany a concussion is not easy to establish, as these symptoms may be from a number of causes. In some instances, athletes may suffer micro-structural damage to white matter tracts in the brain or underlying metabolic changes that impede brain function following a concussion. Both of these mechanisms could lead to mental health-related symptoms depending on the affected structures and functioning of the brain. Researchers have identified potential neurophysiological changes following concussion that may lead to anxi- ety-based symptoms [8, 9]. Both human and rodent studies have supported specific alterations to the amygdala, prefrontal cortex, sensorimotor cortex, and other meta- bolic disruptions following concussion, regions often implicated with emotional regulation [10–13].

Some athletes may instead experience behavioral and emotional responses following their concussion as a result of how they react to the challenges of this "invisible injury" [14]. For instance, an athlete may become frustrated at a lack of overt progress in recovery, lack of control of the rehabilitation process, and isolation from teammates following a concussion. Anxiety post-concussion can result in the context of an exacerbation from pre-injury anxiety, poor psychoeducation regarding concussion, or as a psychological response to the injury and/or removal from sport participation and other lifestyle modifications and restrictions. Concussion may also "fight dirty" and magnify preexisting psychological issues [4]. For instance, a patient with a history of anxiety may experience anxious mood following their concussion, whereas a patient without a history of anxiety may not. In fact, researchers have reported that preexisting psychological disorders are a strong predictor of prolonged symptoms and recovery following a concussion [15]. Risk factors for developing anxiety post-injury such as female gender, higher post-injury symptom reporting including higher emotional symptoms, and a personal or familial history of psychiatric difficulties can all lead to increased risk of developing anxiety post-injury [16]. In fact, a pre-injury history of anxiety has also been reported as a variable associated with longer recovery times [17]. Finally, patients may have unrelated, comorbid, psychological issues that occur concurrently with their concussion, but are not a result of the injury. For example, a patient may develop an adjustment disorder following a move to college that happened to coincide with the timing of their concussion. In this case, although the adjustment disorder may affect an athlete's recovery from concussion, it is not a result of the injury per se.

Anxiety

As described earlier, anxiety is characterized primarily by nervousness, fear, and worry, which can manifest as behavior (e.g., avoidance), cognition (e.g., catastrophizing thoughts), and somatic (e.g., dizziness, upset stomach) responses. Anxiety has also been identified as one of the most prominent psychological symptoms following concussion [18, 19] and can affect cognition, sleep, and lead to other physical symptoms [6, 20]. Prevalence rates of anxiety in the general population range from 4% to 25% in children and adolescents [21]. Researchers have reported that over one-third [22] to 73% [9] of National Collegiate Athletic Association (NCAA) Division I athletes experience state anxiety following a concussion. However, it is likely that most athletes experience these symptoms at a subclinical level that would not meet diagnostic criteria for a clinical anxiety disorder [23]. Regardless, proper identification of these symptoms is of particular interest as they can manifest later in the recovery process and can significantly contribute to prolonged recovery following concussion [8, 24, 25]. Additionally, as alluded to earlier, anxiety symptoms often overlap with other post-concussive symptoms [5, 14, 26], making the management of emotional difficulties following concussion even more challenging and treatment recommendations potentially less effective.

Anxiety and the hypersensitivity of one's symptoms can lead misattributions and the development of avoidance behaviors for provocative activities, situations, and environmental stimuli. These tendencies restrict one's functional exposures and can serve as a catalyst for a feedback loop that leads to further symptom maintenance and general reluctance to engage in the necessary behavioral changes (e.g., hydration, diet, regulated sleep, and exercise) to aid recovery. An example can be drawn from a subset of patients with vestibular impairment following SRC, who have also developed co-occurring anxiety [23, 27, 28]. Research has also found shared neuro-anatomical pathways between the vestibular system and those that subserve anxiety-related conditions [29]. Given both the neuroanatomical connections, discomforting symptoms common with vestibular impairment (e.g., vertigo, dizziness, or mental fogginess), and the tendency for these symptoms to become provoked in complex visual-vestibular environments (e.g., school, work, while driving), patients will often develop an anxiety response. Over time, their anxiety/fear leads to avoidance of these environments and keeps their symptoms at bay and negatively reinforcing anxiety [26]. For example, an athlete with vestibular issues following SRC may find that once returning to conditioning drills during practice (e.g., sprints, dynamic workouts), they begin to experience notable dizziness and subsequent anxiety, leading to them being less willing to return to physical activity the next day for fear of provoking those symptoms again [5].

Given the potential adverse effects of anxiety on concussion outcomes and recovery, early identification is key in order to implement a more targeted treatment plan to mitigate its effects on athletes [6]. The most recent consensus statements on concussion in sport emphasized the importance of properly assessing and managing the emotional sequelae of this injury (e.g., [30]). However, these statements did not provide specific recommendations for assessment or management of anxiety and other mood-related issues following concussion. Based on our clinical experience, we recommend that clinicians conduct a comprehensive clinical interview and exam that includes targeted questions regarding current and premorbid mental health issues and screening batteries in order to characterize the patient's emotional functioning. Most post-concussion test batteries have self-reported symptom scales as part of their protocol that addresses anxiety and other emotional concerns [31]. However, some of these symptoms can be masked and misattributed, given the overlap between certain anxiety symptoms and those common with other physical manifestations of the injury [23]. Therefore, it becomes important to accurately delineate between the potential etiologies. A thorough clinical interview, which includes a biopsychosocial history of the patient, can provide the clinician with the necessary information to assist in further narrowing the contribution of anxiety to the patient's overall symptom presentation. Self-report anxiety can be briefly assessed using the Generalized Anxiety Disorder 7-item [32] which is applicable for high school and college-aged athletes and up. Other anxiety questionnaires such as the Beck Anxiety Inventory (BAI) [33] or the State-Trait Anxiety Inventory (STAI) can also be used to provide more in-depth evaluation of anxiety. More comprehensive measures of psychological functioning and personality, such as the Personality Assessment Inventory (PAI) [34] or the Minnesota Multiphasic Personality Inventory – 2

(MMPI-2) [35], can also be incorporated to determine the severity of an athlete's emotional disturbance, particularly for those with chronic symptoms. A broader measure, the Behavioral Symptom Inventory-18 [36] is an 18-item self-report scale that provides anxiety, somatic, and depression subscales in addition to a global symptom severity score. Regardless of how it is assessed or its origins, anxiety should be identified early in the recovery process so that targeted treatments can be implemented to mitigate the likelihood of prolonged recovery [6]. Finally, more protracted or severe cases of anxiety following concussion may require referral for psychological and/or psychiatric evaluation and use of other treatments including psychopharmacology and psychotherapy.

Depression

Depression is a common affective symptom following concussion, with one in six athletes reporting these symptoms during the first week following injury [15]. Commonly used concussion symptom inventories such as the Post-concussion Symptom Scale and symptom evaluation component of the Sport Concussion Assessment Tool-5 (SCAT-5) include many depression-related items such as difficulty concentrating, fatigue/low energy, sadness, irritability, and trouble falling asleep. Each of these symptoms may occur following a concussion, but they are also components of current diagnostic criteria for major depressive disorder (DSM-5, 2013).

Although the association and overlap in symptoms of concussion and those associated with depression is widely acknowledged, literature examining prospectively the relationship between concussion and depression is sparse. In one study, researchers examined 75 high school and collegiate athletes with a diagnosed concussion using the Beck Depression Inventory-II (BDI-II) and the Immediate Post-concussion Assessment and Cognitive Test and reported subclinical increases in depression scores up to 14 days after concussion [1]. Depression was associated with lower computerized neurocognitive performance on reaction time and visual memory [1]. In another study examining 15 collegiate athletes who sustained musculoskeletal injury matched with 15 athletes who had concussions, researchers (REF) elevated mood disturbance the first couple of weeks post-concussion and a gradual improvement in mood state through the recovery process. However, in both studies, increases in depression were subclinical in severity.

Much like with anxiety, following concussion depression should be evaluated with a combination of clinical interview and exam questions and screening tools. The most common brief screening for depression in the clinical setting is the Patient Health Questionnaire 9-item (PHQ-9). The PHQ is a 9-item questionnaire designed to assess the presence of common symptoms of depression including sadness, loss of interest, and fatigue or loss of energy. Other tools for depression evaluation include the BDI-II, which includes 21 items that assess the severity of depression to help inform potential referrals for moderate to severe levels depression. Finally, the

BSI-18, described earlier, also includes a depression subscale, though it is not validated as a stand-alone subscale in athletes following concussion.

Other Less Common Issues

Malingering

Malingering involves the fabrication or exaggeration of physical symptoms. Malingering is intentional and is usually done for some extrinsic gain such as money from litigation. Although athletes are more likely to minimize or hide concussions symptoms, they may also engage in malingering following this injury. Athletes may malinger for a variety of reasons including as an excuse for performance failure, because of fear or reinjury, or to get out of sport altogether. To date, there are no studies on malingering in athletes, and as such little is known about its occurrence in this population.

Functional Neurological and Somatic Symptom Disorders

Functional neurological disorder, which replaced the term conversion disorder in the Diagnostic and Statistical Manual of Mental Disorders (DSM-5), is associated with medical symptoms which cannot be explained by a medical disorder or a psychological disorder (DSM-5, 2013). This disorder is believed to be associated with a stressful event and the symptoms are not intentional. In our experience, patients may experience concussion precipitated and related symptoms in a manner consistent with this disorder. However, there are only a handful of these patients per year among the 6000 to 7000 patients we see each year in clinic. Actual estimates on the prevalence of functional neurological disorder following concussion are not available. Multiple somatic symptoms associated with functional neurological disorder represent somatic symptom disorder, which was formerly referred to as somatization disorder (DSM-5, 2013).

We believe that a number of factors may contribute to the development of both functional neurological disorder and somatic symptom disorder. A patient's mental health, current stressors, and general coping skills prior to injury likely play a key role in these disorders following concussion. For example, a young American football star quarterback who is under tremendous pressure from his parents to obtain a scholarship, and lacks the ability to cope with this stressor directly, could with no intention develop a functional neurological disorder set of symptoms such as conversion blindness following a concussion. Media attention over deaths in retired athletes associated with neurodegeneration termed "chronic traumatic encephalopathy" (CTE) and cases of second impact syndrome (SIS) which involves a rapid neurological decline and often death following a second brain injury in younger athletes may also serve as stressors associated with these disorders. In addition, potential disability, time away from work, and compensation may be associated with a secondary gain to prolonged recovery from concussion.

There is limited research on functional neurological or somatic symptom disorders and concussion. In one of the only empirical studies in this area, researchers retrospectively examined medical records of 60 patients from an outpatient concussion specialty clinic housed in a neurology clinic at a teaching hospital [37]. These researchers reported that over half (55%) of patients were somaticizing their symptoms. On a subclinical level, researchers have reported that high somaticizers are more likely to have prolonged symptoms and recovery following concussion [38].

Concussion and Suicide

The possible link between concussion and suicide is often discussed in the media following high profile suicides of professional or collegiate athletes. However, research in this area is sparse and limited to population studies looking at suicides retrospectively. For example, researchers examined a health insurance database of 235,000 adults with concussions—from any cause not just sport-related—who did not sustain severe head injury [39]. These researchers reported that the long-term risk of suicide increased threefold among adults who had concussions [39]. In theory, if concussion can result in or exacerbate anxiety and depressed mood, it could influence suicide ideation. To date, however, a clear causal link between the subtle neurophysiological injury in the brain following concussion and suicidal ideation and suicide has not been established and warrants further research.

The CTE Effect: The Effects of Perceived Long-Term Effects of Concussion on Athletes' Mental Health

There is substantial fear surrounding concussion, and it purported association with long-term effects. In fact, these concerns have been identified as the leading issue in lowered participation rates of contact and collisions sports such as American football [40]. In a 2015 poll of over 2000 US adults, 25% stated that they would not let their children play sports because of fear of concussion and its effects [41]. One health concern that has resulted in much of the fear and anxiety surrounding concussion is CTE [42, 43]. Chronic traumatic encephalopathy is considered a chronic, neurodegenerative disease evident in neuropathological (i.e., at autopsy) findings characterized as a tauopathy where hyperphosphorylated tau protein (p-tau) is deposited in clusters in the sulcal depths and around small blood vessels in the form of neurofibrillary tangles, astrocytic tangles, and neuritis [44]. Clinical manifestations of the disease including behavioral, cognitive, and emotional symptoms are quite broad and share common characteristics with other neurological and psychiatric conditions [45]. Moreover, in spite of media and researcher accounts to the contrary, we know little about the prevalence of CTE in the general population or in athletes [46]. However, some researchers have intimated that some contact and collision sport athletes are at risk for CTE, and that there is a direct causal relationship between CTE and concussion and/or repetitive head traumas, such as those that are sustained during a career in collision or contact sports (e.g., football, hockey, soccer) [47]. Given these outcomes and the dramatic deaths of former professional football players that have been amplified by the media [48], current athletes, parents, and others are concerned about their long-term brain health. However, most of the research supporting CTE and its relation to contact sports is full of methodological shortcomings, including selection bias, case series data, and lack of control groups that have led other researchers to question the prevalence of CTE and its association to concussion and other head trauma [49–51].

Although there has not been research examining the association of perceived fear and hysteria surrounding CTE and mental health and other consequences, we observe these concerns every day in our patients and their parents following a concussion. In addition, we know that not participating in sports can also have detrimental health effects on children and result in them missing out on the physical, social, and psychological benefits associated with sport [52]. Until we have better research on the prevalence of CTE and its association and relationship to concussion, we must be careful to balance the fear with education and awareness to minimize potential harmful effects of the hysteria surrounding this issue on athletes' anxiety, depression, and decisions to play sport.

Concurrent Psychological and Other Concussion Profiles

The clinical profile model allows clinicians to determine whether the pattern of reported symptoms and impairment evidence from assessments is consistent with a single or multiple profiles or subtypes [6]. Following a concussion, athletes do not experience anxiety/mood and other mental health symptoms in a vacuum separate from other symptoms and impairment. In fact, more often than not, athletes with a concussion will experience multiple overlapping clinical profiles. Two of the clinical profiles that can co-occur are post-traumatic headache/migraine and anxiety. This comorbidity has been documented in non-concussed populations [27, 53–55, 56, 57]. Therefore, given the compromised neurophysiology following concussion [58, 59], it should not be surprising that this relationship also occurs in concussion clinical profiles. Although stress and anxiety can be triggers for migraines [60], the debilitating, and at times random, nature of the physical symptoms associated with migraine headaches can develop a sense of hyperarousal and anxiety around the onset of the next migraine. Further, avoidance behaviors, which are common with anxiety, can become further reinforced as patients avoid situations or activities that can produce a migraine. This pattern of behavior can serve as a feedback loop that can lead to a more complicated and prolonged recovery from concussion.

Vestibular dysfunction is also believed to be associated with anxiety. Researchers have demonstrated an association of vestibular symptoms and anxiety in a community sample where one-third of primary care patients reported dizziness, anxiety, or both [61]. About one-third of these patients reported both dizziness and anxiety concurrently [61]. With regard to concussion, vestibular and anxiety/mood clinical profiles may both involve overlapping, underlying vestibular and limbic system components of the brain [62]. Dizziness, vertigo, and difficulties with balance associated with vestibular injury such as those that might occur following a concussion are also similar to symptoms of panic attacks. Although the mechanisms of the co-occurrence of vestibular and anxiety symptoms following concussion are unknown, this intuitive connection warrants further research.

Cognitive difficulties are believed to be associated with depression following concussion. Researchers [1] prospectively examined the relationship of sport-related concussion with depression and neurocognitive performance and symptoms among high school and college athletes. They reported that somatic depression was related to slower reaction time at 7 days post-concussion, and lower visual memory scores at 14 days post-concussion. While additional research is needed, these findings echo findings involving non-concussed individuals with clinical depression (REF).

Case Example

In order to conclude this chapter, we wanted to provide an illustration of the anxiety/ mood profile following a concussion using a case study. Daniel is a 17-year-old male ice hockey player who presented for an initial evaluation of a head injury sustained 3 months prior when he was checked from behind during a game causing him to fall forward and striking the right-frontal region of his head (helmeted) off the boards. He then fell backward and sustained a secondary blow to the back of the head off the ice. There was no associated loss of consciousness or post-traumatic amnesia; however, he did report a fair degree of confusion/disorientation, lasting for the rest of the night. He stated that he experienced the following acute symptoms: headaches, dizziness, photo and phonophobia, irritability and emotional changes, sleep difficulties, and noticeable fatigue. He was evaluated by an on-site medical provider and his team athletic trainer and followed up at the local emergency department, who discharged him after neuroimaging was interpreted as normal.

When he had presented to our clinic for his initial evaluation (3 months post-injury), he reported a mild degree of overall improvements in his symptoms and functioning since the day of the injury. Aside from daily headaches, photo and phonophobia, nausea, noticeable dizziness/motion sickness, and mental fogginess, he presented with a notable speech stutter/stammer, which had not been present pre-injury and progressively worsened with increased levels of stress. After further questioning regarding emotional functioning, he reported increased anxiety, constant rumination, and worry about his injury, which were also negatively affecting his sleep. Further, Daniel had missed the first 2 weeks of school after the injury with eventual progression to full-days; however, he endorsed feeling overwhelmed in the classroom and struggled catching up with his missed schoolwork, worsening his mood because of the associated psychosocial stress. On vestibular screening, he became provoked for dizziness and nausea on a number of activities. Computerized neurocognitive testing revealed scores that were below reliable change metrics in comparison to his baseline scores across all assessed domains and a symptoms score of 67 on the PCSS [63], which represents a high overall symptoms severity score. His treatment plan included regulating daily behaviors (e.g., hydration, diet, sleep, and progressive exposures in physical exertion) to address his post-traumatic headaches/migraines, a referral for targeted vestibular physical therapy for his positive VOMS symptom provocation, and appropriate academic accommodations to assist with difficulties at school and in turn, better manage his stress levels. It was concluded that his noticeable speech stutter/stammer was anxiety-related and would improve as he progressed through treatment.

When he returned for his follow-up appointments (3.5 and 4 months post-injury), he noted overall improvements in most of his physical symptoms (e.g., headaches, photo and phonophobia, dizziness) with a positive response to vestibular therapy in just 2 weeks. An additional referral to exertion-based physical therapy felt warranted after his first follow-up appointment, as this provided him with both a guided return to hockey and more importantly, an outlet for further stress relief and subsequent benefits for his emotional functioning. At his second follow-up, while headaches and all other physical symptoms of concussion were minimal and, more notably, not noticed while he was engaged in social outings or with exercise, he continued to struggle with ongoing anxiety and racing thoughts when not engaged in these activities or while in bed at night. His speech stutter/stammer was also still present and would continue to worsen under increased stress and somatic anxiety-based symptoms. It was at this point where a referral for a more formal psychiatric evaluation was made to determine if pharmacological intervention was warranted, at which point, he was prescribed sertraline, anti-depressant, that has been used for mood-related issues post-concussion.

After starting this medication as prescribed and even incorporating a few sessions of outpatient psychotherapy, Daniel returned to our clinic for follow-up (5.5–6 months post-injury). At this time, he had been cleared and discharged from all established physical therapies (e.g., vestibular and exertion) after demonstrating full tolerance to both aerobic and dynamic physical activity as well as successfully passing all elements of exertional testing. More importantly, he endorsed normal emotional functioning and resolution of his anxiety, ruminative thoughts, and improvements in his ability to manage stress. Further, his stutter/stammering speech had fully dissipated, and Daniel had returned to his normal social functioning and had caught up with all of his coursework. He was excited to return to his hockey team in a full capacity and to train with them going forward. This case example highlights the importance and often times difficult task of disentangling the anxiety-related issues that can result with SRC, the multiple presentations of anxiety, and its contribution to protracted recovery. It also shows how targeted treatment for this issue once all other symptoms are managed can provide further relief and a return to normal functional levels once managed.

Conclusion

Mental health-related issues including the anxiety/mood clinical profile are common following concussion. These profiles may have different etiologies, but they share in common an adverse influence on outcomes in athletes following a concussion. As such, early identification of these athletes using a combination of clinical interview/exam and brief assessment tools is warranted. Most depression and anxiety following concussion is at subclinical levels. However, sometimes these issues may become clinical in severity and evolve into more complex phenomena such as functional neurological and somatic symptom disorders, malingering, or suicide in rare cases. Fear and anxiety associated with perceived though not empirically based long-term effects of concussion have likely exacerbated anxiety and mood issues for many athletes following their injury. As highlighted in the case example, anxiety/mood clinical profiles often overlap with other concussion clinical profiles, thereby presenting a substantial challenge to clinicians treating athletes with this injury.

References

1. Kontos AP, Covassin T, et al. Depression and neurocognitive performance after concussion among male and female high school and collegiate athletes. Arch Phys Med Rehabil. 2012;93:1751–6.
2. Langlois JA, Rutland-Brown W, Wal MM. The epidemiology and impact of traumatic brain injury: a brief overview. J Head Trauma Rehab. 2006;21(5):375–8.
3. Collins MW, Kontos AP, Reynolds E, Murawski CD, Fu FH. A comprehensive, targeted approach to the clinical care of athletes following sport-related concussion. Knee Surg Sports Traumatol Arthrosc. 2014;22(2):235-46. https://doi.org/10.1007/s00167-013-2791-6. Retrieved from https://www.ncbi.nlm.nih.gov/pubmed/24337463.
4. Kontos AP, Collins MW. Concussion: A clinical profile approach to assessment and treatment: American Psychological Association. 2018.
5. Sandel N, Reynolds E, Cohen PE, Gillie BL, Kontos AP. Anxiety and mood clinical profile following sport-related concussion: from risk factors to treatment. Sport Exerc Perform Psychol. 2017;6(3):304.
6. Collins MW, Kontos AP, Reynolds E, Murawski CD, Fu FH. A comprehensive, targeted approach to the clinical care of athletes following sport-related concussion. Knee Surg Sports Traumatol Arthrosc. 2014;22(2):235–46.
7. Kontos AP, Elbin RJ, Newcomer Appaneal R, Covassin T, Collins MW. A comparison of coping responses among high school and college athletes with concussion, orthopedic injuries, and healthy controls. Res Sports Med. 2013;21(4):367–79. https://doi.org/10.1080/1543862 7.2013.825801. Retrieved from https://www.ncbi.nlm.nih.gov/pubmed/24067122.

8. Broshek DK, De Marco AP, Freeman JR. A review of post-concussion syndrome and psychological factors associated with concussion. Brain Inj. 2015;29(2):228–37.
9. Turner S, Langdon J, Shaver G, Graham V, Naugle K, Buckley T. Comparison of psychological response between concussion and musculoskeletal injury in collegiate athletes. Sport Exerc Perform Psychol. 2017;6(3):277.
10. Jones NC, Cardamone L, Williams JP, Salzberg MR, Myers D, O'Brien TJ. Experimental traumatic brain injury induces a pervasive hyperanxious phenotype in rats. J Neurotrauma. 2008;25(11):1367–74.
11. Reger ML, Poulos AM, Buen F, Giza CC, Hovda DA, Fanselow MS. Concussive brain injury enhances fear learning and excitatory processes in the amygdala. Biol Psychiatry. 2012;71(4):335–43.
12. Singh R, Savitz J, Teague TK, Polanski DW, Mayer AR, Bellgowan PS, Meier TB. Mood symptoms correlate with kynurenine pathway metabolites following sports-related concussion. J Neurol Neurosurg Psychiatry. 2016;87(6):670–5.
13. van der Horn HJ, Liemburg EJ, Aleman A, Spikman JM, van der Naalt J. Brain networks subserving emotion regulation and adaptation after mild traumatic brain injury. J Neurotrauma. 2016;33(1):1–9.
14. Bloom G, Horton A, McCrory P, Johnston K. Sport psychology and concussion: new impacts to explore. Br J Sports Med. 2004;38(5):519–21.
15. Guerriero RM, Kuemmerle K, Pepin MJ, Taylor AM, Wolff R, Meehan III WP. The association between premorbid conditions in school-aged children with prolonged concussion recovery. J Child Neurol. 2018;33(2):168–73.
16. Ellis MJ, Ritchie LJ, Koltek M, Hosain S, Cordingley D, Chu S, et al. Psychiatric outcomes after pediatric sports-related concussion. J Neurosurg Pediatr. 2015;16(6):709–18.
17. Corwin DJ, Zonfrillo MR, Master CL, Arbogast KB, Grady MF, Robinson RL, et al. Characteristics of prolonged concussion recovery in a pediatric subspecialty referral population. J Pediatr. 2014;165(6):1207–15.
18. Iverson GL, Lange RT. Examination of "postconcussion-like" symptoms in a healthy sample. Appl Neuropsychol. 2003;10(3):137–44.
19. Kashluba S, Paniak C, Blake T, Reynolds S, Toller-Lobe G, Nagy J. A longitudinal, controlled study of patient complaints following treated mild traumatic brain injury. Arch Clin Neuropsychol. 2004;19(6):805–16.
20. Burstein M, Beesdo-Baum K, He J-P, Merikangas K. Threshold and subthreshold generalized anxiety disorder among US adolescents: prevalence, sociodemographic, and clinical characteristics. Psychol Med. 2014;44(11):2351–62.
21. Covassin T, Elbin R, Beidler E, LaFevor M, Kontos AP. A review of psychological issues that may be associated with a sport-related concussion in youth and collegiate athletes. Sport Exerc Perform Psychol. 2017;6(3):220.
22. Yang J, Peek-Asa C, Covassin T, Torner JC. Post-concussion symptoms of depression and anxiety in division I collegiate athletes. Dev Neuropsychol. 2015;40(1):18–23.
23. Kontos AP, Deitrick JM, Reynolds E. Mental health implications and consequences following sport-related concussion: BMJ Publishing Group Ltd and British Association of Sport and Exercise Medicine; 2015.
24. Grubenhoff JA, Currie D, Comstock RD, Juarez-Colunga E, Bajaj L, Kirkwood MW. Psychological factors associated with delayed symptom resolution in children with concussion. J Pediatr. 2016;174:27–32. e21.
25. McCrea M, Broshek DK, Barth JT. Sports concussion assessment and management: future research directions. Brain Inj. 2015;29(2):276–82.
26. Lahmann C, Henningsen P, Brandt T, Strupp M, Jahn K, Dieterich M, et al. Psychiatric comorbidity and psychosocial impairment among patients with vertigo and dizziness. J Neurol Neurosurg Psychiatry. 2015;86(3):302–8.
27. Balaban CD, Jacob RG, Furman JM. Neurologic bases for comorbidity of balance disorders, anxiety disorders and migraine: neurotherapeutic implications. Expert Rev Neurother. 2011;11(3):379–94.

28. Jacob RG, Furman JM. Psychiatric consequences of vestibular dysfunction. Curr Opin Neurol. 2001;14(1):41–6.
29. Furman J, Balaban C, Jacob R, Marcus D. Migraine–anxiety related dizziness (MARD): a new disorder? London: BMJ Publishing Group Ltd; 2005.
30. McCrory P, Meeuwisse W, Dvorak J, Aubry M, Bailes J, Broglio S, et al. Consensus statement on concussion in sport—the 5th international conference on concussion in sport held in Berlin, October 2016. Br J Sports Med. 2017;51(11):838–47.
31. Lovell MR, Iverson GL, Collins MW, Podell K, Johnston KM, Pardini D, et al. Measurement of symptoms following sports-related concussion: reliability and normative data for the post-concussion scale. Appl Neuropsychol. 2006;13(3):166–74.
32. Spitzer RL, Kroenke K, Williams JB, Löwe B. A brief measure for assessing generalized anxiety disorder: the GAD-7. Arch Intern Med. 2006;166(10):1092–7.
33. Beck AT, Epstein N, Brown G, Steer RA. An inventory for measuring clinical anxiety: psychometric properties. J Consult Clin Psychol. 1988;56(6):893.
34. Morey LC. Personality assessment inventory. Odessa: Psychological Assessment Resources; 1991.
35. Butcher JN, Graham JR, Ben-Porath YS, Tellegen A, Dahlstrom WG. MMPI-2: Minnesota multiphasic personality inventory-2. Minneapolis: University of Minnesota Press; 2001.
36. Derogatis LR, Derogati, L. Brief Symptom Inventory (BSI). Administration, scoring, and procedures manual. 2001.
37. Perrine K, Gibaldi J. Somatization in post-concussion syndrome: a retrospective study. Cureus. 2016;8(8):e704.
38. Root JM, Zuckerbraun NS, Wang L, Winger DG, Brent D, Kontos A, Hickey RW. History of somatization is associated with prolonged recovery from concussion. J Pediatr. 2016;174:39-44. e31..
39. Fralick M, Thiruchelvan D, et al. Risk of suicide after a concussion. CMAJ. 2016;188(7):497.
40. Findler P. Should kids play (American) football? J Philos Sport. 2015;42(3):443–62.
41. Poll H. How knowledgeable are Americans about concussions? Assessing and recalibrating the public's knowledge 2015. 2016.
42. Kaye AH, McCrory P. Does football cause brain damage? Med J Aust. 2012;196(9):547.
43. McKee AC, Cantu RC, Nowinski CJ, Hedley-Whyte ET, Gavett BE, Budson AE, et al. Chronic traumatic encephalopathy in athletes: progressive tauopathy after repetitive head injury. J Neuropathol Exp Neurol. 2009;68(7):709–35.
44. McKee AC, Stein TD, Kiernan PT, Alvarez VE. The neuropathology of chronic traumatic encephalopathy. Brain Pathol. 2015;25(3):350–64.
45. Gardner A, Iverson GL, McCrory P. Chronic traumatic encephalopathy in sport: a systematic review. Br J Sports Med. 2013;48(2):84–90.
46. Kuhn AW, Yengo-Kahn AM, Kerr ZY, Zuckerman SL. Sports concussion research, chronic traumatic encephalopathy and the media: repairing the disconnect. London: BMJ Publishing Group Ltd and British Association of Sport and Exercise Medicine; 2016.
47. Mez J, Daneshvar DH, Kiernan PT, Abdolmohammadi B, Alvarez VE, Huber BR, et al. Clinicopathological evaluation of chronic traumatic encephalopathy in players of American football. JAMA. 2017;318(4):360–70.
48. Ward J, Williams J, Manchester S. 111 NFL brains, all but one had CTE New York Times.
49. Iverson GL, Gardner AJ, McCrory P, Zafonte R, Castellani RJ. A critical review of chronic traumatic encephalopathy. Neurosci Biobehav Rev. 2015;56:276–93.
50. Maroon JC, Winkelman R, Bost J, Amos A, Mathyssek C, Miele V. Chronic traumatic encephalopathy in contact sports: a systematic review of all reported pathological cases. PLoS One. 2015;10(2):e0117338.
51. Randolph C. Is chronic traumatic encephalopathy a real disease? Curr Sports Med Rep. 2014;13(1):33–7.

52. Murphy AM, Askew KL, Sumner KE. Parents' intentions to allow youth football participation: perceived concussion risk and the theory of planned behavior. Sport Exerc Perform Psychol. 2017;6(3):230.
53. Brandt J, Celentano D, Stewart W, Linet M, Folstein MF. Personality and emotional disorder in a community sample of migraine headache sufferers. Am J Psychiatry. 1990;147(3):303.
54. Breslau N, Davis GC. Migraine, physical health and psychiatric disorder: a prospective epidemiologic study in young adults. J Psychiatr Res. 1993;27(2):211–21.
55. Breslau N, Schultz L, Stewart W, Lipton R, Welch K. Headache types and panic disorder directionality and specificity. Neurology. 2001;56(3):350–4.
56. Pesa J, Lage MJ. The medical costs of migraine and comorbid anxiety and depression. Headache J Head Face Pain. 2004;44(6):562–70.
57. Wacogne C, Lacoste J, Guillibert E, Hugues F, Le Jeunne C. Stress, anxiety, depression and migraine. Cephalalgia. 2003;23(6):451–5.
58. Giza CC, Hovda DA. The neurometabolic cascade of concussion. J Athl Train. 2001;36(3):228.
59. Giza CC, Hovda DA. The new neurometabolic cascade of concussion. Neurosurgery. 2014;75(suppl_4):S24–33.
60. Kelman L. The triggers or precipitants of the acute migraine attack. Cephalalgia. 2007;27(5):394–402.
61. Yardley L, Owen N, Nazareth I, Luxon L. Prevalence and presentation of dizziness in a general practice community sample of working age people. Br J Gen Pract. 1998;48:1131–5.
62. Sufrinko A, McAllister-Deitrick J, Elbin RJ, Collins MW, Kontos AP. Family History of Migraine Associated With Posttraumatic Migraine Symptoms Following Sport-Related Concussion. J Head Trauma Rehabil. 2048;33(1):7–14. https://doi.org/10.1097/HTR.0000000000000315. Retrieved from https://www.ncbi.nlm.nih.gov/pubmed/28520665.
63. Lovell MR, Collins MW. Neuropsychological assessment of the college football player. J Head Trauma Rehabil. 1998;13(2):9–26.

Chapter 13
Hazing and Bullying in Athletic Culture

Aaron S. Jeckell, Elizabeth A. Copenhaver, and Alex B. Diamond

Introduction

Over the past several decades, substantial attention has been given to occurrences of abuse in sports. Media coverage has fixated on accounts of harassment, bullying, and hazing in the athletic arena. In response, a number of governing bodies and sports medicine societies, including the International Olympic Committee (IOC), the National Collegiate Athletic Association (NCAA), and the American Medical Society for Sports Medicine, have presented position papers affirming that all

A. S. Jeckell (✉)
Department of Psychiatry, Vanderbilt University Medical Center, Nashville, TN, USA

Vanderbilt University School of Medicine, Nashville, TN, USA

Program for Injury Prevention in Youth Sports, Monroe Carell Jr. Children's Hospital at Vanderbilt, Nashville, TN, USA
e-mail: Aaron.Jeckell@vumc.org

E. A. Copenhaver
Vanderbilt University School of Medicine, Nashville, TN, USA

Program for Injury Prevention in Youth Sports, Monroe Carell Jr. Children's Hospital at Vanderbilt, Nashville, TN, USA

Department of Pediatrics, Vanderbilt University Medical Center, Nashville, TN, USA
e-mail: elizabeth.a.copenhaver@vumc.org

A. B. Diamond
Vanderbilt University School of Medicine, Nashville, TN, USA

Program for Injury Prevention in Youth Sports, Monroe Carell Jr. Children's Hospital at Vanderbilt, Nashville, TN, USA

Department of Pediatrics, Vanderbilt University Medical Center, Nashville, TN, USA

Department of Orthopaedics and Rehabilitation, Vanderbilt University Medical Center, Nashville, TN, USA
e-mail: alex.b.diamond@vumc.org

© Springer Nature Switzerland AG 2020
E. Hong, A. L. Rao (eds.), *Mental Health in the Athlete*,
https://doi.org/10.1007/978-3-030-44754-0_13

athletes of any background have the right to engage in sport in a safe and supportive environment [1, 2]. Nonetheless, athlete maltreatment persists across a range of demographic groups. In this chapter, we will examine the complex and multifaceted aspects of both hazing and bullying in sport.

Hazing in Athletic Culture

Hazing is broadly defined as any act against someone joining or maintaining membership to an organization that is humiliating, intimidating, or demeaning, and endangers the health and/or safety of those involved [2, 3]. More specifically, it has been defined as "a secret, private, interpersonal process that reaffirms a hierarchical status difference between incoming and existing group members" [4]. It has the potential to encompass a range of potentially dangerous interactions, including psychological, sexual, and/or physical abuse [5–7]. While in some cases the victim of hazing may willingly engage in these rites, voluntary participation does not change the fact that hazing has occurred [2, 3]. Sexualized hazing is a form of abuse where the encounter includes a sexualized verbal, nonverbal, or physical violation, either with or without consent to engage in the hazing activity [8–10].

Hazing serves as an opportunity for inductees to demonstrate that they are willing to undergo dangerous or humiliating experiences for the opportunity to be included in team culture. It allows junior members of the team to demonstrate subservience and obedience, as well as other intangible traits that senior members may seek in teammates [11, 12]. In sport culture, hazing allows the victims to demonstrate how much they are willing to endure for their group, and what they are willing to sacrifice of themselves [13]. Athletes frequently express a need for an initiation or trial as a "team bonding experience" that serves to indoctrinate new teammates and bring the group together through some kind of transformative experience. Later sections will outline the common false belief that hazing will enhance group cohesion, and by proxy team success [2, 5, 11–14]. Existing team members may feel the need to prove of this level of dedication from new initiates, especially important in full contact sports where injury is common and a teammate can protect others from harm [15]. Athletes who have willingly subjected themselves to hazing have reported that it is endured in order to be accepted or respected by their peers and that it allows them to prove their dedication to the team [8, 16–19]. Hazing in sports often occurs after athletes have already earned membership into a team by demonstrating that they possess the physical and technical abilities necessary to compete [14]. While athletes who are trying out or have established roles on the team are rarely the targets of hazing activities [20].

Bullying in Athletic Culture

In contrast to hazing which is posited to enhance cohesion, bullying is an exclusionary form of treatment that intends to exclude a peer from the group. It is designed to perpetuate an imbalance of power and intends to force undesired prospects to the group margins [21].

Bullying lacks a consensus definition, but can generally be defined as any pattern of physical, verbal, or psychological maltreatment between peers or teammates that has the potential to be harmful or dangerous [22, 23]. Other emphasized criteria include: (1) it is repeated, (2) is deliberate, and (3) is intended to harm the target victim [24]. It notably exists in the absence of any kind of provocation, and similar to hazing is often directed at newer, less experienced, or less skilled members of the team [21]. In the absence of intervention, it may continue until either the target or abuser is removed from the environment. Bullying can include making unreasonable performance demands of the victim, threats to restrict privileges or opportunities, verbal or emotional abuse, excessive or unwarranted criticism, denying or minimizing accomplishments, excessive blame for mistakes, threats or physical violence, harassment via social media, intentional exclusion from team events, or spreading of rumors or demeaning information [25–27]. When bullying occurs in the sports setting, it is often influenced by gender, sexuality, and coaching behaviors. Literature demonstrates that athletes who are members of an organization led by a more authoritarian coaching structure are more likely to engage in bullying and other types of maltreatment [25].

Behavioral Basis

The rite of passage, coming of age ceremony, and many other forms of social initiation have a long history in human culture and across civilizations [28]. These inductions range from benign to brutal, and if successfully navigated can signal an individual's earned membership into a desired group. By design, they are intended to be transformative, characterized by a "destruction/creation" cycle where an old identity is destroyed and a new one is born in the mold of the dominant group [20]. While these rituals have a tendency to take on a self-perpetuating nature wherein the former initiates become perpetrators out of a sense of tradition, they are theorized to serve an important role in the structural formation of their respective cultures [29–31]. Painful and arduous trials that demonstrated the worth and value of a potential inductee into a group are believed to have been tremendously adaptive in the development of early hierarchies, and many of the underlying motivations of these behaviors are applicable to modern team sports [14].

An athletic team has several important corollaries to the groups that have historically participated in hazing practices. Teams often possess a hierarchy based on age, skill, experience, and clearly defined leadership structure (coach and staff, team captain, and assistant captain(s), varsity and junior varsity. The group's success relies on both the success of individuals and their ability to function as a unit. Affiliation with a team may signal an "elite" status demonstrating high social value and may be a highly coveted position. It is both entrance into this hierarchy and positioning within the hierarchy that may prompt forms of maltreatment in sport [11].

Hazing is a hyperbolic and potentially dangerous reinterpretation of traditional initiation rites. This behavior typically occurs for two reasons: (1) to provide the inductee an opportunity to demonstrate that they possess certain intangible qualities that will make them an asset to the team and (2) to serve as an experience that is posited to enhance team cohesion between new and existing members which is in turn believed to improve team success [13, 25]. Hazing is often time-limited, and when these goals are felt to have been achieved may self-terminate until the next batch of recruits are initiated.

Athletic Culture

Aspects of modern athletic culture predispose participants to hazing and bullying behaviors. Because of the widespread perception that participation in sport is a positive "character builder," hazing and bullying in the sports setting allows such behavior to be more widely accepted [32]. Athletes are expected to play through pain, accept orders, make sacrifices for team gains, take risks, and challenge their own limits in order to achieve success on the playing field. They may do so at the cost of other social and academic obligations [12]. While being exposed to hazing, they are expected to demonstrate an ability to endure upsetting or difficult experiences at the perceived gain of acceptance by the group. If an individual is unable or unwilling to participate in hazing rites, they may quickly become the target of bullying. The athletic community is known to be bound by a code of secrecy, as this type of self-governance is nearly always disavowed when exposed [1, 10, 33]. Typically, any violation of this rigid confidentiality structure signals that an individual will not conform to group norms and may be excluded.

In some circumstances, these types of behaviors can deviate toward sexual abuse. In many cultures throughout history, athletes have demonstrated the "standard for hegemonic masculinity" [20, 34]. The most masculine athletes are frequently the most dominant and well respected [20, 34]. Instances of sexual exploitation in both hazing and bullying exist in order to hyper-masculinize the perpetrator by placing him or her in the role of a sexual aggressor and de-masculinize the victim by making them passive and submissive [13]. By forcing the victims into this role, their status at the bottom of the team hierarchy is solidified. Likewise, the aggressor reasserts their dominance in an extreme way and places themselves as superior, one who possesses "status, hostility, control, and dominance" [12, 17, 35].

Bullying and hazing behaviors tend to self-perpetuate, often referred to in a light-hearted way as "tradition". Through social learning, victims of sports-related hazing and bullying come to believe that these types of behaviors are "normal" and an appropriate means of self-governance. In this traditional pattern, victims may eventually become perpetrators as they turn to the same behaviors that they were subjected to upon achieving a status of superiority in their athletic community.

Institutional protection of the abuser is a concerning aspect of sport-related abuse. There are notable instances of high-profile organizations going to great lengths to either protect abusers or attempt to "cover up" instances of hazing or bullying [36–39]. The reasons for this are complex. In some cases, the abuser is a senior or more experienced athlete and may be perceived as more valuable to the team. Protecting the abuser in these instances may result from concern for the

immediate success of the organization. For any individual or institution to acknowledge that abuse has occurred among their athletes also invokes a degree of culpa-
bility and may tarnish reputations. A program may hope to settle these kinds of
issues quietly and internally to avoid possible negative publicity or any legal
implications.

In certain cases of bullying and hazing, the athletic community may feel inclined
to blame the victim. The majority of research into hazing and bullying has been
done on maltreatment in the general population, rather than the athletic community.
Bystanders may hold on to the misconception that if the victim engaged in hazing
willingly, then there should be no blame. Others may continue to see a benefit in
hazing and disregard any issues caused by it. In cases of sexual assault where the
aggressor and victim have a prior or currently close relationship, blame for the
aggressor tends to be diminished compared to an unknown assailant [40]. When
considering that a teammate may perpetrate against a peer, and that some may feel
the abuse has the potential to enhance cohesion, it is very possible that the assault
is viewed as benign and the victim is blamed for describing the behavior as abusive.
Perhaps the biggest factor leading to the perpetuation of hazing is the misconception that hazing is normal or even beneficial [18, 19]. Although it has been demonstrated that hazing, bullying, and other forms of maltreatment impede individual
and team performance, the belief that it is an important part of sport culture persists. In this context, individuals who report the maltreatment are often felt to be
acting against the best interests of the team. In situations where hazing has been
engaged in willingly, some even recommend that victims need to be punished for
their participation [41].

Epidemiology of Hazing

The prevalence of hazing in sport is obscured by a veil of secrecy and hence is difficult to assess. Prevalence is further confounded by the significant variance with
regard to what each individual considers as hazing. What one individual considers a
harmless event and would never be reported may actually be far from it. Many athletes also admit to unwillingness to report any kind of hazing activity. For instance,
80% of National Collegiate Athletic Association (NCAA) athletes described experiencing events that would qualify as hazing. However, only 12% of these athletes
actually felt that they had been hazed [42]. A follow-up study found that 60–95% of
athletes who have been hazed have explicitly stated that they would not report the
hazing event [19, 42]. These findings support the notion that the incidence of hazing
in sports is likely underestimated.

In a study of United States High School students published in 2008, 47% of student athletes endorsed being hazed [19]. Similarly, 42% of NCAA athletes first experienced hazing while still in high school [42]. Other reports indicate that as many as
800,672 high school students are hazed per year, and 25% of those who had been
hazed reported that the first incident occurred before the age of 13 years old [35].

It has also been reported that 55% of US college students who participated in clubs, teams, or other organizations experienced hazing of some degree during their collegiate experience [19].

Risk Factors for Hazing in Sport

Hazing in athletic populations is not limited to any gender, age range, or skill level [22, 43, 44]. Populations who are particularly vulnerable to the various forms of hazing include elite athletes [2, 12, 18, 42], high school athletes [35, 45], those of homosexual or bisexual orientation [12, 46], transgendered athletes [46], athletes with disabilities [1], or those with academic difficulties [35]. Certain team features also predispose groups to hazing practices. Teams where the athlete-leaders behave in a way that defies or challenges the authority of the coaching staff are particularly high risk. Any group that spends prolonged periods of time in an unsupervised team area or locker-room has more opportunities to engage in this type of behavior. Additionally, it has been posited that teams where there is an imbalance of power shifted toward a hyper-masculine authority experience higher rates of hazing.

Factors that have not been demonstrated to correlate with a greater hazing risk include any specific type of sport, the degree of physicality involved in play, or the type of uniform or body coverage [1].

Epidemiology of Bullying in Sport

A lack of standardized definition and a variety of ways to measure bullying have led to a range of reported prevalence rates [47]. Given that intimidation, aggression, and physical aggression have a place in some sports, detecting maltreatment can be particularly complicated [4, 26]. In a 2016 estimate of the general population, it was estimated that one out of every four children will experience bullying [48]. While there has been a considerable amount of study specific to the school environment, data concerning bullying in sports have been limited [49]. In a study of adolescent athletes (average age 14.5 years, 64% female) involved in Canadian team sports, 14% endorsed experiencing bullying in the context of sports, far lower than what is typically seen in the general population [49]. Much of the current existing literature corroborates that adolescent athletes may not engage in bullying as much as their peers, and that athletes who do experience bullying are more likely to be exposed to it in the school yard rather than the locker-room [27, 49, 50]. This is supported by research that identifies participation in team sport as pro-social and enhancing feelings of interconnectedness, community, and decreasing conditions such as anxiety and depression [51–54].

Cyberbullying is an emerging threat of special concern due to its ubiquitous nature, the permanence of the online reputation created, and the difficulty in detection by authority figures limiting their ability to recognize and respond to it.

Cyberbullying has been roughly defined as any form of abuse perpetrated using electronic communication or other forms of online social media [48, 55–57]. This phenomenon has been on the rise, with recent reports of 49% of children experiencing this kind of behavior at some point [48].

Risk Factors for Bullying

There are a number of potential factors that have the potential to put an individual at heightened risk to experience bullying. Lesbian, Gay, Bisexual, and Transgender youths in the general population are a particularly vulnerable group, with as many as 90% experiencing bullying [48]. Homophobia has been linked to sexual abuse and violence in sport [12, 24].

Bullying can also be heavily influenced by gender issues, masculine norms, and the moral atmosphere of the team. It has been reported that the strongest predictor of bullying behavior was whether or not an individual felt that "the most influential male in their life would approve of the bullying behavior" [27]. Individuals who perceive a lower moral atmosphere and demonstrate higher conformity to hegemonic masculine norms are more likely to perceive bullying as an acceptable behavior and engage in it [27].

Recognition of Bullying and Hazing

There are numerous barriers to the accurate and timely detection of hazing and bullying. One of the main barriers is the aforementioned "veil of secrecy" surrounding these events. Disclosure of any kind of abuse or maltreatment may break from expected social norms and may be grounds for expulsion from any group to which admission has been gained. Recent estimates suggest that less than 40% of bullying occurrences are reported to an adult [58]. There are many reasons a victim or bystander may not notify an adult or ask for help. They may experience feelings of helplessness due to the bullying. There is often fear of backlash or threats of repercussions made by the perpetrator. The victim may feel helpless or ashamed. Victims often express feelings of isolation and rejection that may be a barrier to them communicating these issues to peers or adults [24, 25, 49, 59].

Athletes who are being hazed or bullied may be forced to or voluntarily engage in embarrassing or humiliating situations. They may be expected to dress or act in a way that singles them out from other team members. Perhaps they are forced to act in a way that is subservient to senior team members such as cleaning their equipment, carrying gear, or running errands. Junior team members may be expected to greet or acknowledge senior team members in a specific way. Certain hazing practices involve modification of the body by cutting, branding, or tattooing team logos or other images. Athletes may be expected to shave their head or otherwise alter their appearance. Individuals may be expected to participate in activities involving the excess consumption of alcohol, illicit or mind-altering substances, or other materials. Other potential signs of hazing and athlete maltreatment include unexplained injuries or injuries inconsistent with the sport being played, avoidance of certain teammates or locations, fear or avoidance of certain adults, coaches, or other authority figures, difficulty forming appropriate relationships with other teammates, and difficulty trusting other individuals who are part of the team structure [60]. Any behaviors consistent with these practices may be considered hazing or bullying, and therefore abuse, and any individual familiar with their athletes and team culture may be better able to perceive this behavior.

The disclosure of bullying and hazing by both victims and perpetrators is particularly challenging, and team medical personnel may benefit from using a set of questions to help detect such patterns of behavior.

The following questions can be asked to help detect any possible occurrences of hazing [61]:

- Are members of the group engaging in any kind of non-team sanctioned activity that involves a high level of secrecy?
- Are new members to the team under pressure to participate?
- Is there a specific group (rookies, freshmen, particular position group) or type of individual singled out for certain treatment?
- Do existing team members justify the practice as a "tradition"?
- What would outside individuals (coach, athletic director, parents) think about the activities?
- Is anything illegal, dangerous, embarrassing, or incriminating taking place?

Open communication is crucial in the detection and recognition of hazing and bullying. Incidences of bullying can be navigated using questions, such as "Do you feel safe at school or in your neighborhood? Has anyone been hurting, teasing, or harassing you? Are there people who have been making your life more difficult?" Signs of bullying and hazing include [59]:

- Are there unexplained injuries inconsistent with sport participation?
- Is there any lost or destroyed personal property?
- Does the potential victim experience frequent headaches, stomach aches, feel or feign sickness?
- Are there changes in eating habits, sleep patterns, declining grades, or activity level?
- Has there been a sudden avoidance of sport or social activities?

Impact of Bullying and Hazing

The effects of hazing and bullying have been well studied. Many of those who engage in hazing actually hold positive views of their experience. A study of hazing in NCAA athletes found that nearly one-third endorsed feeling a stronger sense of identification with the group as a result of being hazed, while others endorsed a sense of accomplishment or reported feeling "stronger" [18]. Victims of bullying in athletic settings may deny negative feelings toward the perpetrators and feel that the abuser was acting out of beneficence, particularly when the abuser was a coach [26]. A positive response to these negative experiences can be explained in part by dissonance theory. Individuals who undergo an unpleasant experience to gain membership to a group often subconsciously distort their conception of what has been endured. By viewing either the abuse or the group to which membership has been gained in a more positive light, an individual can reconcile that the trauma they have gone through was worthwhile or even helpful [14, 62, 63].

Despite some perceived benefits, meta-analyses on the effects of bullying and hazing demonstrate that victims are at a significantly higher risk of developing serious physical and mental health disorders [8, 25, 64]. These individuals are prone to the development mental disorders including depression, anxiety, posttraumatic stress disorder, eating disorders, and suicidality [8, 56, 65–67]. Specific symptoms range considerably between individuals, but commonly include worsening of self-esteem, aggression toward self or others, interpersonal conflicts, emotional instability, impaired moral judgment and reasoning, delinquency/criminality, overly submissive behaviors, and worsening athletic and/or academic performance [1, 5, 15, 68]. Many individuals will voluntarily withdraw from sports in response to negative experiences. These victims of abuse may demonstrate changes in weight, fluctuating energy levels, or aberrant sleep patterns. Individuals enduring physical and sexual abuse may experience subsequent sexual dysfunction, sustain trauma to their internal or sexual organs, or be exposed to sexually transmitted illnesses [16, 69–73].

There is also abundant research to support considerable damage to teams and organizations due to hazing. There is some evidence for enhanced cohesion between the abuser and victim, though this is often one-sided with the victim harboring significant distrust and resentment [14, 18, 20, 74]. By subdividing a team into smaller units of hazers and victims, overall team unity and cohesion is actually fractured [11, 14]. A series of questionnaires administered to collegiate athletes found participation in hazing was inversely correlated with their perception of team cohesion, and that more appropriate forms of team building were directly correlated with cohesion [14]. Hazing has been demonstrated to promote unification through a "code of silence" among both abusers and victims, whether out of a sense of unity, fear, or other factors, and this has not be shown to enhance other aspects of team cohesion or success [15].

Treatment

A rapid, effective, and appropriate response is the critical first step that should be taken in the event of identified abuse [75, 76]. The victim(s) may still be in a position of potential harm, so removing them or the abuser from further interaction is crucial. By using active and empathic listening, one can safely encourage disclosure of any events that have taken place. The provider should rely on asking open-ended questions and avoiding suggestive, judgmental, or leading lines of questioning. Acknowledge that the victim may experience shame, fear, or guilt, and work toward fostering an environment where the victim knows that they are safe. Provide abundant emotional and psychological support, and understand that what the victim may be experiencing can be difficult and complicated [8, 9]. It can be important to reinforce that what they have experienced is not a healthy part of team sports, nor is it their fault [11, 14]. Denigrating the perpetrator should be avoided, as it has the potential to distort accurate recollection of abuse [8].

Every responsible team should have an established Mental Health-Emergency Action Plan (MH-EAP) that can be applied in situations of abuse or other mental health crises. A MH-EAP should include roles, responsibilities, and plans of action for every member of the team with careful consideration of what resources are available. Contact information for local administrative, emergency, and medical services must be readily available. The MH-EAP should be updated frequently as staff and team members change, and not only reviewed but practiced on a periodic basis [77, 78]. It is important for team members to be knowledgeable about various statues and regulations regarding the duty to report in their respective locale.

Litigating Abuse in Sport

Title IX has served as an important litigation tool in instances of sexual harassment or abuse involved in bullying and hazing. Established in 1972, Title IX states that, "No person in the United States shall, on the basis of sex, be excluded from participation in, be denied the benefits of, or be subjected to discrimination under any education program or activity receiving Federal financial assistance" [79]. It can be applied in any situation where verbal or physical aggression of a sexual nature, disparagement against a victim's gender or sexuality, or any type of sexual assault occurs. This federal civil rights law has been important in challenging institutions and power structured that have created an environment where sexual abuse can exist [20].

As of 2018, 44 out of 50 states have anti-hazing laws [80, 81], though the practice continues to proliferate. Bullying continues to be a major concern, and easy access to the internet and social media has created another venue where abuse can take place [59]. Clearly increasing restrictions of laws and policies are unlikely to have a strong impact on hazing and bullying practices as a majority of states have passed laws and the practice continues to proliferate. As such, additional or stricter rules and regulations would be expected to have limited effect in reducing these kinds of abuse. Efforts should be made to enact a culture shift within the athletic community where hazing is not tolerated. Currently, the NCAA is promoting a zero-tolerance policy including a system for athletes to report abuse is a safe way, and disciplinary actions directed toward abusers. By fostering these structures, the NCAA hopes to mitigate future offenses and provide a groundwork for other organizations to do the same [2, 82].

Prevention

It is the responsibility of coaches, athletic administrators, teammates, and medical teams to foster an environment of emotional support and well-being for athletes entering the team community. In such an environment, hazing, bullying, or other forms of abuse are not condoned and are subject to severe penalties. Players, coaches, and family members should all be educated as to what constitutes healthy and appropriate behaviors, as well as what would be considered an unhealthy or dangerous interaction on or off the field of play [83]. Specifically, care should be given to distinguish the difference between healthy team building and unhealthy hazing rites which can quickly evolve into sexual abuse, substance abuse, and other dangerous behaviors. As bullying has been demonstrated to correlate with per-ceived attitudes of influential male figures, outreach should be made to coaches, fathers, brothers, and elite athletes to help foster a culture where bullying is not tolerated [27].

Parents, coaches, and trainers can benefit from information on the warning signs and symptoms that can manifest in athletes who have been exposed to abuse. Demonstrating that hazing actually harms team cohesion and success is important in changing public opinion about the practice. It is crucial to ensure that all athletes have access to a trusted individual to whom they can disclose any kind of abuse without fear of retribution.

Team sport athletes can always be expected to desire a sense of team cohesion and unity. By providing sufficient opportunities for healthy team building and self-governance, the use of hazing activities or unhealthy team rituals can be dra-matically reduced [82]. Positive experiences that promote respect, team pride, and individual empowerment are proven to enhance team unity and subsequently success [5].

Conclusion

Participation in sport has the potential to impart numerous physical and psychologi-cal benefits for those involved [52, 53, 84]. Unfortunately, bullying and hazing remain a significant problem, being both prolific and having been demonstrated to create lasting damage to participants across all levels of play. While hazing and bul-lying do possess fundamental differences, they are both behaviors defined by abuse of peers and can involve physical, emotional, or sexual abuse, as well as violence and exposure to illicit substances. While some consider hazing to be harmless or beneficial to team cohesion and success, it has been empirically proven to harm both teams and individuals. Bullying, while more universally acknowledged as detrimen-tal, still exists in the absence of appropriate adult supervision and intervention. Treatment for the victims of these kinds of abuses include immediate medical, psy-chiatric, and supportive care as needed. A MH-EAP can be developed specifically for each athletic organization and for any kind of situation. Recognition of the types of athletic environments and risk factors that encourage hazing and bullying is crucial in the implementation of changes that can mitigate these behaviors. Actively engaging the community in a way that demonstrates the tremendous risks associated with hazing and bullying, as well providing education with regard to just how severely teams and individual athletes can be harmed, is essential in the development of an athletic culture where abuse is not tolerated, and athletes can thrive.

References

1. Mountjoy M, Brackenridge C, Arrington M, Blauwet C, Carska-Sheppard A, Fasting K, et al. International Olympic Committee consensus statement: harassment and abuse (non-accidental violence) in sport. Br J Sports Med. 2016;50(17):1019–29.
2. Wilfert M. Building new traditions: hazing prevention in college athletic. Indianapolis: The National Collegiate Athletic Association; 2007.
3. Allan E. "Hazing vs. bullying." StopHazing Web site. [Internet]. Orono: StopHazing.Org; [Cited 2018 March 27]. Available from: https://web.archive.org/web/20150906002200/http://www.stophazing.org/hazing-vs-bullying/.
4. Coakley JJ. Sports in society : issues and controversies. 12th ed. New York: McGraw-Hill Education; 2017. pages cm p.
5. Diamond A, Callahan S, Chain K, Solomon G. Qualitative review of hazing in collegiate and school sports: consequences from a lack of culture, knowledge and responsiveness. Br J Sports Med. 2016;50(3):149–53.
6. Fields S, Collins C, Comstock R. Violence in youth sports: hazing, brawling and foul play. Br J Sports Med. 2010;44(1):32–7.
7. Hoover J, Milner C. Are hazing and bullying related to love and belongingness? Reclaim Child Youth. 1998;7(3):138–41.
8. Marks S, Mountjoy M, Marcus M. Sexual harassment and abuse in sport: the role of the team doctor. Br J Sports Med. 2012;46(13):905–8.
9. Cense M, Brackenridge C. Temporal and developmental risk factors for sexual harassment and abuse in sport. Eur Phys Educ Rev. 2001;7:61–79.
10. Kirby S, Greaves L, Hankivsky O. The dome of silence: sexual harassment and abuse in sport. London: Zed Books; 2000.
11. Johnson J. Through the liminal: a comparative analysis of communitas and rites of passage in sport hazing and initiations. Can J Sociol. 2011;36(3):199–227.
12. Anderson E, McCormack M, Lee H. Male team sport hazing initiations in a culture of decreasing homohysteria. J Adolescent Res. 2012;27(4):427–48.
13. Waldron JJ, Kowalski CL. Crossing the line: rites of passage, team aspects, and ambiguity of hazing. Res Q Exerc Sport. 2009;80(2):291–302.
14. Van Raalte J, Cornelius AE, Linder DE, Brewer BW. The relationship between hazing and team cohesion. J Sport Behav. 2007;30:491.
15. Stirling A, Bridges E, Cruz E, Mountjoy M. Canadian Academy of Sport and Exercise Medicine position paper: abuse, harassment, and bullying in sport. Clin J Sports Med. 2011;21(5):385–91.
16. Waldron JJ, Lynn Q, Krane V. Duct tape, icy hot & paddles: narratives of initiation onto US male sport teams. Sport Educ Soc. 2011;16(1):111–25.
17. Lenskyj HJ. What's sex got to do with it? Analysing the sex and violence agenda in sport hazing practices. Toronto: Candaian Scholars' Press; 2004.

18. Allan E. Hazing in view: college students at risk: initial findings from the national study of student hazing: DIANE Publishing; Collingdale, PA, USA. 2008.
19. Allan E, Madden M. Hazing in view: college students at risk. 2008.
20. Stuart SP. Warriors, Machisom, and Jockstraps: sexually exploitative athletic hazing and title IX in the public school locker room. West N Engl Law Rev. 2013;35(35):377.
21. Ferrington D. Understanding and preventing bullying. Crime Justice. 1993;17:381–458.
22. Stirling AE. Definition and constituents of maltreatment in sport: establishing a conceptual framework for research practitioners. Br J Sports Med. 2009;43(14):1091–9.
23. Hospital BCs. Bullying prevention in sports 2016 [June 28th, 2018]. Available from: http://www.beaumont.edu/childrens/specialties/bullying-support-for-children/.
24. Brackenridge C, Rivers I, Gough B, Llewellyn K. Driving down participation: homophobic bullying as a deterrent to doing sport. In: Aitchison CC, editor. Sport and gender identities masculinities, femininities and sexualities. New York: Routledge; 2007. p. 122–39.
25. Fisher LA, Dzikus L. Bullying in sport and performance psychology. Sport Psychology. 2017.
26. Stirling AE, Kerr GA. Initiating and sustaining emotional abuse in the coach–athlete relationship: an ecological transactional model of vulnerability. J Aggress Maltreat Trauma. 2014;23(2):116–35.
27. Steinfeldt JA, Vaughan EL, LaFollette JR, Steinfeldt MC. Bullying among adolescent football players: role of masculinity and moral atmosphere. Psychol Men Masculinity. 2012;13(4):340–53.
28. Gennep Av. The rites of passage. Chicago: University of Chicago Press; 1960. 198 p.
29. Jones RL. The historical significance of sacrificial ritual: understanding violence in the modern black fraternity pledge process. West J Black Stud. 2000;24:112–24.
30. Weisfeld GE. An ethological view of human adolescence. J Nerv Ment Dis. 1979;167(1):38–55.
31. Nuwer H. Broken pledges : the deadly rite of hazing. Atlanta: Longstreet Press; 1990. 340 p.
32. Rees CR. Bullying and hazing/initiation in schools: how sports and physical education can be part of the problem and part of the solution. N Z Phys Educ. 2010;43(1):24–7.
33. Curry TJ. Reply to "a conversation (Re)analysis of fraternal bonding in the locker room". Sociol Sport J. 2001;18(3):339–44.
34. Donaldson M. What is hegemonic masculinity? Theory Soc. 1993;22(5):643–57.
35. Hoover NCP, Norman J. Initiation rites in American High Schools: a national survey. Alfred University. 2000:26.
36. Razzi V. Hazing horror: Lawsuits allege female athletes at Catholic university forced to simulate sex acts. The College Fix 2015.
37. Gutowski C, St. Clair S. Player charged in Wheaton College hazing 'frustrated' and 'disappointed,' attorney says. The Chicago Tribune 2017.
38. Snyder S. St. Joe's suspends softball team play amid hazing investigation. The Inquirer2015.
39. Gutowski C, St. Clair S. 5 Wheaton College football players face felony charges in hazing incident. The Chicago Tribune2017.
40. Freetly AJH, Kane EW. Men's and women's perceptions of non-consensual sexual intercourse. Sex Roles. 1995;33(11–12):785–802.
41. Taylor AN. Sometimes it's necessary to blame the victim. The Chronicle of Higher Education. 2011.
42. Hoover N. National survey: initiation rites and athletics for NCAA sports teams1999. Available from: http://www.alfred.edu/sports_hazing/docs/hazing.pdf.
43. Parrot A, Cummings N, Marchell TC, Hofher J. A rape awareness and prevention model for male athletes. J Am Coll Heal. 1994;42(4):179–84.
44. Hartill M. Sport and the sexually abused male child. Sport Educ Soc. 2005;10:287–304.
45. Gershel JC, Katz-Sidlow RJ, Small E, Zandieh S. Hazing of suburban middle school and high school athletes. J Adolesc Health. 2003;32(5):333–5.
46. Kirby SL, Demers G, Parent S. Vulnerability/prevention: considering the needs of disabled and gay athletes in the context of sexual harassment and abuse. Int J Sport Exerc Psychol. 2008;6(4):407–26.

47. Gladden RM, Vivolo-Kantor AM, Hamburger ME, Lumpkin CD. Bullying surveillance among youths: uniform definitions for public health and recommended data elements, Version 1.0. Atlanta: National Center for Injury Prevention and Control CfDCaP, and U.S. Department of Education; 2014.
48. Stompoutbullying.org. About bullying and cyberbullying 2016 [June 29th, 2018]. Available from: http://www.stompoutbullying.org/.
49. Evans B, Adler A, Macdonald D, Cote J. Bullying victimization and perpetration among adolescent sport teammates. Pediatr Exerc Sci. 2016;28(2):296–303.
50. Volk AA, Lagzdins L. Bullying and victimization among adolescent girl athletes. Athlet Insight. 2009;11(1):13–31.
51. Boone EM, Leadbeater BJ. Game on: diminishing risks for depressive symptoms in early adolescence through positive involvement in team sports. J Res Adolescence. 2006;16(1):79–90.
52. Dunn AL, Trivedi MH, Kampert JB, Clark CG, Chambliss HO. Exercise treatment for depression: efficacy and dose response. Am J Prev Med. 2005;28(1):1–8.
53. Eime RM, Young JA, Harvey JT, Charity MJ, Payne WR. A systematic review of the psychological and social benefits of participation in sport for children and adolescents: informing development of a conceptual model of health through sport. Int J Behav Nutr Phy. 2013;10:98.
54. Pedersen S, Seidman E. Team sports achievement and self-esteem development among urban adolescent girls. Psychol Women Q. 2004;28(4):412–22.
55. Sampasa-Kanyinga H. Co-occurring cyberbullying and school bullying victimization and associations with mental health problems among Canadian middle and high school students. Violence Vict. 2017;32(4):671–87.
56. Schneider SK, O'Donnell L, Stueve A, Coulter RW. Cyberbullying, school bullying, and psychological distress: a regional census of high school students. Am J Public Health. 2012;102(1):171–7.
57. Smith PK, Mahdavi J, Carvalho M, Fisher S, Russell S, Tippett N. Cyberbullying: its nature and impact in secondary school pupils. J Child Psychol Psychiatry. 2008;49(4):376–85.
58. Robers S, Kemp J, Truman J. Indicators of school crime and safety: 2012. Washington, DC; 2013.
59. stopbullying.gov: U.S. Department of Health and Human Services; [Available from: https://www.stopbullying.gov/.
60. Matthews D. Child abuse sourcebook. Detroit: Omnigraphics; 2004.
61. Signs of hazing and what to do: College of Saint Benedict/Saint John's University; 2018 [Available from: https://www.csbsju.edu/hazing/signs-of-hazing-and-what-to-do.
62. Gerard HB, Mathewson GC. The effects of severity of initiation on liking for a group: a replication. J Exp Soc Psychol. 1966;2:278–87.
63. Aronson E, Mills J. The effects of severity of initiation on liking for a group. J Abnorm Soc Psychol. 1959;59:177–81.
64. Hillberg T, Hamilton-Giachritsis C, Dixon L. Review of meta-analyses on the association between child sexual abuse and adult mental health difficulties: a systematic approach. Trauma Violence Abuse. 2011;12(1):38–49.
65. Rao AL. Athletic suicide - separating fact from fiction and navigating the challenging road ahead. Curr Sports Med Rep. 2018;17(3):83–4.
66. Rao AL, Asif IM, Drezner JA, Toresdahl BG, Harmon KG. Suicide in National Collegiate Athletic Association (NCAA) athletes: a 9-year analysis of the NCAA resolutions database. Sports Health. 2015;7(5):452–7.
67. Rao AL, Hong ES. Understanding depression and suicide in college athletes: emerging concepts and future directions. Br J Sports Med. 2016;50(3):136–7.
68. Newman BM, Lohman BJ, Newman PR. Peer group membership and a sense of belonging: their relationship to adolescent behavior problems. Adolescence. 2007;42(166):241–63.
69. Zierler S, Feingold L, Laufer D, et al. Adult survivors of childhood sexual abuse and subsequent risk of HIV infection. Am J Public Health. 1991;81:572–5.

70. Brackenridge C. "He owned me basically…" Women's experience of sexual abuse in sport. Int Rev Sociol Sport. 1997;32:115–30.
71. Brackenridge C. Spoilsports : understanding and preventing sexual exploitation in sport. London/New York: Routledge; 2001. xvii, 284 p.
72. Brackenridge C, Kirby S. Playing safe: assessing the risk of sexual abuse to elite child athletes. Int Rev Sociol Sport. 1997;32:407–18.
73. Kearney-Cooke A, Ackard D. The effects of sexual abuse on body image, self-image, and sexual activity of women. J Gend Specif Med. 2000;3(6):54–60.
74. Lipkins S. Preventing hazing: how parents, teachers, and coaches can stop the violence: Jossey-Bass; August 25th, 2006.
75. Banyard V, Plante E, Moynihan M. Bystander education: bringing a broader community perspective to sexual violence prevention. J Community Psychol. 2004;32(1):61–79.
76. Darley J, Latané B. Bystander intervention in emergencies: diffusion of responsibility. J Pers Soc Psychol. 1968;8(4):377–83.
77. Lew KM. Emergency action plans 2018 [Available from: https://www.nays.org/resources/more/emergency-action-plans/.
78. Medtronic. Emergency Action Planning Program - E-Learning Module 2015 [Available from: http://www.anyonecansavealife.org/e-learning-module/index.htm.
79. Christensen H, Batterham PJ, Mackinnon AJ, Anstey KJ, Wen W, Sachdev PS. Education, atrophy, and cognitive change in an epidemiological sample in early old age. Am J Geriatr Psychiatry. 2009;17(3):218–26.
80. States with Anti-Hazing Laws.
81. HazingPrevention.org. Hazing Law - Interactive State Map 2018 [Available from: https://hazingprevention.org/home/hazing/statelaws/.
82. Green L. School hazing investigations, reports yield prevention guidelines for schools 2017 [updated September 06, 2017. Available from: https://www.nfhs.org/articles/school-hazing-investigations-reports-yield-prevention-guidelines-for-schools/.
83. Associations NFoSHS. Sexual harassment and hazing: your actions make a difference!
84. Janssen I, Leblanc A. Systematic review of the health benefits of physical activity and fitness in school-aged children and youth. Int J Behav Nutr Phys Act. 2010;7:40.

Chapter 14
Impact of Social Media on Mental Health

Steven K. Poon and Laura E. Sudano

Introduction

Social media, or Social Networking Sites (SNS), hold a near ubiquitous place in the lives of athletes and play a role in forming their identity, mental health, and well-being. While there are certainly benefits of increased networking through online formats, there are potential harms of using social media as well. Athletes are not immune to the pitfalls of using social networking and may gain benefits of its use; however, limited research has examined the impact of social media on athletes' mental health.

Social media is defined as an internet-based service that allows individuals to create, maintain, and share a public or private profile among other users [1]. Social networks allow users to build large following, maintain casual acquaintances over long distances, and can help users stay connected to others during life cycle transitions such as college students moving from home to university settings [2]. This medium is constantly growing, evolving, and becoming more popular. Understanding the role of social networking sites in athletes begins with an understanding of differential usage among age-group peers. The Pew Research Center tracks social media use across demographics in a longitudinal manner, finding that social networking site use is widely distributed and influenced by age and gender [3]. In this study, 68% of participants reported using Facebook, with approximately 75% of active users accessing the site daily. YouTube, which allows users

S. K. Poon (✉)
Sports Medicine Section, Arizona State University Health Services, Arizona State University Athletics, Tempe, AZ, USA
e-mail: steven.poon@asu.edu

L. E. Sudano
Collaborative Care, Family Medicine and Public Health, University of California, San Diego, San Diego, CA, USA
e-mail: lesudano@ucsd.edu

© Springer Nature Switzerland AG 2020
E. Hong, A. L. Rao (eds.), *Mental Health in the Athlete*,
https://doi.org/10.1007/978-3-030-44754-0_14

to upload and share videos and for viewers to respond and leave comments, is used by 73% of respondents.

Patterns of use vastly by age and sex. For example, YouTube is utilized by 94% of 18 to 24-year-olds. This divergence is more drastic in other social media applications (apps) such as Snapchat, which is far more utilized by younger individuals and less commonly used in individuals over the age of 50. In the youngest adult demographic, 78% reported being active with only 7% of the 50-and-over age group endorsing its use. Pinterest, a social networking website used to share arts and crafts based designs, is used by 41% of women compared to 10% of men. The ubiquity of social media use in the younger age groups is represented by the frequency of use – 71% of young adults use Snapchat multiple times per day and 55% use Instagram multiple times per day. A majority (51%) of this age group also report that it would be hard to give up use of social media – another testament to the preeminence of these websites and apps in young adults [3].

In 2016, student-athletes from 1300 universities with varying divisional levels report participating in multiple SNS. These include Facebook (97%), Snapchat, (93%), Instagram (89%), and Twitter (84%). Over 65% of athletes report spending more than 1 hour per day on social media [4]. Social media, specifically SNS, are incorporated more than ever into the athlete's daily routine.

Link Between Social Media and Mental Health Overview

Studies have evaluated the negatives and potential dangers of social media. The increased visibility and availability of athletes combined with the widespread accessibility of social media platforms allows for access to individuals not previously possible. This access introduces the potential of cyberbullying and harassment, and the consequences of exposure to each outcome.

Cyberbullying and Harassment

Peer victimization through cyberbullying increases the risk of suicidal ideation and suicide attempts in children and adolescents [5]. The American Academy of Pediatrics lists cyberbullying, sexting, and depression as potential risks of using social media [6]. The National Collegiate Athletic Association (NCAA) Sport Science Institute's Mind, Body and Sport guide to understanding and supporting student-athlete mental wellness suggests that increased use of social media can increase the likelihood of cyberbullying by fans [7]. Specifically, athletes report receiving negative or threatening messages by fans. This increased interaction with fans can have positive effects on the athlete such as raising mental health awareness; however, social media can result in exacerbation of the sport-related pressure they experience.

Nearly 40% of the US population is estimated to experience online harassment, whether through anonymous websites or social media. The Pew Research Center's 2017 study on the subject provides a window into the prevalence and consequence of online harassment. Among the young adults ranging from 18- to 29-year-old, 67% report being the target of harassment and 41% report being the victim of severe behaviors, defined as physical threats, sustained harassment, stalking, and sexual harassment. Rates of online harassment relate inversely with age, as younger individuals are more likely to be targeted than older individuals [8].

While unwanted digital targeting can occur via text messaging, email, gaming, or other websites, 58% of adults experienced harassment through social media channels. Typically, victims do not know the identity or the source of their harassment, with 54% reporting the source as a stranger. Despite the anonymous origin of the targeting, the consequences are real and tangible. Forty-five percent of those who faced severe forms of harassment reported mental or emotional distress as a result [8].

Sexting involves the sending or receiving of sexually explicit images via digital communication, often through text messages or social media apps. The Pew Research Center study found that 31% of adults received explicit images without consent. In addition, 7% had images shared of themselves without permission. Viewed by age and gender, 53% of women 18-to 29-year-old reported receiving unwanted explicit photographs compared to 26% of women over 30 and 37% of similarly aged men. The frequency and severity of harassment leads directly to the mental and emotional distress of those affected and is too often common with the use of social media [8]. This is an area of concern for providers who take care of younger adult and adolescent populations. The American Academy of Pediatrics recommends that all clinicians broaden their understanding of digital technology, including social media, to provide better care and guidance for patients who face these digital media-associated physical and mental health issues [6].

Depression

Individuals who use social media more actively are noted to have higher rates of depression than those with limited to no use [9]. There is an increased likelihood of depression symptoms associated with more frequent and higher volume social media use across a variety of platforms. The highest quartile of users had between 1.66 and 3.05 times the odds of having depression when compared to the lowest quartile of users [9].

Social networking, while able to create a community of individuals spread across geographic, cultural, and interest differences, also appears to be detrimental to consumers. Studies have reported that use of Facebook, the largest and most widely used SNS, leads to a decline in self-reported life satisfaction [10]. Some studies have explored the negatives of social media including poor relationships, lack of privacy, and damaging social comparisons [11].

A phenomenon of social networking sites seems to be an increase in negative self-perception and other harmful behaviors. Studies show an increase in poor self-image associated with social media use. This trend is attributed to comparisons with others on these SNS [12]. One common area where this manifests is in fitness inspiration. While the presumptive aim of these social media accounts is to motivate others to engage in healthy, active, and exercise-centric lifestyles, users who are exposed to and view these accounts have worse moods, greater body dissatisfaction, and lower self-esteem [13].

Sleep Quality

Studies suggest that the use of social media degrades sleep quality. Poor sleep patterns are associated with depression, poor mental health outcomes, and risk-taking behavior in adolescents [14]. Furthermore, there is a link between poor sleep and the onset or worsening of current mental health diagnoses including depression, anxiety, and mood disorders [15–17]. SNS and apps may be accessed via desktop computer, laptop computer, tablet, or smartphone. Research demonstrates an association between the amount of screen time with reduced sleep duration, decreased quality, and increased sleep onset latency [18–20].

For student-athletes, particularly high school and collegiate level, lack of quality sleep can have particularly detrimental effects on academic and potentially athletic performance. Another potential harm of poor sleep is difficulty processing information outside of the classroom and in sports-focused areas such as learning playbooks and studying game film. As such, physicians should consider dedicating time to address the potential harms of reduced sleep quality due to using social media.

Sleep is essential for recovery, immune system health, injury prevention, and reduction of long-term muscle fatigue. In 2015 the International Olympic Committee (IOC) released a consensus statement recognizing sleep insufficiency as a risk factor for youth athletic development [21]. The American Academy of Sleep Medicine recommendations for sleep in teenagers is 8–10 hours per night but due to many factors, including social networking sites, many fall short of this goal [22]. For athletes, low-quality sleep and shortened duration can increase injury risk. In fact, those who sleep less than 8 hours per night have a relative injury risk 1.7 times that of athletes who slept more than 8 hours per night [23]. Other studies have demonstrated that decreased sleep negatively affects athletic performance measure such as endurance, power, and accuracy while also increasing risk of contracting viral illnesses [24, 25].

Interpersonal Engagement

Social media has also altered the nature of interpersonal relationships. One feature of social media is the ability to share text-based information. As the medium has grown image sharing has also increased. One study showed that users who frequently posted or updated their profile pictures or self-presented images exhibited high levels of narcissism [26].

For athletes, fan engagement is a very powerful use of social media. Some athletes have used SNS for personal brand marketing and direct conversation with [27]. This low barrier for communication also comes with risks such as open hostility or even threats. Multiple studies have sought to understand fan reactions on social media ranging positive (community, camaraderie, passion) to negative (venting, frustration) [28, 29]. Researchers use the concept of BIRG – or "basking in reflected glory" – for positive responses and a feeling of shared success. Meanwhile, negative behaviors are referred to as CORF – "cutting off reflected failure" – where fans seek to distance themselves from unsuccessful athletes or outcomes [29].

One study evaluated Twitter reaction after a college football team lost to its primary rival. Many fans attributed the loss to one individual and the evaluation of messages ranged from supportive to demeaning and, in the worst of cases, threatening [30]. Unfortunately, these instances are not unique. An interview-based study of Division 1 collegiate athletes found that responses to critical messages from fans varied. Some were able to use these messages as motivation while others noted these tweets would adversely affect themselves as well [31].

Benefits of Social Media

A promising utilization for social media is in medical awareness, information dissemination, and direct communication. Studies of SNS and disease-specific searches found that it was an effective tool to connect patients who had similar diagnoses. For example, a 2010 study of Facebook groups focused on diabetes patients found that members were able to ask questions, provide information, and support others but there was also risk of spreading advertisements and potentially fictitious accounts [32].

Exercise and physical activity is often effectively used as part of the treatment plan for mental health disorders [33]. Research suggests that users who engage in social networking sites specifically related to activities like running are more likely to engage and continue with the exercise [34]. Attrition and patient subject loss present difficulties of these studies. Personal engagement, group support, and feedback are strategies to help maintain compliance [35]. Social networking has diversified from online webpages to a variety of websites and personalized applications that have then been used as means for increasing physical activity. When research participants were able to track and compare their own activity ranked among peers, even anonymously, the rate of exercise class attendance increased and stayed higher relative to other promotional and outreach methods [36, 37].

Other newer social media modalities are personalized gaming apps. As the name suggests, gamification is the use of game-related tasks to achieve goals. In the healthcare field, studies have been used for exercise increase, mental health, chronic diseases, and many others. A systematic review found that these studies also noted the benefits in self-esteem, providing positive reinforcement and increasing social support [38]. A trial published in 2017 showed a higher goal attainment rate and compliance when gamification strategies are used within families to increase exercise [39].

Social Media Policies

College athletic departments are responsible for their student-athletes. This age group comprised mostly of 18- to 22-year-olds tends to be the most frequent social media users. A 2011 study found 46% of NCAA Division 1 athletic departments had publicly available social media policies contained within their student-athlete handbook [40]. A similar study in 2015 found 55% of NCAA Division 1 "Power 5" conference member schools had electronically accessible social media policies, while 33% of NCAA Division 2 and 21% of NCAA Division 3 schools did the same [41].

When discussing policies, student-athletes recognized the need and benefit of guidelines but also often express frustration because the policies can be too cumbersome, restrictive, punitive, ineffective, or even ambiguous [42]. The research also suggests that student-athletes, while generally understanding and in favor of these policies, often feel more engaged when they have ownership in co-development of social media guidelines at universities [41].

Conclusion

More research is needed to determine the extent to which social media, or SNS, impacts the mental health of athletes. Current research suggests that physicians and healthcare providers are in a position to advice athletes on the impact of social media on prevalence of cyberbullying and harassment, sleep quality, depression, and risk of injury. Clinicians should be familiar with digital trends in order to provide counseling and care for patients due to any physical and mental health issues stemming from social media. Given the ubiquity of social media and the accessibility the medium provides, providers should be acutely aware of the risk of cyberbullying and harassment with the potential ensuing psychological consequences.

Considerations for future research include incorporating variables such as the developmental age of the athlete, the frequency/intensity/duration of social media use, and specific level of the athlete. Furthermore, since social media is rapidly evolving and adoption rates among young populations continue to increase, frequent updates to research are needed to fully capture the effects of social networking as the medium continues to progress.

References

1. Boyd DM, Ellison NB. Social network sites: definition, history, and scholarship. J Comput Mediat Commun. 2007;13(1):210–30. https://doi.org/10.1111/j.1083-6101.2007.00393.x.
2. Steinfield C, Ellison NB, Lampe C. Social capital, self-esteem, and use of online social network sites: a longitudinal analysis. J Appl Dev Psychol. 2008;29(6):434–45.
3. Social media use in 2018. Pew Research Center, Washington, D.C. March 2018. http://www.pewinternet.org/2018/03/01/social-media-use-in-2018. Accessed 16 May 2018.
4. DeShazo K. 2016 Social media use of student athletes [infographic]. 2016. http://www.fieldhousemedia.net/2016-social-media-use-of-student-athletes-infographic/. Accessed 23 June 2018.
5. van Geel M, Vedder P, Tanilon J. Relationship between peer victimization, cyberbullying, and suicide in children and adolescents: a meta-analysis. JAMA Pediatr. 2014;168(5):435–42.
6. O'Keeffe GS, Clarke-Pearson K. Council on Communications and Media. The impact of social media on children, adolescents, and families. Pediatrics. 2011;127(4):800–4.
7. Bell L, Witford M. Social and environmental risk factors - interpersonal violence and the student-athlete population. In: Brown GT, Hainline B, Kroshus E, Wilfert M, editors. Mind, body, and sport, understanding and supporting student-athlete mental wellness. Indianapolis: NCAA Publications; 2014. p. 86–95.
8. Online harassment 2017. Pew Research Center, Washington, D.C. July 2017. http://www.pewinternet.org/2017/07/11/online-harassment-2017. Accessed 16 May 2018.
9. Lin LY, Sidani JE, Shensa A, Radovic A, Miller E, Colditz JB, et al. Association between social media use and depression among U.S. young adults. Depress Anxiety. 2016;33(4):323–31.
10. Kross E, Verduyn P, Demiralp E, Park J, Lee DS, Lin N, Shablack H, Jonides J, Ybarra O. Facebook use predicts declines in subjective well-being in young adults. PLoS One. 2013;8(8):e69841. https://doi.org/10.1371/journal.pone.0069841.
11. Fox J, Moreland JJ. The dark side of social networking sites: an exploration of the relational and psychological stressors associated with Facebook use and affordances. Comput Hum Behav. 2015;45:168–76. https://doi.org/10.1016/j.chb.2014.11.083.
12. de Vries DA, Kühne R. Facebook and self-perception: individual susceptibility to negative social comparison on Facebook. Personal Individ Differ. 2015;86:217–21. https://doi.org/10.1016/j.paid.2015.05.029.
13. Tiggemann M, Zaccardo M. "Exercise to be fit, not skinny": the effect of fitspiration imagery on women's body image. Body Image. 2015;15:61–7. https://doi.org/10.1016/j.bodyim.2015.06.003.
14. Shochat T, Cohen-Zion M, Tzischinsky O. Functional consequences of inadequate sleep in adolescents: a systematic review. Sleep Med Rev. 2014;18(1):75–87.
15. Pigeon WR, Bishop TM, Krueger KM. Insomnia as a precipitating factor in new onset mental illness: a systematic review of recent findings. Curr Psychiatry Rep. 2017;19(8):44. https://doi.org/10.1007/s11920-017-0802-x.
16. Kalmbach DA, Arnedt JT, Song PX, Guille C, Sen S. Sleep disturbance and short sleep as risk factors for depression and perceived medical errors in first-year residents. Sleep. 2017;40(3) https://doi.org/10.1093/sleep/zsw073.
17. Robillard R, Hermens DF, Lee RS, Jones A, Carpenter JS, White D, et al. Sleep-wake profiles predict longitudinal changes in manic symptoms and memory in young people with mood disorders. J Sleep Res. 2016;25(5):549–55.
18. Woods HC, Scott H. #Sleepyteens: social media use in adolescence is associated with poor sleep quality, anxiety, depression and low self-esteem. J Adolesc. 2016;51:41–9.
19. Levenson JC, Shensa A, Sidani JE, Colditz JB, Primack BA. The association between social media use and sleep disturbance among young adults. Prev Med. 2016;85:36–41.
20. Hale L, Guan S. Screen time and sleep among school-aged children and adolescents: a systematic literature review. Sleep Med Rev. 2015;21:50–8.

21. Bergeron MF, Mountjoy M, Armstrong N, Chia M, Cote J, Emery CA, et al. International olympic committee consensus statement on youth athletic development. Br J Sports Med. 2015;49(13):843–51.
22. Paruthi S, Brooks LJ, D'Ambrosio C, Hall WA, Kotagal S, Lloyd RM, et al. Consensus statement of the american academy of sleep medicine on the recommended amount of sleep for healthy children: methodology and discussion. J Clin Sleep Med. 2016;12(11):1549–61.
23. Milewski MD, Skaggs DL, Bishop GA, Pace JL, Ibrahim DA, et al. Chronic lack of sleep is associated with increased sports injuries in adolescent athletes. J Pediatr Orthop. 2014;34(2):129–33.
24. Watson AM. Sleep and athletic performance. Curr Sports Med Rep. 2017;16(6):413–8.
25. Cohen S, Doyle WJ, Alper CM, Janicki-Deverts D, Turner RB. Sleep habits and susceptibility to the common cold. Arch Intern Med. 2009;169(1):62–7.
26. Moon JH, Lee E, Lee J, Choi TR, Sung Y. The role of narcissism in self-promotion on Instagram. Personal Individ Differ. 2016;101:22–5. https://doi.org/10.1016/j.paid.2016.05.042.
27. Filo K, Lock D, Karg A. Sport and social media research: a review. Sport Manag Rev. 2015;18(2):166–81. https://doi.org/10.1016/j.smr.2014.11.001.
28. Stavros C, Meng MD, Westberg K, Farrelly F. Understanding fan motivation for interacting on social media. Sport Manag Rev. 2014;17(4):455–69. https://doi.org/10.1016/j.smr.2013.11.004.
29. Mudrick M, Miller M, Atkin D. The influence of social media on fan reactionary behaviors. Telematics Inf. 2016;33(4):896–903. https://doi.org/10.1016/j.tele.2016.01.005.
30. Sanderson J, Truax C. "I hate you man!": exploring maladaptive parasocial interaction expressions to college athletes via twitter. J Issues Intercollegiate Athl. 2014; 7:333–51.
31. Browning B, Sanderson J. The positives and negatives of twitter: exploring how student-athletes use twitter and respond to critical tweets. Int J Sport Commun. 2012;5(4):503–21. https://doi.org/10.1123/ijsc.5.4.503.
32. Greene JA, Choudhry NK, Kilabuk E, Shrank WH. Online social networking by patients with diabetes: a qualitative evaluation of communication with Facebook. J Gen Intern Med. 2011;26(3):287–92.
33. Strohle A. Sports psychiatry: mental health and mental disorders in athletes and exercise treatment of mental disorders. Eur Arch Psychiatry Clin Neurosci. 2018; https://doi.org/10.1007/s00406-018-0891-5.
34. Mahan JE III, Seo WJ, Jordan JS, Funk D. Exploring the impact of social networking sites on running involvement, running behavior, and social life satisfaction. Sport Manag Rev. 2015;18(2):182–92. https://doi.org/10.1016/j.smr.2014.02.006.
35. Williams G, Hamm MP, Shulhan J, Vandermeer B, Hartling L. Social media interventions for diet and exercise behaviours: a systematic review and meta-analysis of randomised controlled trials. BMJ Open. 2014;4(2):e003926,2013–003926. https://doi.org/10.1136/bmjopen-2013-003926.
36. Zhang J, Brackbill D, Yang S, Becker J, Herbert N, Centola D. Support or competition? How online social networks increase physical activity: a randomized controlled trial. Prev Med Rep. 2016;4:453–8. https://doi.org/10.1016/j.pmedr.2016.08.008.
37. Zhang J, Brackbill D, Yang S, Centola D. Efficacy and causal mechanism of an online social media intervention to increase physical activity: results of a randomized controlled trial. Prev Med Rep. 2015;2:651–7.
38. Sardi L, Idri A, Fernandez-Aleman JL. A systematic review of gamification in e-health. J Biomed Inform. 2017;71:31–48.
39. Patel MS, Benjamin EJ, Volpp KG, Fox CS, Small DS, Massaro JM, et al. Effect of a game-based intervention designed to enhance social incentives to increase physical activity among families: the BE FIT randomized clinical trial. JAMA Intern Med. 2017;177(11):1586–93.
40. Sanderson J. To tweet or not to tweet: exploring division I athletic departments' social-media policies. Int J Sport Commun. 2011;4(4):492–513. https://doi.org/10.1123/ijsc.4.4.492.

41. Sanderson J, Snyder E, Hull D, Gramlich K. Social media policies within NCAA member institutions: evolving technology and its impact on policy. J Issues Intercollegiate Athl. 2015;8:50–73.
42. Sanderson J, Browning B, Schmittel A. Education on the digital terrain: a case study exploring college athletes' perceptions of social-media training. Int J Sport Commun. 2015;8(1):103–24. https://doi.org/10.1123/ijsc.2014-0063.

Chapter 15
Mental Health in the Pediatric Athlete

Michele LaBotz

Since half of adult mental disorders start before 14 years of age [1], issues that affect the mental health of young athletes have both immediate and long-term consequences. Over half of high school students and one-third of school-age children participate in organized sport [2]. Therefore, any consideration of mental health in children and adolescents needs to be taken into account when they participate as an athlete. The World Health Organization (WHO) states that mental health is more than the absence of mental illness and defines mental health as follows:

> a state of well-being in which every individual realizes his or her own potential, can cope with the normal stresses of life, can work productively and fruitfully, and is able to make a contribution to her or his community [3].

Therefore, it is important to examine not only the effect of sport participation on mental illness but also sport-related impact on the development of optimal mental health and function. This chapter will review relationships between athletic participation and mental health in children and adolescents and will provide guidance on optimizing the sport experience for young athletes with common mental disorders and helping young athletes receive the maximal mental/emotional benefit from sport.

Determinants of the Mental Health Impact of Sport

There is a bidirectional relationship between sports and mental health in adolescents (i.e., sport involvement correlates with improved mental health and vice versa) [4]. However, "sport" is a multifaceted construct containing a variety of factors that exert unique influences on mental health, and generalizations may not be applicable

M. LaBotz (✉)
InterMed, Portland, ME, USA

Tufts University School of Medicine, Boston, MA, USA

© Springer Nature Switzerland AG 2020
E. Hong, A. L. Rao (eds.), *Mental Health in the Athlete*,
https://doi.org/10.1007/978-3-030-44754-0_15

to each individual athletes. Physical activity and sport/team culture are two dominant features of youth sport participation worthy of specific consideration.

Physical Activity

Many parents and caregivers equate sport participation with physical activity. However, sport involvement and physical activity exert independent benefits on mental health [5], and there is growing recognition that many young athletes are not meeting current WHO physical activity recommendations for 60 minutes of moderate to vigorous physical activity (MVPA) per day. A study examining 7–14-year-old athletes in San Diego found that only 24% of these athletes met these recommendations during sport practice [6]. Observations of high school sport practices found significant variability between sports, but overall, athletes were sedentary for about 40% of practice time [7]. Therefore, benefits that accrue with physical activity are not automatically applied to sport.

Mental health impact of time spent specifically in sport practice was explored in a web-based survey of 16–20-year-olds, which examined the dose-response curve between hours spent in sport practice and mental health [8]. Peak mental well-being was reported in athletes training 10.6–17.5 practice hours/week (mean ≈14 hours), and rates of poor well-being increased significantly for athletes with higher and lower volumes of training. This seems to indicate that 2 hours/day of sport involvement supports good mental health, but the authors were not able to quantitate the amount of physical activity during practice, and this web-based survey study lacks the rigor of longitudinal data.

Sport Culture

The Women's Sports Foundation (WSF) examined relationships between adolescent sport participation and health behaviors, academic achievement, and psychological health [9]. Sport participation generally correlated with improvements in these parameters, but there was significant variability between sports. Basketball players fared best on measures of mental well-being. Athletes participating in baseball/softball, soccer, football, tennis, and track and field fared better than their nonathlete peers; however, participants in ice hockey, wrestling and crew fared worse. Substance use patterns often correlate with mental health. A recent systematic review found that a large majority of studies showed positive correlation between sport participation and alcohol use in young adolescent athletes and negative correlation between sports and use of non-cannabis illicit drugs [10]. Use of alcohol, marijuana, and cigarettes were evaluated in the WSF analysis, and overall, there was no relationship between sport participation and use of these substances. However, there were significant differences when separated by sport. Track and field athletes reported lower than average rates of binge drinking and use of cigarettes and marijuana, but ice hockey and lacrosse players were more likely to report all three behaviors.

While this data represents large national surveys, sport culture is highly variable and difficult to assess objectively. Some of this is sport-specific (i.e., team sports are intrinsically different from individual sports). However, sport culture is also dependent upon variables that are often very dynamic. Coaching style, environmental influences, and participant personalities vary widely from one setting to another. Depending upon the team and the individual, the vagaries of sport culture may either enhance or hinder overall mental health in young athletes.

Self-Esteem and Sport

A recent meta-analysis found that physical activity in children and adolescent appears to primarily enhance self-efficacy and physical self-concept, which then generalizes to increased self-esteem [11]. However, a 2014 study illuminates the direct relationship between self-esteem and sport participation [12]. This Canadian study followed 1492 adolescents for 4 years and found that higher self-esteem predicted increases in both sport involvement and enjoyment, and increased sport enjoyment predicted enhancements in self-esteem. However, sport participation itself did not predict changes in self-esteem. This is a key point and indicates that the crux of the relationship between sport and mental well-being appears to be the enjoyment that children and adolescents derive from their sport experience, rather than from participation per se.

> **Key Point**
> Enjoyment is the most important factor mediating the relationship between sport participation and mental health in children and adolescents.

There is significant concern that early sport specialization and intensification excessively focuses young athletes (and the adults who work with them) on performance and achievement, with a subsequent decrease in perceived enjoyment and possible adverse impacts on mental health. This concern is supported by WSF findings of multisport athletes faring better than single sport athletes on multiple measures of mental well-being.

Anxiety

Anxiety appears to be the most prevalent mental health condition in adolescents in the United States with a lifetime prevalence of 38% for females and 26% for males [13]. Of these, 8% reported significant anxiety-related impairment. While multiple

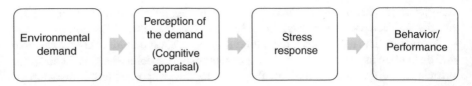

Fig. 15.1 Continuum of anxiety-stress response

studies show beneficial relationships between youth sport participation and anxiety, athletes are not immune. A study in elite adolescent athletes reports 7% with sub-clinical anxiety and 3% meeting clinical criteria for the disorder [14]. The impacts of anxiety on athletes include decreased performance, focus, and concentration, as well as increased risk of injury. A study in collegiate athletes reported a 2.3 relative risk of injury in those with anxiety as compared to their non-anxious peers [15].

One study looking at psychological symptoms in 7th–10th graders found a bidirectional relationship between anxiety and sport [16]. Lower rates of anxiety were reported at baseline among those participating in organized sports, and there was a greater reduction of anxiety symptoms in athletes when reassessed 1 year later. While, overall, these reductions in anxiety symptoms were small, they were greatest among those with highest numbers of baseline symptoms and were not influenced by sex, sport type, or frequency of participation.

Athletes are often less likely to admit to mental health concerns or to seek help for them, and awareness interventions in this population do not appear to show efficacy in changing behavior. When addressing anxiety-related issues in young athletes, providers should consider behavioral-based interventions that affect the anxiety-stress response continuum (Fig. 15.1).

Environmental Demands Anxiety-provoking environments are typically those that assess ability and performance, such as tryouts, showcases, and competitions.

Cognitive Appraisal Cognitive appraisal is the athlete's perception of these environmental demands. Multiple studies indicate that cognitive appraisal appears to mediate much of the benefit of sport participation on anxiety in young athletes, and influencing cognitive appraisal can allow athletes to embrace potentially stressful situations as "challenges" rather than as possible "threats" [17]. This reduces the subsequent stress response and anxiety level. Some determinants of cognitive appraisal in a given situation are intrinsic to the athlete and difficult to change, such as trait anxiety and self-esteem. Other determinants are potentially amenable to intervention and include physical and mental preparation and experience. Acute bouts of aerobic activity as well as overall improvements in cardiovascular fitness lead to less stressful cognitive appraisals. Mental preparation can be enhanced with imagery and "mental rehearsals" that are realistic and focus on self-efficacy and prior success.

Stress Response Some degree of performance-related anxiety is almost universal. Young athletes should understand that the physiologic stress response is normal and can actually enhance performance when appropriately utilized. There is an optimal amount of arousal for each athlete that is associated with performance enhancement [18], and the relationship between sport performance and the physiologic arousal of acute anxiety is best described as an "inverted U" (Fig. 15.2). Suboptimal performance results when physiologic arousal is either too little or too much, and therefore, the focus should be on control of stress and anxiety, rather than elimination. There are multiple techniques for control of performance anxiety, and their effectiveness will vary between individuals. Practice and "trial and error" are needed to help determine which method will work best for a given athlete. Some athletes will do best with techniques directed at reducing the somatic responses to stress while others may prefer those that address the mental component (Table 15.1). Preadolescent athletes may do better with distraction techniques rather than those that focus on positive anticipation [19].

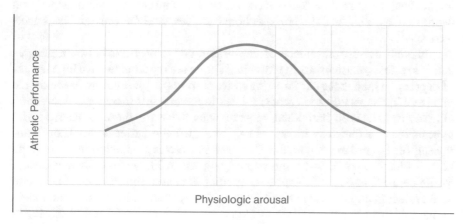

Fig. 15.2 Qualitative representation of athletic performance as a function of physiologic arousal

Table 15.1 Techniques for addressing performance anxiety in young athletes

Somatic/physiologic	Mental/psychological
Progressive muscle relaxation	Mindfulness exercises
Breath control	Pre-performance checklists
Meditation	Visualization/mental practice
Caffeine avoidance	Mental escape/imagery (e.g., music)
Acupuncture/massage	Sensory engagement (e.g., aromatherapy)
Heart rate control (biofeedback via portable monitors)	

Depression

The National Comorbidity Survey-Adolescent Supplement (NCS-A) used parental surveys and adolescent interviews to determine lifetime prevalence of a variety of mental disorders in subjects 13–18 years old in the United States [13]. Of this population, 11.7% met DSM-IV criteria for major depression or dysthymia, and of these, three-fourths reported severe impairment. Parental reports indicate that about 2% of 6–11-year-olds are affected by depression [20].

There is a common perception that sport protects young people from becoming depressed. Although a large Canadian study found that sport participation did not appear to affect depression rates in adolescents [21], at 1-year follow-up, athletes had greater improvements in depression scores as compared to nonathletes, and those who were most depressed gained the most benefit from sport participation. A 2017 meta-analysis analyzed the relationship between depression and physical activity with data from over 89,000 subjects between 8 and 19 years old [22]. More rigorous, longitudinal study methodologies reported weaker impacts of physical activity on depression as compared to cross-sectional studies, and in general, the effects were small.

Although overall prevalence of depression does not differ between athletes and nonathletes, participants in individual sports are reported to have higher rates of depression than those participating in team sports. A German study looking at this issue in almost 200 adolescent athletes found that this increase in depression (11.6% in athletes in individual sports versus 9.5% for those in team sports) appears to be mediated by increased negative attribution after failure (i.e., blaming self for failure) as compared to that seen in athletes competing in team sports [23]. Athletes exposed to hazing or bullying are at higher risk for depression. While depression does not appear to predict increased injury risk [15], several studies document increased rates of depressive symptoms for up to 3 months in young athletes after injury [24]. Athletes with high athletic identity appear to have greater difficulty with post-injury depression, while appropriate social support was protective.

A typical adolescent depressive episode lasts about 9 months, and for the young, depressed athlete, sport participation may either be part of the problem or part of the solution. Many of the same strategies for treatment of depression in mature athletes (see Chap. XX) apply to young athletes as well. Cognitive-behavioral therapy is often the first line of treatment. More severe cases may benefit from medication, although these should be used with caution in the pediatric population due to potential elevation of suicidality. Parents of depressed children should closely monitor their child's response to sport training and competition, and input from teachers or administrators who know the child well may be beneficial.

Overtraining and Burnout

Young athletes who present with symptoms suggesting anxiety or depression should be assessed for possible overtraining or burnout.

Overtraining Syndrome (OTS) Overreaching (OR) and OTS occur when high-intensity training results in the accumulation of physiologic and psychological stress and decrements in athletic performance. Several studies have looked at the prevalence of these issues in young athletes, particularly in swimmers, and it generally appears that about one-third of age-group and junior national athletes have experienced symptoms of OR or OTS at some point in their athletic careers [25]. OTS is the most severe manifestation of this spectrum, and up to 80% of athletes with OTS demonstrate signs of clinical depression [25]. Many athletes initially try to "push through" these symptoms and may experience a downward spiral of decreasing performance and increasing frustration before presenting for medical evaluation. Assessment and treatment of OR and OTS is described elsewhere [25], but full recovery often requires prolonged periods of time away from sport, and the diagnosis is often made in retrospect.

Burnout Athlete burnout occurs when the physiologic and psychological stress of sport participation results in a combination of physical/emotional exhaustion, reduced sense of personal accomplishment, and sport devaluation. Psychological factors (Table 15.2) may play a larger role in burnout in young athletes than in adults, and perfectionism seems to be a significant risk factor [26]. Potential organic underpinnings to presenting symptoms should be appropriately assessed before making a diagnosis of burnout. Treatment often requires time away from sport, correction of any sleep disturbance, and addressing non-sport stressors that create an undue burden for the young athlete. Adequate physical and mental recovery during training is key to burnout prevention (Table 15.3), and supportive coaching appears to be important as well.

Table 15.2 Risk factors for the development of sport-related burnout

Extrinsic	Intrinsic
High training volume/time demands	Perfectionism
Frequent and/or intense competition	Low self-esteem
High performance expectations	Unidimensional self-concept
Authoritarian coaching without significant athlete control in decision-making	Lack of assertiveness
Performance evaluations that are critical rather than supportive	Anxiety-producing cognitive appraisals

Table 15.3 Optimizing recovery in young athletes

Time away from organized sport[a]
1–2 days/week
8–12 weeks/year
(in increments of at least 4 weeks)
Appropriate nutrition
Adequate calories to support training and growth
Carbohydrates to fuel workouts and protect muscle
Protein to build muscle and restore tissue damage
Periodized and varied training
Recovery after hard training sessions
Attention to sport-related limits (e.g., pitch counts)
Address non-sport-related stressors
Family, social, academic
Adequate sleep
6–12 years old: 9–12 hours/night
13–18 years old: 8–10 hours/night

[a]Exploration of recreation and physical activity opportunities outside of organized sport should be encouraged and prevents fitness loss.

Attention Deficit Hyperactivity Disorder (ADHD)

ADHD is marked by inattention, hyperactivity, and/or impulsivity that is developmentally inappropriate for age; 8.5% of parents reported on the National Health Interview Survey having a child who received an ADHD diagnosis [20]. Physical activity and sport participation are widely touted as improving problem behaviors and enhancing academic achievement in children with ADHD [27]. The greatest benefit has been shown for mixed exercise programs that include MVPA, outdoor activity, and activity on at least 5 days/week [28, 29].

However, ADHD can present challenges for children participating in sport, and athletes with this disorder often suffer from adverse performance and interpersonal experiences in sport [30]. The majority of children with ADHD appear to demonstrate some degree of motor skill deficit, and between 30% and 50% meet criteria for developmental coordination disorder (DCD) [31]. Motor issues are often more pronounced in boys than in girls, and while mild motor impairments will often normalize with medication use, more severe impairments will tend to persist in spite of treatment [32]. Those who meet criteria for DCD may benefit from task-oriented physical therapy to improve motor skills [33].

Activity choice may be a key component to successful participation by children with ADHD. Structured sports activities appear to confer greater benefit both in terms of skill development and behavioral modification as compared to more loosely organized settings [34]. Activities that require greater degrees of attention (e.g., outfield in baseball, soccer or hockey goalie) may be particularly challenging for children with ADHD. However, some athletic endeavors may benefit from the unpredictability and impulsivity that may be seen in athletes with ADHD (e.g., wrestling or basketball point guard). In these cases, some athletes may decide to forego medication "coverage" during practice and/or game (see Chapter XX for further discussion on medication use). Some families are hesitant to share an ADHD diagnosis with sport coaches, but athletes often benefit from open communication with coaching staff.

Conduct and Oppositional Defiant Disorder

Children and adolescents with conduct disorder (CD) and oppositional defiant disorder (ODD) demonstrate a pattern of ignoring rules and social norms and demonstrating little regard for the basic rights of others. A national parent survey study reported a history consistent with CD or ODD in almost 6.2% of boys and 3.0% of girls between 3 and 17 years old [20]. However, the NCS-A interview study found much higher prevalence numbers in 13–18 years old with 12.6% meeting criteria for ODD and 6.8% for CD [13].

Sport participation, or other highly structured activity, decreases CD-related antisocial behaviors during adolescence [35]. However, sport participation may create several challenges for children with ODD or CD. Several studies have suggested that children with CD or ODD tend to have delays in motor development, which may be problematic for sports that require high degrees of motor skill or coordination [32]. Although there is some concern that participation in contact or power sports (e.g., football, wrestling) may increase risk of antisocial behaviors, a recent meta-analysis suggests that it is the sporting context and culture, rather than sport per se, that determines the impact of participation on socialization and behavior [35]. Prosocial behavior is promoted in athletic programs with characteristics outlined in Table 15.4.

CD and ODD are widely regarded as precursors to adult antisocial behavior, but sport participation may mitigate that progression. A 2015 prospective longitudinal study examined the effects of extracurricular activities in high school on

Table 15.4 Program characteristics that promote prosocial behaviors in children with conduct and oppositional defiant disorders	
	Training and competition
	Highly structured
	Expectations and consequences
	Consistent, predictable
	Positive reinforcement
	Timely, concrete, specific
	Opportunities to practice social skills
	Develop positive relationships with peers and adults
	Understand that home life is often chaotic
	High rates of parental substance abuse and antisocial behavior

the association between CD and adult antisocial behavior [36]. High school sport participation slightly decreased the association between adolescent CD and adult antisocial behavior ($\beta = 0.24$) as compared to those who participated in non-sport activity ($\beta = 0.42$) or those who did not participate in any extracurricular activity ($\beta = 0.50$).

Resources for Parents and Coaches

Unfortunately, youth and high school coaches are often relatively untrained in best practices for coaching athletes with mental illness and creating programs that foster optimal mental health. Parents and caregivers may need to advocate for additional training. The following resources may help coaches develop a supportive and positive sport environment:

- The Positive Coaching Alliance: https://positivecoach.org/coaches/
- National Federation of State High School Associations (NFHS): https://ww2.nfhslearn.com/home/coaches
- United States Olympic Committee's free "How to Coach Kids" mobile application and website: https://howtocoachkids.org

Parents can find guidance through the NFHS (https://ww2.nfhslearn.com/home/parents) as well as the Healthy Sport Index (http://healthysportindex.com).

References

1. World Health Organization. Adolescent mental health (fact sheet). 2018. http://www.who.int/news-room/fact-sheets/detail/adolescent-mental-health. Accessed 1 Nov 2018.
2. Centers for Disease Control and Prevention. Youth risk behavior survey data. 2017. Available at: http://www.cdc.gov/yrbs. Accessed 1 Nov 2018.
3. World Health Organization. Mental health: a state of well-being (fact sheet). 2014. http://www.who.int/features/factfiles/mental_health/en/. Accessed 1 Nov 2018.
4. Vella SA, Swann C, Allen MS, et al. Bidirectional associations between sport involvement and mental health in adolescence. Med Sci Sports Exerc. 2017;49:687–94. https://doi.org/10.1249/MSS.0000000000001142.
5. Tajik E, Abd Latiff L, Adznam SN, Awang H, Yit Siew C, Abu Bakar AS. A study on level of physical activity, depression, anxiety and stress symptoms among adolescents. J Sports Med Phys Fitness. 2017;57:1382–7. https://doi.org/10.23736/S0022-4707.16.06658-5.
6. Leek D, Carlson JA, Cain KL, et al. Physical activity during youth sports practices. Arch Pediatr Adolesc Med. 2011;165(4):294–9. https://doi.org/10.1001/archpediatrics.2010.252.
7. Kanters M, Edwards M, Casper J, McKenzie T, Bocarro J, Carlton T, Suau L. Physical activity report. Healthy Sport Index. http://healthysportindex.com/report/physical-activity/. Accessed 1 Nov 2018.
8. Merglen A, Flatz A, Belanger RE, Michaud PA, Suris JC. Weekly sport practice and adolescent well-being. Arch Dis Child. 2014;99(3):208–10. https://doi.org/10.1136/archdischild-2013-303729.

9. Zarrett N, Veliz P, Sabo D. Teen sport in America: why participation matters. East Meadow: Women's Sports Foundation; 2018. https://www.womenssportsfoundation.org/research/article-and-report/recent-research/teen-sport-in-america/. Accessed 1 Nov 2018.

10. Kwan M, Bobko S, Faulkner G, Donnelly P, Cairney J. Sport participation and alcohol and illicit drug use in adolescents and young adults: a systematic review of longitudinal studies. Addict Behav. 2014;39:497–506. https://doi.org/10.1016/j.addbeh.2013.11.006.

11. Lubans D, Richards J, Hillman C, Faulkner G, Beauchamp M, Nilsson M, Kelly P, Smith J, Raine L, Biddle S. Physical activity for cognitive and mental health in youth: a systematic review of mechanisms. Pediatrics. 2016;138:e20161642. https://doi.org/10.1542/peds.2016-1642.

12. Adachi PJC, Willoughby TJ. It's not how much you play, but how much you enjoy the game: the longitudinal associations between adolescents' self-esteem and the frequency versus enjoyment of involvement in sports. J Youth Adolesc. 2014;43:137–45. https://doi.org/10.1007/s10964-013-9988-3.

13. Merikangas KR, He JP, Burstein M, Swanson SA, Avenevoli S, Cui L, Benjet C, Georgiades K, Swendsen J. Lifetime prevalence of mental disorders in U.S. adolescents: results from the National Comorbidity Survey Replication – Adolescent Supplement (NCS-A). J Am Acad Child Adolesc Psychiatry. 2010 Oct;49(10):980–9. https://doi.org/10.1016/j.jaac.2010.05.017.

14. Weber S, Puta C, Lesinski M, Bagriel B, Steidten T, Bar KJ, Herbsleb M, Granacher U, Gabriel HW. Symptoms of anxiety and depression in young athletes using the Hospital Anxiety and Depression Scale. Front Physiol. 2018;9:182. https://doi.org/10.3389/fphys.2018.00182.

15. Li H, Moreland JJ, Peek-Asa C, Yang J. Preseason anxiety and depressive symptoms and prospective injury risk in collegiate athletes. Am J Sports Med. 2017;45:2148–55. https://doi.org/10.1177/0363546517702847.

16. Azevedo Da Silva M, Singh-Manoux A, Brunner EJ, Kaffashian S, Shipley MJ, Kivimäki M, Nabi H. Bidirectional association between physical activity and symptoms of anxiety and depression: the Whitehall II study. Eur J Epidemiol. 2012;27:537–46. https://doi.org/10.1007/s10654-012-9692-8.

17. Williams SE, Carroll D, Veldhuijzen van Zanten JJ, Ginty AT. Anxiety symptom interpretation: a potential mechanism explaining the cardiorespiratory fitness-anxiety relationship. J Affect Disord. 2016;193:151–6. https://doi.org/10.1016/j.jad.2015.12.051.

18. Gould D, Krane V. The arousal–athletic performance relationship: current status and future directions. In: Horn TS, editor. Advances in sport psychology. Champaign: Human Kinetics Publishers; 1992. p. 119–42.

19. Vassilopoulos SP, Brouzos A, Tsorbatzoudis H, Tziouma O. Is positive thinking in anticipation of a performance situation better than distraction? An experimental study in preadolescents. Scand J Psychol. 2017;58:142–9. https://doi.org/10.1111/sjop.12355.

20. Centers for Disease Control and Prevention. Mental Health Surveillance Among Children — United States, 2005–2011. MMWR. 2013;62:1–35.

21. Brière FN, Yale-Soulière G, Gonzalez-Sicilia D, Harbec MJ, Morizot J, Janosz M, Pagani LS. Prospective associations between sport participation and psychological adjustment in adolescents. J Epidemiol Community Health. 2018;72:575–81. https://doi.org/10.1136/jech-2017-209656.

22. Korczak DJ, Madigan S, Colasanto M. Children's physical activity and depression: a meta-analysis. Pediatrics. 2017;139:e20162266. https://doi.org/10.1542/peds.2016-2266.

23. Nixdorf I, Frank R, Beckmann J. Comparison of athletes' proneness to depressive symptoms in individual and team sports: research on psychological mediators in junior elite athletes. Front Psychol. 2016;7:893. https://doi.org/10.3389/fpsyg.2016.00893.

24. Sabato TM, Walch TJ, Caine DJ. The elite young athlete: strategies to ensure physical and emotional health. Open Access J Sports Med. 2016;7:99–113. https://doi.org/10.2147/OAJSM.S96821.

25. Meeusen R, Duclos M, Foster C, Fry A, Gleeson M, Nieman D, Raglin J, Rietjens G, Steinacher J, Urhausen A, European College of Sport Science, American College of Sports Medicine.

Prevention, diagnosis, and treatment of the overtraining syndrome: Joint consensus statement of the European College of Sport Science and the American College of Sports Medicine. Med Sci Sports Exerc. 2013;45:186–205. https://doi.org/10.1249/MSS.0b013e318279a10a.

26. DiFiori JP, Benjamin HJ, Brenner J, Gregory A, Jayanthi N, Landry GL, Luke A. Overuse injuries and burnout in youth sports: a position statement from the American Medical Society for Sports Medicine. Clin J Sport Med. 2014;24:3–20. https://doi.org/10.1097/JSM.0000000000000060.

27. Putukian M, Kreher JB, Coppel DB, Glazer JL, McKeag DB, White RD. Attention deficit hyperactivity disorder and the athlete: an American Medical Society for Sports Medicine position statement. Clin J Sport Med. 2011;21:392–401. https://doi.org/10.1097/JSM.0b013e3182262eb1.

28. Ng QX, Ho CYX, Chan HW, Bong BZJ, Yeo WS. Managing childhood and adolescent attention deficit/hyperactivity disorder (ADHD) with exercise: a systematic review. Complement Ther Med. 2017;34:123–8. https://doi.org/10.1016/j.ctim.2017.08.018.

29. Nazeer A, Mansour M, Gross KA. ADHD and adolescent athletes. Front Public Health. 2014;2:46. https://doi.org/10.3389/fpubh.2014.00046.

30. Lee H, Dunn JC, Holt NL. Youth sport experiences of individuals with attention deficit/hyperactivity disorder. Adapt Phys Activ Q. 2014;31:343–61. https://doi.org/10.1123/apaq.2014-0142.

31. Kaiser ML, Schoemaker MM, Albaret JM, Geuze RH. What is the evidence of impaired motor skills and motor control among children with attention deficit hyperactivity disorder (ADHD)? Systematic review of the literature. Res Dev Disabil. 2015;36C:338–57. https://doi.org/10.1016/j.ridd.2014.09.023.

32. Damme TV, Simons J, Sabbe B, van West D. Motor abilities of children and adolescents with a psychiatric condition: a systematic literature review. World J Psychiatry. 2015;5:315–29. https://doi.org/10.5498/wjp.v5.i3.315.

33. Preston N, Magallón S, Hill LJ, Andrews E, Ahern SM, Mon-Williams M. A systematic review of high quality randomized controlled trials investigating motor skill programmes for children with developmental coordination disorder. Clin Rehabil. 2017;31(7):857–70. https://doi.org/10.1177/0269215516661014.

34. Altszuler AR, Morrow AS, Merrill BM, Bressler S, Macphee FL, Gnagy EM, Greiner AR, Coxe S, Raiker JS, Coles E, Pelham WE Jr. The effects of stimulant medication and training on sports competence among children with ADHD. J Clin Child Adolesc Psychol. 2017;19:1–13. https://doi.org/10.1080/15374416.2016.1270829.

35. Spruit A, van Vugt E, van der Put C, van der Stouwe T, Stams GJ. Sports participation and juvenile delinquency: a meta-analytic review. J Youth Adolesc. 2016;45:655–71. https://doi.org/10.1007/s10964-015-0389-7.

36. Samek DR, Elkins IJ, Keyes MA, Iacono WG, McGue M. High school sports involvement diminishes the association between childhood conduct disorder and adult antisocial behavior. J Adolesc Health. 2015;57(1):107–12. https://doi.org/10.1016/j.jadohealth.2015.03.009.

Chapter 16
Pathological Exercise

Jessica Knapp and Ashwin L. Rao

Introduction

Sport participation has gradually increased over time and has been greatly affected by health policy changes such as the landmark Title IX, which has permitted the participation of more female athletes. Sport participation, compared with physical activity alone, has numerous socioeconomic, educational, and health benefits, with few risks. For those athletes with mental health or self-esteem concerns, disordered eating and pathological exercise are potentially negative outcomes which must be considered, particularly in sports with aesthetic considerations. These benefits and risks may be related to various sport-related drives for a specific body type such as drive for thinness, muscularity, and leanness. Identifying factors that enhance the beneficial aspects of sport participation and limit the risks is important for improving the overall health and well-being of athletes.

Many sports suggest an ideal body image to which athletes may ascribe improved performance [1–3]. The desire for certain body images has been described as a drive for thinness, a drive for muscularity, and a drive for leanness [4–7]. In particular, the drive for thinness is strongly linked to disordered eating in both the general population and athlete population [8]. The drive for muscularity describes a desire to have a muscular physique and has been linked to disordered eating in nonathlete males, but not in nonathlete females [8]. In bodybuilders, drive for muscularity may be

J. Knapp (✉)
Sports Medicine MAHEC Family Medicine, Asheville, NC, USA
e-mail: Jessica.knapp@mahec.net

A. L. Rao
Department of Family Medicine and Section of Sports Medicine, University of Washington, Seattle, WA, USA

UW Husky Athletics and Seattle Seahawks, Seattle, WA, USA
e-mail: ashwin@uw.edu

© Springer Nature Switzerland AG 2020
E. Hong, A. L. Rao (eds.), *Mental Health in the Athlete*,
https://doi.org/10.1007/978-3-030-44754-0_16

linked to disordered eating but is potentially mediated by body dysmorphia [9]. The drive for leanness is the desire to have a thin but muscular build [7]. There have been limited studies on drive for muscularity and drive for leanness in the female athlete population. Body image drives are likely to have a strong influence in supporting both disordered eating and exercise. Pathological exercise represents the pursuit of physical training, resulting in excessive exercise that has harmful consequences.

Prevalence

Studies regarding pathological exercise are limited in number and quality, and hence, diagnostic criteria are not well defined or validated to date. Observational studies identify exercise addiction rates of 0.3–0.5% in the general population, while rates are higher for athletes and regular exercises, ranging from 2% to 23% [10–13]. Sport-specific prevalence appears to vary widely, based on factors that include gender, age, sport-specific weight requirements, personality type, and ethnicity. Adolescence appears to be a period of great risk for the development of addictive behaviors, and exercise addiction is no exception [14]. Those involved in endurance sports (i.e., track and cross-country, crew) and sports with defined weight expectations (wrestling) are more likely to demonstrate disordered exercise behaviors targeting weight reduction due to the pressures imposed by their sport. In many instances, disordered exercise behaviors accompany disordered eating behaviors. One study has shown that nearly 21% of individuals with disordered eating also exhibited pathological exercise patterns [15]. Thus, these eating and exercise behaviors should be considered together when engaging the at-risk athlete.

Exploring Increased Rates of Exercise Addiction in Athletes

The increased rate of pathological exercise behaviors in athletes has several potential explanations. There is an overlap in traits that foster high performance and traits associated with eating disorders: perfectionism, increased exercise levels, and desire to please others. This may represent an inherent psychological reason for the increased rates of disordered exercise and eating. Another explanation is that the athlete perceives improved performance from a certain body type and attempts to achieve this "ideal," which consequently can lead to restrictive eating behaviors or increased exercise.

The athlete driven by desire to improve performance may go to extreme measures as suggested by "Goldman's dilemma." Goldman's dilemma was a question posed in the 1980s to Olympic athletes of whom the majority responded that they would take an unknown substance if it would guarantee a gold medal but results in early death [16]. When repeated in the general population, the question was posed, and the ultimate goal was "achieves the highest level in one's field," and the majority responded that they would not accept such a substance [17]. This high-lights the difference between the elite athlete and the nonathlete regarding a drive to succeed by any means available.

Performance thinness and appearance thinness have both been theorized to explain the drive for thinness in female athletes [18, 19]. Performance thinness is the idea that performance is enhanced with lower body fat and lower body weight, as in a distance runner. The desire to improve performance could be the impetus for muscularity and leanness as well, in that a muscular build or lean build may improve performance as a weight lifter or tennis player [3]. Appearance thinness, on the other hand, is the idea that in aesthetic sports there is a desire to be thin if it is per-ceived to help one's score, as in figure skating and gymnastics. Appearance thinness is not a factor in most sports, but does suggest the influence of societal standards of beauty [18]. It has been suggested that a dichotomy develops in athletes between the feminine and masculine self or sport self [2, 3, 20]. This tension is often com-pounded by the cultural standards of beauty and femininity contrasting with the masculine features of sports, competition, and muscularity that develop with train-ing. Perhaps if this tension increased and the athlete's self-esteem suffered, then there might be an increase in behaviors that lead to disordered eating and exercise. Additionally, if the athlete used extreme methods to attain the ideal body image as suggested by Goldman's dilemma, then this could lead to an increase in disordered eating rates or increased exercise rates.

Pathological Exercise

Pathological exercise is an umbrella term for two concepts of exercise addiction or dependence and exercise compulsive behaviors. Primary pathological exercise is described as addictive in notion, while secondary pathological exercise is more likely compulsive [21]. Compulsive exercise occurs to the exclusion of other activi-ties and for which the person is aware of potential negative consequences. Exercise addiction or dependence is conceptualized in the same vein as other addictions with the tolerance and withdrawal. Pathological exercise is often secondary to or a symp-tom of disordered eating and when it is compulsive in nature. Neither concept is present in the Diagnostic and Statistical Manual of Mental Disorders-V (DSM-V). Exercise addiction or dependence is difficult to manage because unlike substance addiction, exercise is viewed as a positive behavior in Western culture and not rec-ognized as something that requires intervention unless it happens to be paired with disordered eating [22]. Pathological exercise could also be viewed as a tool to achieve performance goals and ideal body image for their sport.

Exercisers with orthorexia, perfectionism, disordered eating, and high athletic identity are at risk for compulsive aspects of pathological exercise [23–25]. Athletes of both genders have higher rates of compulsive exercise as well, when compared to the general nonathletic population [26]. Studies suggest that compulsive exercise may be a symptom of disordered eating and possibly a purging behavior [27].

Additionally, individuals with disordered eating behaviors may exercise excessively in an attempt to manage depression and anxiety symptoms [28]. As with those athletes with disordered eating, athletes who compulsively exercise have an increased risk for bone stress injury and other similar negative health outcomes [29].

When examining the addiction aspect of pathological exercise, there is an association with disordered eating, orthorexia, use of performance-enhancing drugs, low self-esteem, anxiety, perfectionism, high achievement, increased rate of injury, and decreased health-related quality of life [24, 30–34]. Higher rates of exercise addiction or dependence are seen in males, young adult exercisers, adults doing vigorous physical activity, and athletes with disordered eating behavior [35, 36]. Surprisingly, exercise volume was not found to associate with exercise addiction in a study of collegiate athletes [37].

The impact of gender on the prevalence of pathological exercise remains difficult to ascertain. A study by Cunningham et al. found that men and women are at equal risk for pathological exercise. Men were more likely to have primary and addictive pathological exercise, while women were more likely to have secondary and compulsive pathological exercise. This is potentially due to the higher rates of disordered eating in females and the link between compulsive exercise and disordered eating [21].

Screening for Disordered Eating, Eating Disorders, and Pathological Exercise

Determining pathological exercise behaviors in athletes is challenged by the increased exercise requirements in this population, whose exercise volume is expected to be higher than that of the general population. Further, there is paucity validated tools to screen athletes for exercise disorders. Hence, screening protocols for pathological exercise require additional care in interpretation. Depending on the sport, high volumes of exercise may not be considered pathological, and the athlete may interpret survey questions differently from a nonathlete.

The Compulsive Exercise Test (CET) is a reliable and validated test in collegiate and adolescent exercisers, adults and adolescents with eating disorder, and across cultures [38–43]. A version of the CET was developed for detecting eating disorders in female athletes, the Compulsive Exercise Test in Athletes (CET-A) [44]. There are five factors in the test: rule-driven behavior, weight control, mood improvement, lack of exercise enjoyment, and exercise rigidity. This female-athlete-specific tool is an interesting use of an exercise test to screen for disordered eating as well. Another tool is the Exercise Dependence Scale (EDS), validated and reliable across cultures [45–47]. This scale focuses on the criteria of dependence and addiction with the following factors of withdrawal, continuance, tolerance, lack of control, reduction, time, and intention. The Exercise Addiction Inventory (EAI) is a reliable and valid tool to screen athletes, offering an option to screen young athletes through the Exercise Addiction Inventory-Youth (EAI-Y) [21, 48–50]. It was developed to be a shorter screening tool for ease of administration in the office and remains a popular tool for screening athletes.

A number of additional screening tools have been used to attempt to evaluate for pathological exercise. The Godin Leisure-Time Exercise Questionnaire, the Exercise Dependence Scale-21, the Exercise Addiction Inventory, the Compulsive Exercise Test, the Obligatory Exercise Questionnaire, the Commitment to Exercise Scale, and an exercise-specific adaptation of the Dimensional Obsessive-Compulsive Scale were recently found to provide similar results in ascertaining addictive versus compulsive exercise behaviors [21].

How to Manage Athlete

When disordered eating is present, the provider should consider screening for pathological exercise, and conversely if pathological exercise is suspected or present, screening for disordered eating should be considered. In the case of pathological exercise in the presence or absence of disordered eating, the provider should explore other mental health concerns such as anxiety or depression. A recent study of disordered eating in patients indicated that those with concomitant pathological exercise improved by reducing exercise volume [51]. Further, these patients had an improvement in compulsiveness scores when they developed other non-exercise coping strategies for depression and anxiety symptoms. This is important to consider when treating athletes with disordered eating. Current eating disorder guidelines for the general population suggest exercise restriction during treatment with gradual reintroduction of healthy exercise habits [52].

Management of the athlete with pathological exercise is best done as an interdisciplinary team. This team should include primary care team physician, certified athletic trainers, psychologists, coaching staff, and a nutritionist [53]. The primary care team physician should be the team lead to coordinate care and management return to play decisions. While screening methods are not currently universally applied, the primary care physician should consider screening tests for pathological exercise and eating behaviors for all incoming and returning athletes. There is not currently an established return to play guideline for pathological exercise, but one could consider the return to play guidelines used for the management of athletes with female athlete triad or relative energy [54, 55].

Conclusion

The aesthetic or athletic drive to a certain body image or body type may lead to increased rates of pathological exercise in the athletic population. In turn, pathological exercise may contribute to increased rates of disordered eating among athletes, though such associations need to be clarified. While current practices of most institutions do not include routine screening for disordered eating or pathological exercise patterns, screening tools are available and should be considered for all new or returning athletes. While there are no established guidelines for the management of pathological exercise in athletes, the provider should consider treatment schemes employed for female athlete triad or relative energy deficiency, given the strong links between disordered eating and exercise addiction.

References

1. Martinsen M, Bratland-Sanda S, Eriksson AK, Sundgot-Borgen J. Dieting to win or to be thin? A study of dieting and disordered eating among adolescent elite athletes and non-athlete controls. Br J Sports Med. 2010;44(1):70–6.
2. Krane V, Choi P, Baird S, Aimar C, Kauer K. Living the paradox: female athletes negotiate femininity and muscularity. Sex Roles. 2004;50(5/6):315–29.
3. Steinfeldt J, Carter H, Benton E, Stienfeldt M. Muscularity beliefs of female college student-athletes. Sex Roles. 2011;64:543–54.
4. Garner DM, Olmsted MP, Bohr Y, Garfinkel PE. The eating attitudes test: psychometric features and clinical correlates. Psychol Med. 1982;12(4):871–8.
5. McCreary DR, Sasse DK. An exploration of the drive for muscularity in adolescent boys and girls. J Am Coll Heal. 2000;48(6):297–304.
6. McCreary DR, Sasse DK, Saucier DM, Dorsch KD. Measuring the drive for muscularity: factorial validity of the drive for muscularity scale in men and women. Psychol Men Masculinity. 2004;5(1):49–58.
7. Smolak L, Murnen SK. Drive for leanness: assessment and relationship to gender, gender role and objectification. Body Image. 2008;5(3):251–60.
8. Kelley CC, Neufeld JM, Musher-Eizenman DR. Drive for thinness and drive for muscularity: opposite ends of the continuum or separate constructs? Body Image. 2010;7(1):74–7.
9. Goldfield GS, Blouin AG, Woodside DB. Body image, binge eating, and bulimia nervosa in male bodybuilders. Can J Psychiatr. 2006;51(3):160–8.
10. Mónok K, Berczik K, Urbán R, et al. Psychometric properties and concurrent validity of two exercise addiction measures: a population wide study. Psychol Sport Exerc. 2012;357:739–4.
11. Griffiths MD, Urbán R, Demetrovics Z, et al. A cross-cultural re-evaluation of the Exercise Addiction Inventory (EAI) in five countries. Sports Med Open. 2015;357:5.
12. Griffiths MD, Szabo A, Terry A. The Exercise Addiction Inventory: a quick and easy screening tool for health practitioners. Br J Sports Med. 2005;39(6):e30.
13. Tsai J, Huh J, Idrisov B, Galimov A, Espada JP, Gonzálvez MT, Sussman S. Prevalence and co-occurrence of addictive behaviors among Russian and Spanish youth. J Drug Educ Subst Abuse Res Prevent. 2017;46(1–2):32–46.
14. Griffiths MD. Gambling and gaming addictions in adolescence. Leicester: British Psychological Society/Blackwells; 2002.
15. Lichtenstein MB, Griffiths MD, Hemmingsen SD, Stoving RK. Exercise addiction in adolescents and emerging adults - validation of a youth version of the Exercise Addiction Inventory. J Behav Addict. 2018;7(1):117–25.
16. Goldman B, Bush P, Klatz R. Death in the locker room. London: Century; 1984. p. 32.
17. Connor JM, Mazanov J. Would you dope? A general population test of the Goldman dilemma. Br J Sports Med. 2009;43(11):871–2.
18. Johnson C, Powers P, Dick R. Athletes and eating disorders: the National Collegiate Athletic Association Study. Int J Eat Disord. 1999;26:179–88.
19. Powers P, Johnson C. Small victories: prevention of eating disorders among athletes. Eating Disorders: The Journal of Treatment and Prevention. 1996;4:364–7.

20. Royce W, Gebelt G, Duff R. Female athletes: being both athletic and feminine. Athl Insight Online J Sport Psychol. 2003;5(1):47–61.
21. Cunningham HE. Pearman S,3rd, Brewerton TD. Conceptualizing primary and secondary pathological exercise using available measures of excessive exercise. Int J Eat Disord. 2016;49(8):778–92.
22. Lichtenstein MB, Emborg B, Hemmingsen SD, Hansen NB. Is exercise addiction in fitness centers a socially accepted behavior? Addict Behav Rep. 2017;6:102–5.
23. Turton R, Goodwin H, Meyer C. Athletic identity, compulsive exercise and eating psychopathology in long-distance runners. Eat Behav. 2017;26:129–32.
24. Oberle CD, Watkins RS, Burkot AJ. Orthorexic eating behaviors related to exercise addiction and internal motivations in a sample of university students. Eat Weight Disord. 2018;23(1):67–74.
25. Egan SJ, Bodill K, Watson HJ, Valentine E, Shu C, Hagger MS. Compulsive exercise as a mediator between clinical perfectionism and eating pathology. Eat Behav. 2017;24:11–6.
26. Goodwin H, Haycraft E, Meyer C. Disordered eating, compulsive exercise, and sport participation in a UK adolescent sample. Eur Eat Disord Rev. 2016;24(4):304–9.
27. Taranis L, Meyer C. Associations between specific components of compulsive exercise and eating-disordered cognitions and behaviors among young women. Int J Eat Disord. 2011;44(5):452–8.
28. Cunningham HE, Pearman S, Brewerton TD. Conceptualizing primary and secondary pathological exercise using available measures of excessive exercise. Int J Eat Disord. 2016;49(8):778–92.
29. Duckham RL, Peirce N, Meyer C, Summers GD, Cameron N, Brooke-Wavell K. Risk factors for stress fracture in female endurance athletes: a cross-sectional study. BMJ Open. 2012;2(6) https://doi.org/10.1136/bmjopen-2012-001920. Print 2012.
30. Cook B, Engel S, Crosby R, Hausenblas H, Wonderlich S, Mitchell J. Pathological motivations for exercise and eating disorder specific health-related quality of life. Int J Eat Disord. 2014;47(3):268–72.
31. Hale BD, Diehl D, Weaver K, Briggs M. Exercise dependence and muscle dysmorphia in novice and experienced female bodybuilders. J Behav Addict. 2013;2(4):244–8.
32. Buck K, Spittler J, Reed A, Khodaee M. Psychological attributes of ultramarathoners. Wilderness Environ Med. 2018;29(1):66–71.
33. Mooney R, Simonato P, Ruparelia R, Roman-Urrestarazu A, Martinotti G, Corazza O. The use of supplements and performance and image enhancing drugs in fitness settings: a exploratory cross-sectional investigation in the United Kingdom. Hum Psychopharmacol. 2017;32(3) https://doi.org/10.1002/hup.2619.
34. Lichtenstein MB, Christiansen E, Elklit A, Bilenberg N, Stoving RK. Exercise addiction: a study of eating disorder symptoms, quality of life, personality traits and attachment styles. Psychiatry Res. 2014;215(2):410–6.
35. Costa S, Hausenblas HA, Oliva P, Cuzzocrea F, Larcan R. The role of age, gender, mood states and exercise frequency on exercise dependence. J Behav Addict. 2013;2(4):216–23.
36. Bratland-Sanda S, Martinsen EW, Rosenvinge JH, Ro O, Hoffart A, Sundgot-Borgen J. Exercise dependence score in patients with longstanding eating disorders and controls: the importance of affect regulation and physical activity intensity. Eur Eat Disord Rev. 2011;19(3):249–55.
37. Szabo A, Vega Rde L, Ruiz-BarquIn R, Rivera O. Exercise addiction in Spanish athletes: investigation of the roles of gender, social context and level of involvement. J Behav Addict. 2013;2(4):249–52.
38. Taranis L, Touyz S, Meyer C. Disordered eating and exercise: development and preliminary validation of the compulsive exercise test (CET). Eur Eat Disord Rev. 2011;19(3):256–68.
39. Goodwin H, Haycraft E, Taranis L, Meyer C. Psychometric evaluation of the compulsive exercise test (CET) in an adolescent population: links with eating psychopathology. Eur Eat Disord Rev. 2011;19(3):269–79.
40. Formby P, Watson HJ, Hilyard A, Martin K, Egan SJ. Psychometric properties of the Compulsive Exercise Test in an adolescent eating disorder population. Eat Behav. 2014;15(4):555–7.

41. Swenne I. Evaluation of the Compulsive Exercise Test (CET) in adolescents with eating disorders: factor structure and relation to eating disordered psychopathology. Eur Eat Disord Rev. 2016;24(4):334–40.
42. Meyer C, Plateau CR, Taranis L, Brewin N, Wales J, Arcelus J. The compulsive exercise test: confirmatory factor analysis and links with eating psychopathology among women with clinical eating disorders. J Eat Disord. 2016;4:22-016-0113-3. eCollection 2016.
43. Sauchelli S, Arcelus J, Granero R, Jimenez-Murcia S, Aguera Z, Del Pino-Gutierrez A, et al. Dimensions of compulsive exercise across eating disorder diagnostic subtypes and the validation of the Spanish version of the compulsive exercise test. Front Psychol. 2016;7:1852.
44. Plateau CR, Arcelus J, Meyer C. Detecting eating psychopathology in female athletes by asking about exercise: use of the compulsive exercise test. Eur Eat Disord Rev. 2017;25(6):618–24.
45. Sicilia A, Gonzalez-Cutre D. Dependence and physical exercise: Spanish validation of the Exercise Dependence Scale-Revised (EDS-R). Span J Psychol. 2011;14(1):421–31.
46. Costa S, Cuzzocrea F, Hausenblas HA, Larcan R, Oliva P. Psychometric examination and factorial validity of the Exercise Dependence Scale-Revised in Italian exercisers. J Behav Addict. 2012;1(4):186–90.
47. Shin K, You S. Factorial validity of the Korean version of the exercise dependence scale-revised. Percept Mot Skills. 2015;121(3):889–99.
48. Griffiths MD, Szabo A, Terry A. The exercise addiction inventory: a quick and easy screening tool for health practitioners. Br J Sports Med. 2005;39(6):e30.
49. Sicilia A, Alias-Garcia A, Ferriz R, Moreno-Murcia JA. Spanish adaptation and validation of the Exercise Addiction Inventory (EAI). Psicothema. 2013;25(3):377–83.
50. Lichtenstein MB, Christiansen E, Bilenberg N, Stoving RK. Validation of the exercise addiction inventory in a Danish sport context. Scand J Med Sci Sports. 2014;24(2):447–53.
51. Weinstein A, Maayan G, Weinstein Y. A study on the relationship between compulsive exercise, depression and anxiety. J Behav Addict. 2015;4(4):315–8.
52. Noetel M, Dawson L, Hay P, Touyz S. The assessment and treatment of unhealthy exercise in adolescents with anorexia nervosa: a Delphi study to synthesize clinical knowledge. Int J Eat Disord. 2017;50(4):378–88.
53. Bergeron MF, Mountjoy M, Armstrong N, Chia M, Cote J, Emery CA, et al. International Olympic Committee consensus statement on youth athletic development. Br J Sports Med. 2015;49(13):843–51.
54. De Souza MJ, Nattiv A, Joy E, Misra M, Williams NI, Mallinson RJ, et al. 2014 female athlete triad coalition consensus statement on treatment and return to play of the female athlete triad: 1st international conference held in San Francisco, California, May 2012 and 2nd international conference held in Indianapolis, Indiana, May 2013. Br J Sports Med. 2014;48(4):289-2013-093218.
55. Mountjoy M, Sundgot-Borgen J, Burke L, Carter S, Constantini N, Lebrun C, et al. The IOC relative energy deficiency in sport clinical assessment tool (RED-S CAT). Br J Sports Med. 2015;49(21):1354.

Chapter 17
The Cellular and Physiological Basis of Behavioral Health After Mild Traumatic Brain Injury

Laura L. Giacometti, Lauren A. Buck, and Ramesh Raghupathi

The Centers for Disease Control and Prevention estimates that in the United States alone, there are more than 3 million traumatic brain injury (TBI)-related hospital visits per year [2]. There has been an increase in clinical and preclinical concussion research over the past two decades due in part to the attention on sports-related brain injuries and those sustained by military personnel during active combat. Organizations such as the Concussion Legacy Foundation, the Headway Foundation, and the Brain Trauma Foundation have also actively promoted public education on the incidence, signs, and symptoms of concussions. Concussions are a type of mild TBI caused either by direct traumatic force to the head or as a result of indirect or rotational forces which cause the brain to move within the skull (e.g., whiplash) leading to changes in brain function. Immediately following mild TBI, commonly reported symptoms include headache, dizziness, nausea, vomiting, difficulty maintaining balance, blurred vision, and disrupted motor coordination. In addition, mild TBI may lead to post-traumatic amnesia accompanied by confusion, disorientation, and attentional deficits [1]. These symptoms usually resolve within 7–10 days although sleep disruptions, difficulty with reasoning, and trouble concentrating continue to persist anywhere from a few weeks to years after the injury. Together, these symptoms make mild TBI a condition that is often hard to recognize and even more difficult for society to understand [2].

L. L. Giacometti · L. A. Buck
Department of Pharmacology and Physiology, College of Medicine, Drexel University, Philadelphia, PA, USA
e-mail: llk34@drexel.edu; lap352@drexel.edu

R. Raghupathi (✉)
Department of Neurobiology and Anatomy, College of Medicine, Drexel University, Philadelphia, PA, USA

Coatesville Veteran's Administration Medical Center, Coatesville, PA, USA
e-mail: rr79@drexel.edu

© Springer Nature Switzerland AG 2020   211
E. Hong, A. L. Rao (eds.), *Mental Health in the Athlete*,
https://doi.org/10.1007/978-3-030-44754-0_17

Table 17.1 Behavioral outcomes following TBI in rodents

Behavior	Test	Species	References
Spatial learning/memory	Morris water maze	Mouse, rat	[3]
Working memory	Radial arm water maze	Mouse	[4]
	Y-maze, T-maze	Mouse	[4]
	Novel object recognition	Mouse	[5]
Depression	Forced swim test	Mouse	[6, 7]
	Passive avoidance test	Mouse	[6, 7]
Anxiety	Open field test	Mouse	[7]
	Elevated plus maze	Mouse	[6]
	Elevated zero maze	Mouse	[4]
Locomotion	Rotarod	Mouse	[3, 4]
Post-traumatic headache	Facial allodynia	Mouse, rat	[8–11]
	Photophobia	Mouse	[8]

A number of animal models have been developed to study the complexity of behavioral changes that occur following mild TBI. Most of these animal models utilize rats and mice and, up until relatively recently, focused almost exclusively on males. Animal models replicate some aspects of the biomechanical forces at play during a TBI as well as some of the behavioral deficits; however, no one model can recreate all aspects of TBI. The criteria for defining an animal model of TBI as "mild" also vary greatly and can be based on lack of lesion, cell death, or overt pathological change or the transient nature of cognitive deficits, although many mild TBI models report evidence of cell death, axonal injury, and persistent cognitive deficits. Immediately after injury, apnea time, loss of righting reflex, and presence of fractures and/or hematoma are all reported as acute indicators of injury severity. As in humans, TBI is characterized in animals using various methods including physiological, behavioral, and cognitive measures (Table 17.1). Despite these limitations, animal models of mild TBI have successfully recreated many of the behavioral deficits of human TBI as well as provide some insight into the underlying mechanisms. Some of these mechanisms included cell death, axonal injury, inflammation, and neurotransmitter dysfunction. This chapter will summarize the effects of mild TBI in rodents on measures of depression, anxiety, post-traumatic headache, sleep dysfunction, and substance abuse as well as explore the potential role of cellular alterations that may shed light on the mechanisms underlying these behavioral changes.

Behavioral Deficits Following Mild TBI

Depression-Like Behavior

Depression-like behavior in animal models is evaluated using various tests; some of the most common include the forced swim test, tail suspension test, and sucrose preference test. Both the forced swim test and tail suspension test use immobility as a measure of behavioral despair, while the sucrose preference test is considered a measure of anhedonia [12–17]. As depression-like behaviors can be observed in one behavioral test, but not others, it is important to utilize more than one test of depression. Depression-like behaviors have been observed following mild TBI in rats and mice as early as 24–72 h following injury and up to 90 days [6, 7, 18, 19]. There is some suggestion that mice subjected to mild TBI are more vulnerable to depression-like behavior; mice sustaining a mild (but not moderate or severe) injury exhibited an increase in immobility in the tail suspension test at 13 days post-injury [20]. Sex and age also appear to be contributing factors to vulnerability of exhibiting depression-like behavior as female, but not male, rats subjected to mild TBI during adolescence exhibited an increase in depression-like behavior in the forced swim test at 20 days post-injury [21].

Anxiety-Like Behavior

Anxiety-related behaviors can be measured using a variety of behavioral tests including the elevated plus maze, open field test, and light/dark box. The aforementioned tests are all based on the idea that an anxious rodent will spend more time in dark, enclosed spaces than open, bright spaces. Alterations in anxiety-related behaviors following mild TBI have been observed up to 30 days post-injury [22]. Adult male rats subjected to mild TBI demonsrated an exhibited increased latency in completing a structured task 6-days post-injury [23].

Sleep Disturbances

Sleep disturbances are also a particularly common symptom following TBI but appear to be most prevalent after a mild TBI [24]. Types of TBI-induced sleep disturbances include increased latency to fall asleep, irregular sleep-wake patterns, and insomnia [25–28]. Moderate TBI in both adult male mice and rats has been shown to result in reduced wakefulness up to 29 days post-injury [29–31]. As sleep plays an essential role in consolidation of memory and can contribute to depression-like behavior, it is not surprising that impairments in novel object recognition memory and depression-like behaviors were observed in rats exhibiting disrupted sleep-wake cycles [31].

Post-traumatic Headache

One of the symptoms of headache is facial allodynia, wherein patients have heightened sensitivity to touch in their face and around the head. In rodents, von Frey filaments can be used to determine a pain threshold [8, 9]. Another common symptom of headache is photosensitivity or photophobia measured by the light/ dark box test [8, 32] wherein animals with photosensitivity would spend less time in the light chamber. More recently, the mouse grimace scale was developed wherein pain levels are measured in rodents by grading certain aspects of facial expression in a manner similar to that in human infants and those unable to vocally express themselves [33, 34]. Multiple studies have clearly demonstrated the presence of facial allodynia following mild TBI in both male mice and rats, using it as a surrogate measure of PTH [8–10]. Even after the resolution of TBI-induced facial allodynia, rats demonstrated a pronounced sensitivity to a known headache trigger such as glyceryl trinitrate (GTN) [10]. Facial hypersensitivity to both hot and cold modalities using an orofacial operant task has been documented in female rats subjected to mild TBI [11].

Substance Abuse

TBI has been associated with an increased risk for substance abuse disorders. Interestingly, moderate TBI in male mice induced greater sensitivity to ethanol and decreased ethanol self-administration at 2 weeks post-injury [35]. Following mild TBI, however, it has been observed that female, but not male, mice injured as adolescents, but not adults, exhibited increased self-administration of ethanol [36]. Adolescent female mice subjected to mild TBI also exhibited an increase in conditioned place preference for ethanol, which was not observed in male mice, suggesting that female mice found ethanol more rewarding following injury [36].

Repetitive Mild TBI

As having sustained a concussion increases the likelihood of sustaining subsequent concussions, a number of models of repetitive mild TBI have been developed. These models vary greatly, however, in terms of species used, age, injury type and severity, interval between injuries, and injury frequency. *There is a general consensus, however, that the shorter the interval between injuries, the greater the pathological damage and behavioral deficits* [37, 38]. Repetitive injuries have the potential to unmask behavioral deficits that were not present with a single mild TBI. Adult male rats exhibited a depression-like phenotype in the FST and an anxiety-like phenotype in the EPM only after five mild TBIs, but not one or three [39]. In other behaviors, repetitive injury does not simply exacerbate or prolong behavioral deficits compared to a mild TBI but results in a different type of deficit. Following a single mild TBI during adolescence, female rats exhibited an increase in immobility in the forced swim test but a decrease following repetitive mild TBI [21].

Mechanisms of Behavioral Deficits Following Mild TBI

Cell Death

Cell death following TBI in humans has long been considered a major mechanism of behavioral dysfunction. Cell death has been observed in various brain regions of post-mortem tissue following TBI including the cortex, hippocampus, and thalamus [40–43]. This has been recapitulated in multiple animal models of TBI as well [44–48]. Loss of gamma-aminobutyric acid (GABA) interneurons at 7 days has been observed following mild TBI in adolescent male rats, which corresponded to the presence of anxiety-related behaviors at 7 days [22]. Other studies have seen a reduction in the number of hypocretin (HCRT)-positive neurons in the lateral hypothalamus from 6 to 29 days post-injury, corresponding to sleep-wake disturbances [30, 31].

In addition, apoptotic signaling cascades have been implicated in behavioral deficits following TBI. The β-isoform of the serine threonine kinase, glycogen synthase kinase (GSK)-3, which has been linked to apoptosis, has been implicated in depression-like behavior following mild TBI. Adult male mice subjected to mild TBI exhibited an increase in phosphorylation of GSK-3β, and protein kinase B, which phosphorylates GSK-3β to inhibit its activity. β-Catenin, which is phosphorylated by GSK-3β, was also increased following injury, but this increase was due to an accumulation of the active, dephosphorylated form of β-catenin. Inhibition of GSK3-β phosphorylation 30 min prior to mild TBI using lithium or L803-mts prevented the depression-like phenotype 24 h post-injury. However, prolonged memory impairment has been observed in the absence of cell death, suggesting that cell death is not always sufficient to explain behavioral deficits following TBI [49].

Traumatic Axonal Injury

The stretching of axons is believed to result in unregulated flow of ions, resulting in increased intracellular calcium, triggering a cascade of events resulting in degradation of cytoskeletal proteins, which in some axons can lead to the formation of retraction bulbs and eventual disconnection [50–52]. Impaired axonal transport (IAT) is also observed in some axons following TBI. Accumulations of β-amyloid precursor protein (APP), which is transported via fast axonal transport both anterogradely and retrogradely, are used as a surrogate marker of IAT [52]. In addition, the retrogradely transported neuronal tracer, Fluoro-Gold, has been used to show evidence of impaired retrograde transport in the corpus callosum up to 14 days post-injury following mild TBI in the adult male mouse [53]. It has been suggested that IAT is the underlying basis for deficits in spatial learning; however, APP accumulation in the absence of spatial learning deficits and spatial learning deficits in the absence of APP accumulation have both been observed following TBI [7, 37].

Microglial Activation

Microglia, the resident immune cells of the brain, become activated following TBI as evidenced by morphological changes from a thin elongated resting or "ramified" state to a large, rounded "amoeboid" shape with little to no visible processes. Microglia serve to phagocytose clear cellular debris and promote repair though upregulation of neurotrophic factors and anti-inflammatory cytokines [54]. Within hours following mild TBI in the micro pig, microglial processes have been shown to closely interact with the proximal aspect of injured axons, a region which is typically associated with remodeling, suggesting that microglia may participate in this remodeling [55]. However, microglia, when chronically activated, can also further contribute to neurodegeneration and cell death through upregulation of pro-inflammatory cytokines and chemokines and reactive oxygen species to promote oxidative stress [54]. Thus, microglial activation following mild TBI is complex and can be both beneficial and detrimental.

Microglial activation has been observed following mild TBI in adult male rats, as evidenced by an increase in ionized calcium-binding adaptor molecule 1 (Iba-1) in the corpus callosum and thalamus up to 15 days post-injury [56]. Following moderate-severe TBI in mice, female mice exhibited a much less pronounced microglial response than male mice up to 3 days post-injury but reached similar levels by 7 days post-injury, suggesting that females may exhibit a more delayed microglial response following TBI [57]. Following repetitive mild TBI, unmasking of behavioral deficits corresponded to a significant increase in ED1-labeled activated microglia in the injured cortex [39].

Inflammation has also emerged as a potential modulator of dopaminergic signaling alterations following TBI and has also been implicated in ethanol self-administration deficits following mild TBI. Male adolescent mice subjected to mild TBI exhibited increased self-administration of ethanol and increased ED1-labeled activated microglia in the ventral tegmental area and nucleus accumbens shell, which were ameliorated by the administration of the anti-inflammatory, minocycline [58].

Astrocytic Reactivity

Following TBI, astrocytes become reactive, undergoing morphological changes and upregulating glial fibrillary acidic protein (GFAP) [59]. Astrocytes can form a protective scar around injured tissue, preventing further damage to the adjacent tissue, and promote restoration of blood-brain barrier integrity [60]. Astrocytes also release matrix metalloproteases which aid in the removal of damaged tissue [61]. However, astrocytes also play detrimental roles following TBI [62]. Astrocytes normally function to remove excess extracellular glutamate through the astrocytic glutamate transporters, GLT-1 and GLAST, thus preventing excitotoxicity [63]. Following

TBI, however, GLT-1 and GLAST are downregulated, thus further contributing to excitotoxicity [64]. Although the majority of the research elucidating the role of astrocytes in TBI has been in the context of moderate-severe TBI, astrocytic reactivity has been observed in the corpus callosum and thalamus of adult male rats at 15 days following mild TBI, as indicated by an increase in GFAP immunoreactivity, suggesting that reactive astrocytes are also active players in mild TBI [56].

Neurotransmitter Dysfunction

TBI results in extensive neuronal depolarization as measured by large increases in extracellular potassium and subsequent nonspecific neurotransmitter release [65]. Increases in extracellular glutamate, aspartate, γ-aminobutyric acid (GABA), acetylcholine, dopamine, and norepinephrine have been observed [66–69]. Using microdialysis, glutamate and aspartate were shown to increase rapidly following moderate-severe injury, peaking within 10 minutes and remaining elevated for up to 1 hour [69]. The magnitude of this increase also increased with increasing injury severity [69]. Interestingly, tissue levels of dopamine in the cortex have been shown to decrease at 1 hour and remain decreased up to 2 weeks following moderate-severe TBI while remaining elevated for hours in the striatum and hypothalamus [66]. Following mild TBI, however, tissue dopamine levels remain elevated in the striatum for up to 36 hours, suggesting that injury severity affects not only magnitude but also duration of neurotransmitter alterations following TBI [70].

Depression-like behavior following TBI in adult male rats, which was associated with fluctuations in dopamine and its metabolites, 3,4-dihydroxyphenylacetic acid (DOPAC) and homovanillic acid (HVA), was ameliorated by chronic administration of amantadine, which increases dopamine release and blocks dopamine uptake [71]. Similarly, brain-injured mice exhibited reductions in extracellular hypocretin (HCRT) levels in the hippocampus and hypothalamus and increases in HCRT-positive neurons in the lateral hypothalamus measured using microdialysis which corresponded with increased wake bouts during the dark phase and decreased length of wake bouts at 3 days post-injury [29].

This disruption in neurotransmitter signaling is also believed to result in alterations in receptor binding and expression. Moderate TBI in the adult rat resulted in decreased NMDA receptor binding in the hippocampus up to 3 h and in layers V and VI of the cortex up to 24 h post-injury [72]. Following TBI in the adult male rat, increased expression of the dopamine D1 receptor, but not D2 receptor, has been observed up to 3 days post-injury [73]. In contrast, at 15 days following a moderate injury in the adult male rat, when spatial learning memory deficits were observed, muscarinic cholinergic receptors exhibited increased binding affinity in the hippocampus and cortex [74]. More recently, female rats, which received a mild TBI as adolescents, exhibited decreased D2 receptor immunoreactivity in the striatum at 7 weeks post-injury [75]. Together, these studies suggest that the timing and direction of receptor density and expression alterations following TBI are complex and depend on the neurotransmitter system being evaluated.

In addition to receptor changes, alterations in neurotransmitter synthesis and uptake have been observed following TBI. Activity of tyrosine hydroxylase (TH), the rate-limiting enzyme in dopamine synthesis, decreases in the striatum and cortex beginning at 1 week post-injury and remained decreased until 4 weeks post-injury [76]. In the PFC, alterations in TH activity are more dynamic, increasing from days 3 to 14 and decreasing at 4 weeks [77]. The dopamine transporter, DAT, is decreased in the cortex and striatum beginning at 1 week and up to 4 weeks following moderate TBI in the adult male, but not female, rat [78]. Following mild TBI in the adolescent female rat, however, a decrease in DAT immunoreactivity in the striatum was observed at 7 weeks [75].

Downstream signaling cascades can also be altered following disruption of neurotransmitter signaling. An increase in the phosphorylated form of dopamine- and cAMP-regulated phosphoprotein (DARPP-32) in the striatum was observed in male rats who exhibited an increase in self-administration of ethanol following mild TBI, as well as an inability to show a further increase in phospho-DARPP-32 after acute ethanol administration, which was observed in sham-injured rats [35].

Conclusions

The etiology of each incidence of mild TBI can vary from direct or indirect traumatic force to the brain to forces generated by explosions [2]. Not surprisingly, so can the symptomology of MTBI vary, with vastly different changes in cognition, mood, and personality among all patients [2]. Moreover, males sustain higher rates of mild TBI than women although more women report symptoms associated with mild TBI [79]. Commonly reported symptoms included fatigue, poor memory, headache, frustration, and depression, for which women report significantly more headache occurrences [79]. In fact, gender may be a significant risk factor for chronic complications following mild TBI [79, 80]. Although clinically validated animal models have advanced the understanding of the functional consequences of TBI, they are not without their limitations. Structural differences between rodent and human brains may result in differential behavioral and physiological outcomes following mild TBI [81]. It is also important to note that outcomes using the same injury device can vary between rodent species and strain, suggesting that even small differences in physiology can lead to changes in the pathophysiology of mild TBI. Additionally, most preclinical studies use anesthetized animals which can complicate interpretations of TBI-induced alterations in brain function associated with behavioral dysfunction [82]. Despite these limitations, the wealth of preclinical models in both sexes should be advantageous in determining mechanistic causes for mild TBI-induced behavioral dysfunction, with a potential goal of developing targeted therapies that can be translated to the clinic.

References

1. Rao VV, Vaishnavi S. The traumatized brain. Baltimore: Johns Hopkins University Press; 2015.
2. Heim LR, Bader M, Edut S, Rachmany L, Baratz-Goldstein R, Lin R, et al. The invisibility of mild traumatic brain injury: impaired cognitive performance as a silent symptom. J Neurotrauma. 2017;34(17):2518–28.
3. Yu S, Kaneko Y, Bae E, Stahl CE, Wang Y, van Loveren H, et al. Severity of controlled cortical impact traumatic brain injury in rats and mice dictates degree of behavioral deficits. Brain Res. 2009;1287:157–63.
4. Luo J, Nguyen A, Villeda S, Zhang H, Ding Z, Lindsey D, et al. Long-term cognitive impairments and pathological alterations in a mouse model of repetitive mild traumatic brain injury. Front Neurol. 2014;5:12.
5. Chen H, Chan YL, Nguyen LT, Mao Y, de Rosa A, Beh IT, et al. Moderate traumatic brain injury is linked to acute behaviour deficits and long term mitochondrial alterations. Clin Exp Pharmacol Physiol. 2016;43(11):1107–14.
6. Milman A, Rosenberg A, Weizman R, Pick CG. Mild traumatic brain injury induces persistent cognitive deficits and behavioral disturbances in mice. J Neurotrauma. 2005;22(9):1003–10.
7. Tweedie D, Milman A, Holloway HW, Li Y, Harvey BK, Shen H, et al. Apoptotic and behavioral sequelae of mild brain trauma in mice. J Neurosci Res. 2007;85(4):805–15.
8. Daiutolo BV, Tyburski A, Clark SW, Elliott MB. Trigeminal pain molecules, allodynia, and photosensitivity are pharmacologically and genetically modulated in a model of traumatic brain injury. J Neurotrauma. 2016;33(8):748–60.
9. Elliott MB, Oshinsky ML, Amenta PS, Awe OO, Jallo JI. Nociceptive neuropeptide increases and periorbital allodynia in a model of traumatic brain injury. Headache. 2012;52(6):966–84.
10. Bree D, Levy D. Development of CGRP-dependent pain and headache related behaviours in a rat model of concussion: implications for mechanisms of post-traumatic headache. Cephalalgia. 2018;38(2):246–58.
11. Mustafa G, Hou J, Tsuda S, Nelson R, Sinharoy A, Wilkie Z, et al. Trigeminal neuroplasticity underlies allodynia in a preclinical model of mild closed head traumatic brain injury (cTBI). Neuropharmacology. 2016;107:27–39.
12. Porsolt RD, Anton G, Blavet N, Jalfre M. Behavioural despair in rats: a new model sensitive to antidepressant treatments. Eur J Pharmacol. 1978;47(4):379–91.
13. Porsolt RD, Bertin A, Jalfre M. Behavioral despair in mice: a primary screening test for antidepressants. Arch Int Pharmacodyn Ther. 1977;229(2):327–36.
14. Porsolt RD, Le Pichon M, Jalfre M. Depression: a new animal model sensitive to antidepressant treatments. Nature. 1977;266(5604):730–2.
15. Steru L, Chermat R, Thierry B, Simon P. The tail suspension test: a new method for screening antidepressants in mice. Psychopharmacology. 1985;85(3):367–70.
16. Katz RJ. Animal model of depression: pharmacological sensitivity of a hedonic deficit. Pharmacol Biochem Behav. 1982;16(6):965–8.
17. Willner P, Towell A, Sampson D, Sophokleous S, Muscat R. Reduction of sucrose preference by chronic unpredictable mild stress, and its restoration by a tricyclic antidepressant. Psychopharmacology. 1987;93(3):358–64.
18. Shapira M, Licht A, Milman A, Pick CG, Shohami E, Eldar-Finkelman H. Role of glycogen synthase kinase-3beta in early depressive behavior induced by mild traumatic brain injury. Mol Cell Neurosci. 2007;34(4):571–7.
19. Washington PM, Forcelli PA, Wilkins T, Zapple DN, Parsadanian M, Burns MP. The effect of injury severity on behavior: a phenotypic study of cognitive and emotional deficits after mild, moderate, and severe controlled cortical impact injury in mice. J Neurotrauma. 2012;29(13):2283–96.
20. Schwarzbold ML, Rial D, De Bem T, Machado DG, Cunha MP, dos Santos AA, et al. Effects of traumatic brain injury of different severities on emotional, cognitive, and oxidative stress-related parameters in mice. J Neurotrauma. 2010;27(10):1883–93.

21. Wright DK, O'Brien TJ, Shultz SR, Mychasiuk R. Sex matters: repetitive mild traumatic brain injury in adolescent rats. Ann Clin Transl Neurol. 2017;4(9):640–54.
22. Almeida-Suhett CP, Prager EM, Pidoplichko V, Figueiredo TH, Marini AM, Li Z, et al. Reduced GABAergic inhibition in the basolateral amygdala and the development of anxiety-like behaviors after mild traumatic brain injury. PLoS One. 2014;9(7):e102627.
23. Meyer DL, Davies DR, Barr JL, Manzerra P, Forster GL. Mild traumatic brain injury in the rat alters neuronal number in the limbic system and increases conditioned fear and anxiety-like behaviors. Exp Neurol. 2012;235(2):574–87.
24. Mahmood O, Rapport LJ, Hanks RA, Fichtenberg NL. Neuropsychological performance and sleep disturbance following traumatic brain injury. J Head Trauma Rehabil. 2004;19(5):378–90.
25. Ouellet N, Morris DL. Sleep satisfaction of older adults living in the community: identifying associated behavioral and health factors. J Gerontol Nurs. 2006;32(10):5–11.
26. Ayalon L, Borodkin K, Dishon L, Kanety H, Dagan Y. Circadian rhythm sleep disorders following mild traumatic brain injury. Neurology. 2007;68(14):1136–40.
27. Parcell DL, Ponsford JL, Rajaratnam SM, Redman JR. Self-reported changes to nighttime sleep after traumatic brain injury. Arch Phys Med Rehabil. 2006;87(2):278–85.
28. Ponsford JL, Ziino C, Parcell DL, Shekleton JA, Roper M, Redman JR, et al. Fatigue and sleep disturbance following traumatic brain injury--their nature, causes, and potential treatments. J Head Trauma Rehabil. 2012;27(3):224–33.
29. Willie JT, Lim MM, Bennett RE, Azarion AA, Schwetye KE, Brody DL. Controlled cortical impact traumatic brain injury acutely disrupts wakefulness and extracellular orexin dynamics as determined by intracerebral microdialysis in mice. J Neurotrauma. 2012;29(10):1908–21.
30. Thomasy HE, Febinger HY, Ringgold KM, Gemma C, Opp MR. Hypocretinergic and cholinergic contributions to sleep-wake disturbances in a mouse model of traumatic brain injury. Neurobiol Sleep Circadian Rhythms. 2017;2:71–84.
31. Skopin MD, Kabadi SV, Viechweg SS, Mong JA, Faden AI. Chronic decrease in wakefulness and disruption of sleep-wake behavior after experimental traumatic brain injury. J Neurotrauma. 2015;32(5):289–96.
32. Harris HM, Carpenter JM, Black JR, Smitherman TA, Sufka KJ. The effects of repeated nitroglycerin administrations in rats; modeling migraine-related endpoints and chronification. J Neurosci Methods. 2017;284:63–70.
33. Langford DJ, Bailey AL, Chanda ML, Clarke SE, Drummond TE, Echols S, et al. Coding of facial expressions of pain in the laboratory mouse. Nat Methods. 2010;7(6):447–9.
34. Miller AL, Leach MC. The mouse grimace scale: a clinically useful tool? PLoS One. 2015;10(9):e0136000.
35. Lowing JL, Susick LL, Caruso JP, Provenzano AM, Raghupathi R, Conti AC. Experimental traumatic brain injury alters ethanol consumption and sensitivity. J Neurotrauma. 2014;31(20):1700–10.
36. Weil ZM, Karelina K, Gaier KR, Corrigan TE, Corrigan JD. Juvenile traumatic brain injury increases alcohol consumption and reward in female mice. J Neurotrauma. 2016;33(9):895–903.
37. Longhi L, Saatman KE, Fujimoto S, Raghupathi R, Meaney DF, Davis J, et al. Temporal window of vulnerability to repetitive experimental concussive brain injury. Neurosurgery. 2005;56(2):364–74; discussion -74.
38. Meehan WP 3rd, Zhang J, Mannix R, Whalen MJ. Increasing recovery time between injuries improves cognitive outcome after repetitive mild concussive brain injuries in mice. Neurosurgery. 2012;71(4):885–91.
39. Shultz SR, Bao F, Omana V, Chiu C, Brown A, Cain DP. Repeated mild lateral fluid percussion brain injury in the rat causes cumulative long-term behavioral impairments, neuroinflammation, and cortical loss in an animal model of repeated concussion. J Neurotrauma. 2012;29(2):281–94.
40. Kotapka MJ, Graham DI, Adams JH, Gennarelli TA. Hippocampal pathology in fatal nonmissile human head injury. Acta Neuropathol. 1992;83(5):530–4.
41. Ross DT, Graham DI, Adams JH. Selective loss of neurons from the thalamic reticular nucleus following severe human head injury. J Neurotrauma. 1993;10(2):151–65.

42. Maxwell WL, Dhillon K, Harper L, Espin J, MacIntosh TK, Smith DH, et al. There is differential loss of pyramidal cells from the human hippocampus with survival after blunt head injury. J Neuropathol Exp Neurol. 2003;62(3):272–9.
43. Minambres E, Ballesteros MA, Mayorga M, Marin MJ, Munoz P, Figols J, et al. Cerebral apoptosis in severe traumatic brain injury patients: an in vitro, in vivo, and postmortem study. J Neurotrauma. 2008;25(6):581–91.
44. Rink A, Fung KM, Trojanowski JQ, Lee VM, Neugebauer E, McIntosh TK. Evidence of apoptotic cell death after experimental traumatic brain injury in the rat. Am J Pathol. 1995;147(6):1575–83.
45. Raghupathi R, Conti AC, Graham DI, Krajewski S, Reed JC, Grady MS, et al. Mild traumatic brain injury induces apoptotic cell death in the cortex that is preceded by decreases in cellular Bcl-2 immunoreactivity. Neuroscience. 2002;110(4):605–16.
46. Hicks RR, Smith DH, Lowenstein DH, Saint Marie R, McIntosh TK. Mild experimental brain injury in the rat induces cognitive deficits associated with regional neuronal loss in the hippocampus. J Neurotrauma. 1993;10(4):405–14.
47. Fukuda K, Aihara N, Sagar SM, Sharp FR, Pitts LH, Honkaniemi J, et al. Purkinje cell vulnerability to mild traumatic brain injury. J Neurotrauma. 1996;13(5):255–66.
48. Tashlykov V, Katz Y, Volkov A, Gazit V, Schreiber S, Zohar O, et al. Minimal traumatic brain injury induce apoptotic cell death in mice. J Mol Neurosci. 2009;37(1):16–24.
49. Lyeth BG, Jenkins LW, Hamm RJ, Dixon CE, Phillips LL, Clifton GL, et al. Prolonged memory impairment in the absence of hippocampal cell death following traumatic brain injury in the rat. Brain Res. 1990;526(2):249–58.
50. Saatman KE, Creed J, Raghupathi R. Calpain as a therapeutic target in traumatic brain injury. Neurotherapeutics. 2010;7(1):31–42.
51. Kampfl A, Posmantur RM, Zhao X, Schmutzhard E, Clifton GL, Hayes RL. Mechanisms of calpain proteolysis following traumatic brain injury: implications for pathology and therapy: implications for pathology and therapy: a review and update. J Neurotrauma. 1997;14(3):121–34.
52. Buki A, Povlishock JT. All roads lead to disconnection?--traumatic axonal injury revisited. Acta Neurochir. 2006;148(2):181–93; discussion 93-4.
53. Creed JA, DiLeonardi AM, Fox DP, Tessler AR, Raghupathi R. Concussive brain trauma in the mouse results in acute cognitive deficits and sustained impairment of axonal function. J Neurotrauma. 2011;28(4):547–63.
54. Loane DJ, Byrnes KR. Role of microglia in neurotrauma. Neurotherapeutics. 2010;7(4):366–77.
55. Lafrenaye AD, Todani M, Walker SA, Povlishock JT. Microglia processes associate with diffusely injured axons following mild traumatic brain injury in the micro pig. J Neuroinflammation. 2015;12:186.
56. Hylin MJ, Orsi SA, Zhao J, Bockhorst K, Perez A, Moore AN, et al. Behavioral and histopathological alterations resulting from mild fluid percussion injury. J Neurotrauma. 2013;30(9):702–15.
57. Villapol S, Loane DJ, Burns MP. Sexual dimorphism in the inflammatory response to traumatic brain injury. Glia. 2017;65(9):1423–38.
58. Karelina K, Nicholson S, Weil ZM. Minocycline blocks traumatic brain injury-induced alcohol consumption and nucleus accumbens inflammation in adolescent male mice. Brain Behav Immun. 2018;69:532–9.
59. Baldwin SA, Scheff SW. Intermediate filament change in astrocytes following mild cortical contusion. Glia. 1996;16(3):266–75.
60. Bush TG, Puvanachandra N, Horner CH, Polito A, Ostenfeld T, Svendsen CN, et al. Leukocyte infiltration, neuronal degeneration, and neurite outgrowth after ablation of scar-forming, reactive astrocytes in adult transgenic mice. Neuron. 1999;23(2):297–308.
61. Falo MC, Fillmore HL, Reeves TM, Phillips LL. Matrix metalloproteinase-3 expression profile differentiates adaptive and maladaptive synaptic plasticity induced by traumatic brain injury. J Neurosci Res. 2006;84(4):768–81.

62. Laird MD, Vender JR, Dhandapani KM. Opposing roles for reactive astrocytes following traumatic brain injury. Neurosignals. 2008;16(2–3):154–64.
63. Anderson CM, Swanson RA. Astrocyte glutamate transport: review of properties, regulation, and physiological functions. Glia. 2000;32(1):1–14.
64. Rao VL, Baskaya MK, Dogan A, Rothstein JD, Dempsey RJ. Traumatic brain injury down-regulates glial glutamate transporter (GLT-1 and GLAST) proteins in rat brain. J Neurochem. 1998;70(5):2020–7.
65. Hayes RL, Jenkins LW, Lyeth BG. Neurotransmitter-mediated mechanisms of traumatic brain injury: acetylcholine and excitatory amino acids. J Neurotrauma. 1992;9(Suppl 1):S173–87.
66. McIntosh TK, Yu T, Gennarelli TA. Alterations in regional brain catecholamine concentrations after experimental brain injury in the rat. J Neurochem. 1994;63(4):1426–33.
67. Nilsson P, Hillered L, Ponten U, Ungerstedt U. Changes in cortical extracellular levels of energy-related metabolites and amino acids following concussive brain injury in rats. J Cereb Blood Flow Metab. 1990;10(5):631–7.
68. Katayama Y, Becker DP, Tamura T, Hovda DA. Massive increases in extracellular potassium and the indiscriminate release of glutamate following concussive brain injury. J Neurosurg. 1990;73(6):889–900.
69. Faden AI, Demediuk P, Panter SS, Vink R. The role of excitatory amino acids and NMDA receptors in traumatic brain injury. Science. 1989;244(4906):798–800.
70. Shen H, Harvey BK, Chiang YH, Pick CG, Wang Y. Methamphetamine potentiates behavioral and electrochemical responses after mild traumatic brain injury in mice. Brain Res. 2011;1368:248–53.
71. Tan L, Ge H, Tang J, Fu C, Duanmu W, Chen Y, et al. Amantadine preserves dopamine level and attenuates depression-like behavior induced by traumatic brain injury in rats. Behav Brain Res. 2015;279:274–82.
72. Miller LP, Lyeth BG, Jenkins LW, Oleniak L, Panchision D, Hamm RJ, et al. Excitatory amino acid receptor subtype binding following traumatic brain injury. Brain Res. 1990;526(1):103–7.
73. Kobori N, Dash PK. Reversal of brain injury-induced prefrontal glutamic acid decarboxylase expression and working memory deficits by D1 receptor antagonism. J Neurosci. 2006;26(16):4236–46.
74. Jiang JY, Lyeth BG, Delahunty TM, Phillips LL, Hamm RJ. Muscarinic cholinergic receptor binding in rat brain at 15 days following traumatic brain injury. Brain Res. 1994;651(1–2):123–8.
75. Karelina K, Gaier KR, Weil ZM. Traumatic brain injuries during development disrupt dopaminergic signaling. Exp Neurol. 2017;297:110–7.
76. Shin SS, Bray ER, Zhang CQ, Dixon CE. Traumatic brain injury reduces striatal tyrosine hydroxylase activity and potassium-evoked dopamine release in rats. Brain Res. 2011;1369:208–15.
77. Kobori N, Clifton GL, Dash PK. Enhanced catecholamine synthesis in the prefrontal cortex after traumatic brain injury: implications for prefrontal dysfunction. J Neurotrauma. 2006;23(7):1094–102.
78. Wagner AK, Chen X, Kline AE, Li Y, Zafonte RD, Dixon CE. Gender and environmental enrichment impact dopamine transporter expression after experimental traumatic brain injury. Exp Neurol. 2005;195(2):475–83.
79. Ahman S, Saveman BI, Styrke J, Bjornstig U, Stalnacke BM. Long-term follow-up of patients with mild traumatic brain injury: a mixed-method study. J Rehabil Med. 2013;45(8):758–64.
80. Yilmaz T, Roks G, de Koning M, Scheenen M, van der Horn H, Plas G, et al. Risk factors and outcomes associated with post-traumatic headache after mild traumatic brain injury. Emerg Med J. 2017;34(12):800–5.
81. Xiong Y, Mahmood A, Chopp M. Animal models of traumatic brain injury. Nat Rev Neurosci. 2013;14(2):128–42.
82. Wojnarowicz MW, Fisher AM, Minaeva O, Goldstein LE. Considerations for experimental animal models of concussion, traumatic brain injury, and chronic traumatic encephalopathy-these matters matter. Front Neurol. 2017;8:240.

Chapter 18
Mental Health Treatment Engagement of Athletes: Self-Determination Theory as a "Prescription for Excellence"

Paul C. Furtaw

Introduction

Athletes are known to experience mental health issues at significant rates, whether as a by-product of their participation in sport-related activities (secondary to injury, competitive pressures, perfectionism, etc.) [13] or due to issues external to sports participation (biological predispositions, environmental stressors, trauma and loss, etc.) [22]. When athletes experience such concerns, timely receipt of mental health care allows them to reclaim their personal well-being and athletic functioning and protects against further intensification of symptoms and chronic impairment. For this reason, it is imperative that athletes' mental health concerns are identified promptly through proper screening by their physician [11, 21] and result in equally rapid referral to qualified mental health providers [18], ideally physically co-located and operationally integrated with sports medicine. One of the most critical factors in successful mental health treatment engagement is timeliness of scheduling [2, 18].

However, given the nature of athletic identity and role socialization (often characterized as one of traditional, idealized, or even extreme masculinity) [4, 8, 12], significant personal and social barriers must first be surmounted if an athlete is to engage in treatment willingly. The sports medicine professional's active management of the referral process, drawing upon pertinent knowledge, skills, and attitudes, will foster maximum buy-in and confidence on the part of the athlete regarding the pursuit of mental health care [9, 21]. Otherwise, an athlete will face formidable barriers to mental health treatment engagement in the form of stereotypical beliefs, social stigma and self-stigma, and resulting doubt, defensiveness, and avoidance.

P. C. Furtaw (✉)
Department of Psychiatry, School of Osteopathic Medicine, Rowan University,
Mt. Laurel, NJ, USA
e-mail: furtaw@rowan.edu

© Springer Nature Switzerland AG 2020
E. Hong, A. L. Rao (eds.), *Mental Health in the Athlete*,
https://doi.org/10.1007/978-3-030-44754-0_18

Self-Determination Theory as a Basis for Understanding Human Behavior

Self-determination theory (SDT) [5], as a dominant theory of motivation and behavior over the past several decades, is frequently utilized to explain the dynamics of athletic excellence and well-being [3, 10, 14]. It also can be a basis for conceptualizing athletes' responses to their own psychological distress. In summary, SDT states that human beings are guided by three foundational psychological needs, consisting of relatedness, competence, and autonomy. These needs, while not explicitly present in the manifest nature of one's goal-directed actions, are almost always at the core of what allows one to experience sufficient satisfaction in the midst of one's daily activities. These core needs, when realized, provide value distinct from the extrinsic motivations present in the surrounding environment.

Barriers to Successful Mental Health Treatment Engagement

Barriers to engagement in mental health treatment are multifaceted in nature, stemming from individual, interpersonal, and systemic components. Together, they will often manifest in an athlete's ambivalence, minimization, and avoidance of his or her mental health-related concerns. More specifically, athletes, like human beings in general, can possess stereotypical beliefs about mental illness and its treatment, anticipated social stigma and self-stigma (i.e., internalized shame) regarding one's own mental functioning, and fear of the potential negative consequences of engagement in mental health treatment.

Mental Health Stereotypes With respect to athletes' stereotypical beliefs regarding mental health issues and their treatment, there is close consistency with broader misconceptions in society, including the framing of mental health and illness as dichotomous, rather than existing along a continuum. More specifically, mental illness is often portrayed as a function of moral deficiency, weakness of character, or emotional vulnerability. Thus, athletes understandably fear being viewed in all-or-nothing terms (i.e., crazy, lazy, stupid, or bad). Not surprisingly, the athletic ideal of mental toughness, emotional restraint, self-reliance, and even invincibility leaves little room to acknowledge one's mental challenges [4, 8, 9, 12].

Athletes may also harbor misconceptions regarding the nature of mental health treatment, including the notion that the process requires in-depth exploration of one's past history, harsh confrontation of unwelcome and potentially overwhelming emotions, or wholesale adoption of an alien worldview espoused by a treating mental health professional. While athletes may fear being labeled or pathologized, they may also look down on mental health professionals as out of touch with the realm of athletic performance [4]. Additionally, athletes may fear disclosing of personal information to the mental health professional, especially if concerns exist about whether the therapist's allegiance lies more so with key stakeholders (coach, family member, ownership, etc.) and thereby run counter to the athlete's best interests.

An additional aspect of athletic identity that appears incongruent with counseling values is that athletes may privilege "doing" over "feeling" or "thinking." As such, athletes may view the life of the mind as a "black box" that is best left unexamined. Athletes may fear "loss of their mojo" if they dare to examine the inner workings of the apparatus that fuels their drive to achieve excellence. The elaborate superstitions espoused by some of the world's most accomplished athletes belie the lack of an explicit understanding of the relationship between mind and performance. At the same time, athletes exhibit an intense desire for control over their "mental game."

Given athletes' potential bias against introspection, it is not surprising to encounter distrust or even denigration of mental health services and the professionals who provide those services. Athletes, like the public more generally, may hold pejorative misconceptions of the mental health professional as psychologically intrusive, controlling, or even manipulative – "you just want to get inside my head – you're probably analyzing me right now."

These combined factors conspire to form a powerful impediment to utilization of mental health care by athletes. Unless the sports medicine professional is prepared to bridge the divide between the perception and the reality of mental health treatment, athletes may forestall mental health services, if not avoid them altogether, rather than risk threats to perceived mastery.

Stigma and Shame Compounding athletes' misunderstanding of the nature of mental health treatment, athletes may fear judgment and devaluation by their fellow athletes, coaches, or the general public. Because the conceptualization of mental health versus illness is so closely associated with notions of personal agency, an individual's self-worth can be undermined by any combination of distressing emotions, mental conflict, and dysfunctional behaviors.

Athletes are especially vulnerable to internalization of a negative self-image as a by-product of anticipated social stigma, in part because their identities are predicated on a presumption of competence, fortitude, and imperturbability. Particularly in the presence of an authority figure such as a coach or sports medicine professional, athletes may fear devaluation. Given the importance of social affirmation of human beings' identity as a condition of psychological survival, the prospect of negative appraisal by those whose opinions matter can seriously undermine one's sense of belonging. As such, athletes have historically refrained from disclosing to others their emotional suffering, unfortunately often to the detriment of their sport performance, not to mention personal well-being. The stigma of mental health for athletes is a topic that is further discussed in another chapter in this book.

Negative Outcomes No different than any other human being, athletes will refrain from help seeking if it results in an unfavorable risk-reward ratio [12]. To the extent that athletes have uncertainty as to how counseling could improve their functioning (fueled also by unflattering caricatures of therapists and clients in the popular media), athletes may question the wisdom of risking negative fallout from peers, family, coaches, etc. were those individuals to learn of an athlete's mental health treatment status.

Athletes may also fear that the nature of mental health treatment will be interminable, whether remaining on medications for "the rest of their life" or having to attend counseling indefinitely. The presumption of chronicity also speaks to the athlete's fear of losing a sense of competence and control. Together, these concerns speak to the importance that the athlete ascribes to self-determination and personal agency, in contrast to the role of passive care recipient.

An Applied Motivational Model of Effective Treatment Engagement

As described previously, self-determination theory proposes three key components of intrinsic motivation, including (1) the need for relatedness, (2) the need for competence, and (3) the need for individual autonomy [5]. From this perspective, to capitalize on an athlete's motivation for mental health treatment, one should look for opportunities to enhance the athlete's well-being by satisfying these primary motives (each representing a core psychological need). There is a range of strategies that a sports medicine professional may deploy in order to harness the "action potential" of these motives (see Table 18.1). These strategies adhere to the three conceptual clusters noted above, as follows: (1) relationship-based (relatedness), (2) knowledge-based (competence), and (3) action-based (autonomy).

Relationship-Based Strategies A relationship-based approach to mental health treatment engagement emphasizes the human need for interpersonal connection and belonging. By far, the most aversive element when contemplating mental health treatment is the perceived social cost. Given the pejorative attributions often directed at persons experiencing mental distress, the athlete may anticipate social distancing and ostracization. The physician can actively combat this expectation by promoting solid rapport with the athlete [21]. Even more powerfully, the physician can convey a sense of respect for the athlete as an individual actively pursuing physical and mental excellence, rather than as an impaired, passive recipient of another's clinical expertise.

By positioning the athlete as an active partner in his or her own care, it is that much easier to leverage a strong working relationship between the athlete and the mental health provider. The physician should endorse the expertise of the mental health professional as a specialist while simultaneously affirming the athlete's social legitimacy as the central member of a team assembled in the service of the athlete's own peak performance. This can be communicated concretely by endorsing prior positive treatment outcomes achieved through the coordinated efforts of physician, mental health professional, and athlete. By virtue of the physician's active and explicit endorsement of the athlete's membership in the peak performance triad

Table 18.1 An SDT-informed logic model of athlete mental health treatment engagement

	Key intrinsic motives for human behavior		
	Relatedness "We've all got 'mental stuff.' I'm no different from my peers."	**Competence** "I understand what's going on in my head. I can conquer my demons."	**Autonomy** "I alone call the shots. I'm in charge of my mental game."
Adaptive mindsets >>	Social legitimacy and belonging (as function of athletic identity/role)	Cognizance of the nature of mental functioning and behavior change	Ownership of one's mental functioning and enhancement
Impediments >>	Social stigma and self-stigma (shame and self-blame)	Stereotypes and superstitions (ignorance and naivete)	Selflessness and stasis (doubt, defensiveness, and denial)
Catalysts >>	*Relationship-based* Rapport and partnering	*Knowledge-based* Reframing and psychoeducation	*Action-based* "Change Talk" and stepwise experimentation
Interventions >>	Enhance identification with one's athletic peers ("same here") and universality of mental struggles Normalize help seeking as striving for mental excellence Promote positive prognosis (track record of mental health/behavior change outcomes)	Demystify the "black box" of psychological functioning *Mental well-being involves the following:* learning and growth process partnerships with mental experts skill/performance enhancement reclaiming one's mental agency	Model "change" values, including athlete self-awareness, flexibility, and agency Cost-benefit analysis for change Readiness for implementation Conduct "thought experiments" Recruitment of change resources

[6, 7, 12], the athlete does not have to disavow the presence of mental struggles in order to preserve his or her social status and self-worth. Ultimately, this offers the athlete the opportunity to not only embrace change but also experience him- or herself as the co-author of that same change process, rather than feeling incapable, pathologized, abnormal, deficient, or otherwise disenfranchised.

Knowledge-Based Strategies The second element that can be a resource for treatment engagement is the opportunity for the physician to provide psychoeducation (sometimes defined as "mental health literacy") [1, 9, 16, 17, 20]. The physician must convey to the athlete a means of understanding the mental landscape that the athlete is wishing to navigate in the service of enhanced well-being and peak performance. The athlete benefits from an appreciation that mental functions can be decipherable, amenable to change, and ultimately a source of motivation, confidence, and poise. Because the emphasis is on mastery and self-awareness, not pathology, the athlete can embrace the reparative nature of the therapy process, not unlike what they would experience were they to undergo physical rehabilitation after a more traditional injury.

It is easier for the athlete to tolerate mental distress and attenuate strong maladaptive impulses when he or she can understand that thoughts, feelings, and behaviors have an intrinsic functional relationship to one another. Self-acceptance forms the motivational basis to "befriend" and ultimately master one's "mental game," rather than disavow the existence of so-called maladaptive thoughts and feelings (which only fuel shame and self-loathing). When the athlete absolves him- or herself of wholesale blame for mental suffering, while still taking responsibility for his or her mental rebound and growth, this obviates the need for additional defensiveness and acting out and attenuates anxiety and depression.

Action-Based Strategies Given the emphasis on autonomy, action-based treatment engagement strategies align well with the Transtheoretical Model (TTM) of behavior change and its concept of readiness therein [19]. The stages of change in TTM include *contemplation*, *preparation*, and *implementation* as three key stages. In order to embrace treatment, the athlete must relinquish a stance of pseudo-agency whereby control over one's psychological distress is obtained through disavowal and avoidance. Instead, the physician assists the athlete to take assertive ownership of the change process by actively and explicitly considering the need for change, potential positive or negative consequences of change, obstacles and facilitators of change, and one's overall readiness to initiate change at the present moment. Depending on the athlete's position along the readiness continuum, the physician can propose perspectives and tasks to promote the athlete's readiness for treatment engagement.

Based on the athlete's sense of social legitimacy as an individual in pursuit of excellence and his or her cognizance of the nature of one's mental experience, the athlete can be assisted in committing to change. The physician may use motivational interviewing techniques [15] to elicit "change talk." For example, the athlete can be prompted to identify at what point along a continuum of severity and impact they would be sufficiently motivated to seek formal professional assistance to change their situation (e.g., "What would cause you sufficient concern to cause you to want to do something about how you're feeling right now?"). Most individuals have a bottom line at which point further impact becomes a "deal breaker" for business as usual. This functions to delineate a finite threshold for taking action. The physician could alternately encourage the athlete to imagine how his or her life might be different without the mental issue being present, as well as ask the athlete to establish the relative benefit of such an outcome.

The physician could also promote an openness to an attitude of incremental experimentation, to insure the athlete experiences any change efforts as tolerable due to their finite nature, with an emphasis on "testing the waters," rather than having to make a broad and irrevocable commitment to behavior change. Similarly, the physician can highlight the pragmatic feasibility of small gains and "low-hanging fruit," (i.e., behavioral improvement that requires the least investment of effort or is most amenable to modification). These efforts can be further encouraged by emphasizing how little is truly at stake ("What do you have to lose by trying? Life will be happy to refund your misery").

Conclusion

Athletes may have a need for timely, effective mental health treatment to maintain well-being and attenuate the risk of impaired mental and physical performance. Unfortunately, social stigma, stereotypes, and avoidance of one's distress can interfere with successful treatment engagement on the part of the athlete, especially given the performance pressures athletes face. Sports medicine professionals are uniquely positioned to assist athletes by offering a "prescription for excellence" which frames mental health services in the context of "whole person" peak performance [12] (i.e., mind and body as an integrated and high-achieving singular entity). As such, the sports medicine provider can help the athlete embrace the opportunity for mental health treatment enthusiastically in the spirit of enhanced relatedness, competence, and autonomy.

References

1. Breslin G, Shannon S, Haughey T, Donnelly P, Leavey G. A systematic review of interventions to increase awareness of mental health and well-being in athletes, coaches and officials. Syst Rev. 2017;6:177. https://doi.org/10.1186/s13643-017-0568-6.
2. Byatt N, Levin LL, Ziedonis D, Moore Simas TA, Allison J. Enhancing participation in depression care in outpatient perinatal care settings: a systematic review. Obstet Gynecol. 2015;126(5):1048–58. https://doi.org/10.1097/AOG.0000000000001067.
3. Chang WH, Chang J-H, Chen LH. Mindfulness enhances change in athletes' Well-being: the mediating role of basic psychological needs fulfillment. Mindfulness. 2018;9(3):815–23. https://doi.org/10.1007/s12671-017-0821-z.
4. Daltry R, Milliner K, James TC. Understanding gender differences in collegiate student-Athletes' help-seeking behaviors and attitudes toward counseling. Int J Sport Soc Ann Rev. 2018;9(1):11–21.
5. Deci EL, Ryan RM. The 'what' and 'why' of goal pursuits: human needs and the self-determination of behavior. Psychol Inq. 2000;11(4):227–68. https://doi.org/10.1207/S15327965PLI1104_01.
6. Donohue B, Chow GM, Pitts M, Loughran T, Schubert KN, Gavrilova Y, et al. Piloting a family-supported approach to concurrently optimize mental health and sport performance in athletes. Clin Case Stud. 2015;14(3):159–77. https://doi.org/10.1177/1534650114548311.
7. Gavrilova Y, Donohue B, Galante M. Mental health and sport performance programming in athletes who present without pathology: a case examination supporting optimization. Clin Case Stud. 2017;16(3):234–53. https://doi.org/10.1177/1534650116689302.
8. Gucciardi DF, Hanton S, Fleming S. Are mental toughness and mental health contradictory concepts in elite sport? A narrative review of theory and evidence. J Sci Med Sport. 2017;20(3):307–11.
9. Herring SAea. Psychological issues related to injury in athletes and the team physician: a consensus statement. Med Sci Sports Exerc. 2006;38(11):2030–4. https://doi.org/10.1249/mss.0b013e31802b37a6.
10. Kipp LE, Weiss MR. Social influences, psychological need satisfaction, and well-being among female adolescent gymnasts. Sport Exerc Perform Psychol. 2013;2(1):62–75. https://doi.org/10.1037/a0030236.
11. Klein MC, Ciotoli C, Chung H. Primary care screening of depression and treatment engagement in a University Health Center: a retrospective analysis. J Am Coll Heal. 2011;59(4):289–95.

12. Kroshus E. Stigma, coping skills, and psychological help seeking among collegiate athletes. Athl Train Sports Health Care J Pract Clin. 2017;9(6):254–62.
13. Mann BJ, Grana WA, Indelicato PA, O'Neill DF, George SZ. A survey of sports medicine physicians regarding psychological issues in patient-athletes. Am J Sports Med. 2007;35(12):2140–7.
14. McLoughlin G, Fecske CW, Castaneda Y, Gwin C, Graber K. Sport participation for elite athletes with physical disabilities: motivations, barriers, and facilitators. Adapt Phys Act Q. 2017;34(4):421–41. https://doi.org/10.1123/apaq.2016-0127.
15. Miller WR, Rose GS. Toward a theory of motivational interviewing. Am Psychol. 2009;64(6):527–37. https://doi.org/10.1037/a0016830.
16. Neal TL, Diamond AB, Goldman S, Klossner D, Morse ED, Pajak DE, et al. Inter-association recommendations for developing a plan to recognize and refer student-athletes with psychological concerns at the collegiate level: an executive summary of a consensus statement. J Athl Train (Allen Press). 2013;48(5):716–20.
17. Neal TL, Diamond AB, Goldman S, Liedtka KD, Mathis K, Morse ED, et al. Interassociation recommendations for developing a plan to recognize and refer student-athletes with psychological concerns at the secondary school level: a consensus statement. J Athl Train (Allen Press). 2015;50(3):231–49.
18. Pace CA, Gergen-Barnett K, Veidis A, D'Afflitti J, Worcester J, Fernandez P, et al. Warm handoffs and attendance at initial integrated behavioral health appointments. Ann Fam Med. 2018;16(4):346–8. https://doi.org/10.1370/afm.2263.
19. Prochaska JO, DiClemente CC, Norcross JC. In search of how people change: applications to addictive behaviors. Am Psychol. 1992;47(9):1102–14. https://doi.org/10.1037/0003-066X.47.9.1102.
20. Sebbens J, Hassmén P, Crisp D, Wensley K. Mental Health in Sport (MHS): improving the early intervention knowledge and confidence of elite sport staff. Front Psychol. 2016;7:911. https://doi.org/10.3389/fpsyg.2016.00911.
21. Trojian T. Depression is under-recognised in the sport setting: time for primary care sports medicine to be proactive and screen widely for depression symptoms. Br J Sports Med. 2016;50(3):137–9.
22. Wolanin A, Hong E, Marks D, Panchoo K, Gross M. Prevalence of clinically elevated depressive symptoms in college athletes and differences by gender and sport. Br J Sports Med. 2016;50(3):167–71.

Chapter 19
Mindfulness Approaches to Athlete Well-Being

Mike Gross

In recent years, the psychological construct of mindfulness has gained increased attention in the field of sport psychology. Prior to the year 2000, a search criteria of "mindfulness and sports" in the database PsycInfo resulted in only one publication. Since that time, the same search criteria result in 298 publications (e.g., book chapters, peer-reviewed journal articles, and dissertations). This increase in mindfulness-based sport psychology research publications coincides with the development of several mindfulness-based interventions created specifically for athletes such as the Mindfulness-Acceptance-Commitment (MAC; [1]) approach, Mindful Sport Performance Enhancement (MSPE; [2, 3]), and Mindfulness Meditation Training for Sport (MMTS; [4]). More broadly, the term mindfulness has started to become commonplace in athletics. There have been stories in popular media outlets such as ESPN and Sports Illustrated [5, 6] discussing the growth of mindfulness among elite athletes and teams. This has led to eye-catching headlines such as "Meditation, mindfulness, and the rise of the baseball shrinks" [7] and attention-grabbing stories about championship-level teams such as Pete Carroll's Seattle Seahawks, Phil Jackson's Los Angeles Lakers and Bulls, and Joe Maddon's Chicago Cubs using mindfulness training with seemingly remarkable success. Even meditation apps have made news in the sports world as it was reported in March 2018 that Headspace (a popular meditation app) agreed to a partnership with the National Basketball Association (NBA).

The rise in popularity of mindfulness training among athletes comes on the heels of a significant increase in research-based mindfulness publications in the clinical psychology literature since the 1990s. For frame of reference, in the year 1990, there were only five mindfulness research publications, and by the year 2016, there were 692 [8]. This number has only continued to grow, and a vast body of research has demonstrated the effectiveness of mindfulness-based

M. Gross (✉)
Princeton University, Princeton, NJ, USA
e-mail: mg46@princeton.edu

© Springer Nature Switzerland AG 2020
E. Hong, A. L. Rao (eds.), *Mental Health in the Athlete*,
https://doi.org/10.1007/978-3-030-44754-0_19

interventions (MBIs) for a wide range of mental and physical health concerns, all of which can impact athletes. Research on MBIs for mental health concerns has demonstrated their effectiveness for reducing anxiety and depression [9], eating pathology [10], insomnia [11], and substance use [12]. MBIs have also been shown to be beneficial for physical health concerns such as chronic pain [13] and immune functioning [14, 15].

Given the competitive nature of sports and the desire for athletes to gain a "mental edge," it is more common to see a news article discuss how the development of mindfulness can help athletes improve some aspect of performance than it is to see it connected to mental health. For example, it is not uncommon to see articles talk about how mindfulness can help athletes reduce distraction, execute under pressure, and decrease anxiety in high-pressure situations. Despite some notable limitations such as small sample sizes, sole reliance on self-report measures, lack of randomization, and suboptimal controls, the sport psychology research literature does support some of these claims. Research on mindfulness for sport performance has evidenced its effectiveness in a number of areas including improving concentration [16], increasing mindful awareness and attention [17], increasing state flow [2], decreasing sport-related worry [18], greater attention to task-relevant information [19], and improving sport performance [16, 20–22].

Viewing mindfulness as a "technique" or "method" to help athletes improve sport performance or gain a mental edge is a limited perspective on the potential for mindful-based approaches. Extrapolating from the growing body of research on mindfulness, this chapter will focus on how MBIs can benefit the overall psychological well-being of athletes, not just their sport performance. First, this chapter will define mindfulness and address common misconceptions associated with it. What follows will be a breakdown of the core mechanisms targeted by MBIs and how addressing these areas, which are thought to underlie mental health concerns, can be of benefit to athletes.

What Is Mindfulness?

The word mindfulness conjures up various meanings and images for different people, and this can be problematic when explaining mindfulness to athletes. As such, to describe mindfulness, it often can be helpful to first address misconceptions. Mindfulness is not emptying the mind, attaining enlightenment, changing the content of thoughts and feelings to be more positive, turning off thoughts, or a religious practice. Mindfulness *is not* relaxation training, and this is an important point to make when describing mindfulness to athletes because it is a frequent misconception. Relaxation may be a byproduct of engaging in some form of mindfulness training, but it definitely is not an inherent goal. Lastly, mindfulness is not solely meditation. Rather, mindfulness is an awareness that arises as Kabat-Zinn [23] describes through "paying attention in a particular way; on purpose, in the present moment, and nonjudgmentally" (p. 4).

Mindfulness can be thought of as a way of being, rather than a specific practice (e.g., meditation). This way of being is characterized by nonjudgmental acceptance of one's moment-by-moment experience, increased awareness, a present moment focus, openness, curiosity, kindness, and compassion. A mindfulness exercise such as a 15-minute meditation on breath can be used to help cultivate this way of being, in the same way that bicep curls can be used to develop a larger bicep muscle. However, doing 15 minutes of meditation per day will likely not be enough to develop a mindful way of being if outside of the meditation an athlete is living their life mindlessly. Similarly, an athlete is unlikely to get in good playing shape for the season if they exercise daily but also eat fast food for every meal. As such, the cultivation of mindfulness can be developed in all our moments. We can eat mindfully, shower mindfully, stretch mindfully, communicate mindfully, read mindfully, walk mindfully, and so on.

Based upon this premise, a good question to explore with athletes is "are you living your life mindlessly or mindfully?" For example, a student-athlete at a university could walk mindlessly to class (e.g., head buried in their smartphone, worrying about an upcoming game, dwelling on a mistake made in yesterday's practice) or mindfully (e.g., noticing the sensations of the air against the skin, feeling the movement of the arms and legs, and bringing attention back to the present moment whenever the mind drifts off into the future or past). As stated by Kabat-Zinn [24], "the real meditation is how you live your life," and the remainder of this chapter will discuss how cultivating this way of being can be beneficial to the overall well-being of athletes, specifically as they deal with sport-specific stressors.

Mindfulness and Sport-Related Stress

The life of an athlete can often involve dealing with a significant amount of stressors. In particular, there are several sport-related stressors that can impact the overall psychological well-being of athletes [25]. A range of sport-specific stressors have been identified including time demands, coping with injury, loss of status/playing time, opportunities for failure, negative relationships with coaches and teammates, performance pressures, career transitions and termination, and overtraining/burnout [25–28]. Although these stressors can have a deleterious effect upon on athlete's psychological functioning and mental health, there has historically been a stigma in sports that athletes need to demonstrate strength and toughness in the face of issues that impact their mental well-being. This perhaps was best stated in a recent TED Talk about dealing with depression and an eating disorder given by University of Southern California (USC) women's volleyball player Victoria Garrick. In this talk, she stated, "Why? Why did it take me so long to acknowledge and accept my illness? And I realized the culture that we live in as athletes does not make it easy for us to honor this. If you think about it… the culture of athletics preaches – "Where there is a will there is a way," "The best don't rest," "Unless you puke, faint or die keep going." "Mental illness is associated with weakness. To appear weak is the last thing an athlete wants."

Fortunately, thanks to athletes like Victoria Garrick, in recent years, a growing conversation surrounding the topic of mental health and athletes has arose. There has been an increased effort to identify athletes who may benefit from accessing resources related to mental health, efforts to normalize help-seeking among athletes, and greater attempts at fostering a health-promoting environment that supports the mental well-being of athletes [29]. There have also been several examples of elite athletes such as Michael Phelps, Brandon Marshall, Allison Schmitt, Imani Boyette, DeMar DeRozan, and Kevin Love opening up about mental health concerns such as anxiety, depression, eating disorders, substance use, and bipolar disorder. Even coaches have come forward, such as Cleveland Cavalier's coach Tyronn Lue. In a recent interview, Lue described that anxiety was the reason he did not coach several games in the second half of the 2017–2018 season [30].

As the importance of mental health awareness has grown among athletes, sport psychologists have been hired in steadily increasing numbers to work at Division I universities and colleges with a primary responsibility of helping athletes deal with mental health concerns. At the highest levels of sport, a greater emphasis is being placed upon athlete mental health, and this was perhaps most notably made clear when the National Basketball Players Association (NBPA) hired a Director of Mental Health and Wellness in May 2018. Given this growing awareness and due to the fact that athletes confront several unique stressors specific to their sport participation that have the potential to impact their psychological well-being, identifying interventions that may buffer stress is an important consideration for those working with athletes. From a theoretical standpoint, the literature suggests that MBIs should be beneficial for helping athletes deal with stress and enhancing overall psychological well-being (e.g., [16]). This makes sense considering that a substantial body of literature has demonstrated that MBIs can help a number of different populations manage stress more effectively and improve psychological well-being [31–33].

To date, there have been very few studies with athlete samples that have demonstrated the effectiveness of MBIs for mental health-related concerns and well-being. Gross et al. [20] conducted a randomized control trial (RCT) comparing the MAC approach to traditional psychological skills training (PST) among a sample of female college athletes and found that the MAC was effective in reducing psychological symptoms, behavioral difficulties, and emotional distress. In another study, using a sample of college athletes from a wide range of sports, it was found that MSPE may be an effective intervention to prevent the escalation of depressive symptoms [34]. In addition, a recent study found that a five-session mindfulness-based program led to reduced anxiety and increased well-being among a sample of university athletes [35].

Although there is a small body of research that appears to suggest that MBIs could be beneficial for the psychological well-being of athletes, it is also important to explore the mechanisms by which mindfulness can foster change. In other words, understanding *how* mindfulness can work to improve the psychological functioning of athletes is necessary and essential. As such, what follows will be an exploration of three processes believed to be associated with change in MBIs and how these processes can be used specifically to help athletes deal with stress and potentially improve well-being. The three processes are cognitive defusion, present moment focus, and acceptance. As will be described, these processes do not operate in isolation but rather interact with one another to help promote mindfulness.

Cognitive Defusion

A common misconception about mindfulness is that it entails attaining a state of nonthinking or cultivating positive thoughts. Neither is true. Rather, the intention of mindfulness practice is *to develop a moment-by-moment awareness of the process of thinking*. In other words, mindfulness involves developing the ability to observe the process of thinking itself without getting caught up in the content of those thoughts. A frequently used analogy to highlight this point is to view thoughts as if they are cars passing on the highway or clouds floating through the sky. In taking this approach, it is necessary to view thoughts just as thoughts, rather than the truth or absolute facts. In presentations to athletes, the author of this chapter will frequently state, "Just because you think it does not mean it's true." For example, if a child is mad at their mom for not letting them have ice cream for dessert, they may think "I hate my mom." Just because they think that does not mean it is true. In a very similarly way, if a football player has all the signs of depression and thinks "I cannot tell anyone about this because everyone will think I am weak," just because he thinks that doesn't mean it is true. In addition to emphasizing this point, exploring the costs (e.g., not seeking help) of buying into this type of thought would also be important to address.

The approach described above is known as cognitive defusion. The term cognitive defusion comes from the Acceptance and Commitment Therapy (ACT; [36]) literature, a third-wave behavioral therapy which emphasizes mindfulness and acceptance. The target of cognitive defusion is not to alter the content of thinking, but rather to change our relationship with thoughts. By contrast, when we fuse with the content of thoughts, particularly when unhelpful, there is an increased risk for the development and maintenance of mental health issues [37]. For example, if an athlete suffers an injury and during the rehabilitation process has thoughts such as "My teammates don't want me around anymore," "Nobody cares about me," and "I'll never recover from this" *and buys into them*, then there may be an increased risk for avoidance behaviors (e.g., pulling away from teammates, lack of rehabilitation adherence) that could lead to the development of a depressive episode. As noted by Hayes, Strosahl, and Wilson [38], "Suffering occurs when people so strongly believe the literal contents of their mind that they become fused with their cognitions" (p. 20). However, if an athlete is taught through mindfulness training to simply observe those thoughts as nothing more than passing mental events, then the potential for avoidance and mental health concerns may decrease. Yet, this approach typically does not take place in an athletic context because athletes and those working with them are often socialized from an early age to believe that eliminating "negative" thoughts is necessary in order to function optimally. As such, the injured athlete described above may attempt to fix, control, or eliminate unhelpful thoughts, and this approach may be reinforced by others who know the athlete through using phrases such as "don't think about that" or making reassuring comments such as "everybody on the team cares about you." Although well-meaning, this approach can often reinforce the idea that changing the content of thoughts is necessary for symptom improvement. To provide another example, a swimmer with anorexia nervosa (an eating disorder characterized by being underweight) may think "I look ugly in my bathing suit, I need to lose weight" or "Everybody is looking at my legs, they must be thinking how fat they are." Telling this swimmer "you look great the way you are" or even worse "you are already so thin, you actually need to gain weight" would not be helpful. Rather, it would likely be more effective to help the swimmer see those thoughts as the "eating disorder story" and to change their relationship with that story so it no longer leads to eating disordered behaviors (i.e., food restriction) that maintain their condition.

To introduce cognitive defusion to an athlete, a strategy used by this chapter's author is to compare the mind to a sportscaster. Similar to a sportscaster, the mind is constantly analyzing, judging, commenting, criticizing, predicting, dwelling, and so on. If we are watching a sporting event and do not like what the sportscaster is saying, we can hit the mute button or perhaps turn to another station with a different announcer. However, the same approach does not work for our thoughts. We cannot hit the mute button on our thoughts. Nor can we easily "change the station," and efforts to do so may actually be problematic. Research suggests that attempts to suppress or eliminate unwanted thoughts can often lead to an increase in the frequency and intensity of the very thoughts we are attempting to avoid [39]. As noted by the mindfulness expert Jon Kabat-Zinn in his book *Full Catastrophe Living* [24], "trying to suppress thoughts will only result in greater tension and frustration and more problems, not in calmness, insight, clarity, and peace" (p. 66). This notion was reinforced in an interview with basketball superstar and known meditator Kobe Bryant when he stated, "When my 'obnoxious roommate' knocks on the door in my head, I've found it's better just to let him in. If you try to tune him out, he just bangs louder. If you let him in, he sits down, watches TV and shuts up."

In contrast to attempting to fix, control, or eliminate thoughts, the mindfulness approach suggests that our thoughts will just come and go if we simply allow them to. This requires that athletes put in the necessary mental repetitions to shift attention away from trying to fight or control the "sportscaster mind" and toward developing the "observing mind." The observing mind is characterized by simply watching thoughts come and go without judgment or getting caught up in them, the same way an individual could observe a sunset. There are several mindfulness exercises such as sitting meditations (e.g., breath meditation, body scan, meditation of sound, leaves on a stream) and cognitive defusion strategies that can help develop this ability. Given cognitive defusion can be difficult, particularly initially, to fully comprehend, this author recommends athletes to check out YouTube videos that discuss this concept. For example, searching "changing perspective headspace" on YouTube offers an excellent description of defusion. However, the practice of cognitive defusion is best understood experientially (e.g., through actually practicing it), rather than intellectually. As such, below are a few ways to promote defusion:

- Put the following words in front of your thought – "My mind is telling me that….." or "I notice my mind is having the thought that….":
  - Doing this type of exercise creates distance between yourself and your thoughts. Try it out: "My mind is telling me that I am never going to return from this injury" versus "I am never going to be able to return from this injury." The first one promotes defusion and can help an athlete realize that a thought is just a thought, not the literal truth. This can seem unnatural at first, so it is recommended to practice it many times throughout the day. It is also recommended to keep in mind that if the thought arises – "this technique doesn't work for me," you really should be rephrasing that as "my mind is telling me this technique doesn't work for me."
- Sing your thoughts to a popular tune or say them in a funny voice (not aloud):
  - An athlete can start to become less fused with thoughts when they say something like "Everyone on the team hates me" in the voice of Stewie from Family Guy or a Minion from Despicable Me. Or sing that phrase to the tune of Happy Birthday. This should be done in your mind, not aloud.
- Be aware, acknowledge, and do an attentional shift:
  - The idea here is to first notice (awareness) when you are fused with a particular thought. In doing so, you step out of automatic pilot and the ongoing narrative in your mind. When you notice and acknowledge you are caught up in unhelpful thinking, you can then use your senses to shift your attention back into the present moment. A great way to do that is to check in with all your senses. Notice one thing you see. Notice one thing you feel. Notice one thing you smell. Notice one thing you hear. The idea is to notice when you are caught up in unhelpful thinking, acknowledge it, and gently shift your attention back into the present moment. You may need to do this over and over and over again, but consider it weight training for the mind.
- Remind yourself that thoughts do not guide behavior:
  - A quick exercise that can be done with athletes is to have them think in silence the thought "I can't raise my hand, I can't raise my hand," over and over again. And then, ask them to raise their hand. This highlights the point that even though your mind is saying something that does not mean it is true or that you have to obey its direction. Problem is we often reinforce thoughts when we buy into them and let them guide our behavior. For example, it is quite common to get home from work or wake up in the morning and the mind to say something like "I cannot exercise today. I am just too tired. I just do not feel like it." When you listen to those thoughts and do not go exercise, then those types of thoughts only grow stronger and will take more control over your behavior. Remember you control your behavior, not the words of your mind.

Present Moment Awareness

The second core mechanism targeted by mindfulness that can benefit athletes is present moment awareness. Present moment awareness involves attending to current experience rather than worrying about the future or ruminating about past events. Much easier said than done. So often, we, as human beings, live our lives caught up in distraction and mind wandering that we do not fully connect to the present moment. Research has found that a "wandering mind is an unhappy mind," [40] and unfortunately, our minds wander approximately between a third and a half of our waking lives [41]. The development of present moment awareness has been associated with a number of benefits including lower levels of anxiety and depression [42], lower levels of perceived stress [43], and improved well-being [37].

The nature of being an athlete carries with it a litany of material that can distract attention away from being fully present. Athletes may frequently worry about the future – upcoming performances, fear of reinjury, concern about losing a starting position, concern about an intense practice happening later in the day, fear about being called in for a difficult conversation with the coach, concerns about a burdensome travel schedule, and pondering their post-career future. There is also plenty of opportunity to think about the past such as replaying a past performance, dwelling on a perceived slight such as not being chosen as captain or given "enough minutes," replaying an injury, brooding on a loss, and reflecting on perceived failures or mistakes. Often when the mind drifts into these places, it can be problematic and detrimental to an athlete's overall psychological well-being. As such, athletes may benefit from learning mindfulness strategies to help promote present moment awareness. As noted by Kaufman, Glass, and Pineau [44], "seizing opportunities to reconnect with the present moment is the essential work that may allow participants (athletes) to derive benefits from MSPE for athletic performance and everyday life" (p. 92).

A central component of mindfulness involves flexibility of attention and developing the ability to consciously direct attention on various aspects of experience as desired [45]. It can be important to emphasize to athletes that attention is trainable and can be built through mindfulness exercises. As part of training present moment awareness, it is necessary to focus first on awareness itself. Essentially, it is not possible to bring attention back to the moment if an athlete is unaware that the mind has wandered. So, the first step is to help athletes actively notice when the mind has wandered and where it has gone. Once an athlete develops the ability to catch the wandering mind, then the next step is to bring attention back into the present moment.

There are ways to do this through formal and informal mindfulness exercises. For example, the MAC protocol includes a formal mindfulness exercise called the brief centering exercise in which athletes are prompted to pay attention to different aspects of their experience (breath, sounds, bodily sensations) and when the mind wanders to simply bring attention back to these objects of awareness [1]. A similar exercise is a sitting breath meditation which is part of many MBIs, such as MSPE which offers a 9-minute sitting breath meditation to athletes in session 1 of its protocol [44]. In this exercise, the breath is used as an anchor to ground attention in the present moment, and the instruction is to notice whenever the mind wanders from the breath and when it does (as it will over and over and over again) to return attention back to the breath. Each time the mind wanders and attention is brought back to the breath, it can be considered a mental repetition to help build and sculpt the muscle of attention. Common concerns that athletes express when doing this type of formal meditation is "I don't feel like I am doing it right" or "I am not good at this meditation stuff." This makes sense given that this is a population that is frequently striving to excel. However, meditation is a form of non-striving, and efforting to "get it right" will only serve as an impediment to progress. As such, athletes should be reminded that as long as they are noticing when the mind wanders and returning back to the breath (even if it is for just one second) and doing that repeatedly, then that is all that is necessary.

Informal mindfulness exercises can include doing any activity mindfully. As an example, the MAC protocol includes a "Washing a Dish" mindful exercise in which athletes are instructed to pay attention to their various senses while they wash a dish. As another way to teach this concept, athletes can attend to various aspects of their experience while playing a sport such as having a softball player feel the sensations that arise from the contact of the bat or glove against the hand. Or a basketball player can hear the sound of the bouncing ball or sneakers against the floor. It is the hope that through these types of exercises, athletes will grasp the idea that there exist several ways to ground attention in the present moment, and the key is to practice both formally and informally on a daily basis.

Fortunately, there are a number of resources available to help athletes develop present moment awareness. A frequently recommended app is Headspace because it has specific meditations for sport and uses an engaging approach to teach mindfulness. Another useful meditation app is 10% Happier, and this app features the opportunity to learn more about mindfulness from some of the world's most accomplished mindfulness teachers. There are also free resources available online for guided meditations. For example, a google search of UC San Diego health and mindfulness audio connects to a page that has several guided meditations.

Acceptance

MBIs emphasize acceptance of internal processes such as thoughts and emotions. From the perspective of mindfulness, there are no right or wrong thoughts or emotions, but rather, it is the struggle to have the "right" thoughts and emotions that cause a great deal of suffering and interference with functioning. As such, MBIs aim to change an individual's relationship with their internal processes to become more open, accepting, allowing, and loving. This requires the *willingness* to remain in contact with rather than avoid internal experiences. Acceptance should not be viewed as giving up or resignation, but rather the willingness to be with discomfort. This is often what is required to grow in both sport and life.

With mindfulness training, athletes can learn that judging, suppressing, and pushing away thoughts and emotion are not effective strategies. All of those strategies can be classified as experiential avoidance which stands in contrast to acceptance and is defined as "the phenomenon that occurs when a person is unwilling to remain in contact with particular private experiences (e.g., bodily sensations, emotions, thoughts, memories, behavioral predispositions) and takes steps to alter the form or frequency of these events and the contexts that occasion them" ([46], p. 1156). In the short term, experiential avoidance can be effective in ameliorating discomfort; however, when used rigidly and inflexibly over the long term, it can have very detrimental effects and psychological consequences. Experiential avoidance has been associated with a wide range of psychopathological problems and correlates with psychological symptoms across diagnostic categories [47]. Further, individuals with higher levels of experiential avoidance tend to experience reduced emotionally positive life experiences, life satisfaction, meaningful life experiences, and fewer positive day-to-day events [48].

That said, it is quite possible that the very nature of being an athlete within an emotionally inhibitive athletic context may impact an athlete's relationship with so-called "negative" internal experiences. Although in some athletic contexts there is an evolving understanding and acceptance of mental health in recent years, the culture of athletics can often send several messages to athletes centered around the notion that they should be mentally and physically "tough." Therefore, an athlete may start to internalize such beliefs feeling they need to portray confidence, positivity, and mental toughness. Mankad, Gordon, and Wallman [49] highlighted this point in a study which qualitatively examined nine injured athletes' perceptions of the emotional climate of their sporting environment during their long-term rehabilitation process. The athletes surveyed in this study reportedly engaged in suppressive coping strategies and avoidance behaviors due to fear that they would be negatively evaluated by coaches and teammates had they fully disclosed their emotional distress. Although this study had a small sample size, it provides some evidence that the athletic context is one in which athletes are encouraged to inhibit rather than disclose their emotional distress. This is problematic considering inhibiting thoughts and emotions associated with an acute injury can be psychologically detrimental and maintain trauma-related symptoms. As such, for injury and other sport-related stressors, a mindful approach that encourages approaching difficult or unpleasant experiences with openness and interest, rather than avoidance and suppression, is emphasized.

This chapter's author often introduces a three-step approach for those dealing with emotional discomfort using the following instructions:

Step 1: Notice It Notice sensations of anxiety (or other forms of emotional discomfort) in the body. Perhaps certain body parts – the hands, feet, jaw, toes, and forehead – are clenched/tight. Let a spotlight zoom in on where you are carrying tension in your body (i.e., grip on the golf club, bat, racket, etc.). With openness and curiosity, observe the sensations of anxiety in your body and the thoughts/images associated with it. Remember you are separate from your thoughts and feelings. You are not anxiety. You are the audience, the observer, and the watcher of your emotional experience, not the emotional experience itself. In this sense, you can observe anxiety for what it really is – a cluster of thoughts, emotions, and physiological sensations – that can be viewed without judgment as passing internal states. Nothing more, nothing less.

Step 2: Name It Once you notice emotional discomfort in the body, you can then name it. "This is anxiety," "This is frustration," or "Here is anxiety," "Here is frustration." You can also name the thoughts associated with emotional discomfort such as "there is judging," "there is doubt," "there is self-criticism," or "there is impatience."

Step 3: Make Space for It With practice, you can learn to put out the red carpet for anxiety rather than fighting to make it walk the plank. It is already here, why fight it? Just make room for it. If it is already here, why not greet it with kindness, compassion, and openness. When anxiety or other forms of emotional discomfort arise, perhaps you can imagine an emoji waving hello or a welcome mat. Imagine creating space within you as vast as a golf course and just opening up to whatever is there to be experienced. You may not like it but you can make space for it.

Ultimately, the capacity to be mindful entails accepting whatever is coming up in that moment even if it is painful or difficult and taking an attitude of curiosity and openness toward it.

Conclusion

The above review was intended to describe how targeting core processes common to MBIs can be used to help promote athlete well-being. To date, only a few studies have explored the effectiveness of MBIs for athlete well-being, and these studies have been limited by issues such as small sample sizes. A number of questions remain about how to best implement MBIs for athlete well-being; for example, how many sessions are needed, and how often and for how long should an athlete meditate to get the most benefit? Based on the growing clinical psychology literature on mindfulness, it does make conceptual sense that MBIs would be beneficial for athlete well-being. This chapter author hypothesizes that athletes who can become less fused with cognitions and establish greater connection to the present moment and are more accepting of the full range of human thoughts and emotions would derive benefits from MBIs. Further research is necessary to assess to what degree these core processes impact athlete well-being, if some processes are more valuable to address than others, and what other processes would be beneficial to target.

Fortunately, as athletes have become more forthcoming about mental health issues, there has also been an observable growth in the use of MBIs among an athletic population. Even over the course of writing this chapter, more and more professional athletes have come forward to publicly reveal their struggles with mental health concerns. It does appear that the stigma surrounding mental health and athletes is decreasing, although it certainly remains a significant and ongoing issue that needs to be addressed in the athletic environment. If the trend continues in the direction of a decrease in mental health stigma, there likely will be an increase in athletes seeking mental health treatment. For example, it was over a decade ago that Watson [50] found that student-athletes are less willing than nonathletes to seek mental health treatment. However, in a recent study, Barnard [51] found that student-athletes were just as likely as nonathletes to seek mental health treatment. Barnard [51] concluded that although the generalizability of the findings is a limitation, this may provide some indication that over time, the gap between help-seeking behavior of athletes and nonathletes has decreased. If that is true, it is important that sport psychologists and other sport medicine professionals working with athletes are aware of and understand interventions that are efficacious and effective. As contended in this chapter, more research is definitely needed, and the potential benefit of MBIs offers promise for the future of improving athlete well-being.

References

1. Gardner FL, Moore ZE. The psychology of human performance: the mindfulness-acceptance-commitment approach. New York: Springer; 2007.
2. Kaufman KA, Glass CR, Arnkoff DB. Evaluation of Mindful Sport Performance Enhancement (MSPE): a new approach to promote flow in athletes. J Clin Sport Psychol. 2009;3:334–56.
3. Kaufman KA, Glass CR. Mindful Sport Performance Enhancement: a treatment manual for archers and golfers. Unpublished manuscript, The Catholic University of America, Washington, DC; 2006.
4. Baltzell A, Akhtar VL. Mindfulness Meditation Training for Sport (MMTS) intervention: impact of MMTS with division I female athletes. J Happiness Well Being. 2014;2(2):160–73.
5. Joyner MJ. Get healthy in 2016: how meditation, sleep and more can calm your mind. 2016. Website. https://www.si.com/edge/2016/02/25/getting-healthy-in-2016-mental-training-sleep-meditation-mindfulness. Accessed 11 Jan 2018.
6. Roenigk A. Settle Seahawks use unusual techniques in practice. 2013. Website. https://www.espn.com/nfl/story/_/id/9581925/seattle-seahawks-use-unusual-techniques-practice-espn-magazine. Accessed 11 Jan 2018.
7. Foley M. Meditation, mindfulness, and the rise of the baseball shrinks. 2017. Website. https://www.ozy.com/the-huddle/meditation-mindfulness-and-the-rise-of-baseball-shrinks/76525. Accessed 11 Jan 2018.
8. Black DS. Mindfulness journal publications by year, 1980–2016. Website. https://goamra.org/resources/. Accessed 11 Jan 2018.
9. Hofmann SG, Sawyer AT, Witt AA, Oh D. The effect of mindfulness-based therapy on anxiety and depression: a meta-analytic review. J Consult. 2010;78(2):169–83.
10. Wanden-Berghe RG, Sanz-Valero J, Wanden-Berghe C. The application of mindfulness to eating disorders treatment: a systematic review. Eat Disord. 2011;19(1):34–48.
11. Gong H, Ni C, Liu Y, Zhang Y, Su W, Lian Y, et al. Mindfulness meditation for insomnia: a meta-analysis of randomized controlled trials. J Psychosom Res. 2016;89:1–6.
12. Sancho M, De Gracia M, Rodriguez RC, Mallorqui-Bague N, Sanchez-Gonzalez J, Trujols J, et al. Mindfulness-based interventions for the treatment of substance and behavioral addictions: a systematic review. Front Psych. 2018;9:95.

13. Hilton L, Hempel S, Ewing BA, Apaydin E, Xenaiks L, Newberry S, et al. Mindfulness meditation for chronic pain: systematic review and meta-analysis. Ann Behav Med. 2017;51(2):199–213.
14. Black DS, Slavich GM. Mindfulness meditation and the immune system: a systematic review of randomized controlled trials. Ann N Y Acad Sci. 2016;1373(1):13–24.
15. Davidson RJ, Kabat-Zinn J, Schumacher J, Rosenkranz M, Muller D, Santorelli S, et al. Alterations in brain and immune function produced by mindfulness meditation. Psychosom Med. 2003;65:564–70.
16. Gardner FL, Moore ZE. A Mindfulness-Acceptance-Commitment (MAC) based approach to athletic performance enhancement: theoretical considerations. Behav Ther. 2004;35:707–23.
17. Schwanhausser L. Application of the mindfulness-acceptance-commitment (MAC) protocol with an adolescent springboard diver: the case of Steve. J Clin Sport Psychol. 2009;3:377–95.
18. DePetrillo L, Kaufman K, Glass C, Arnkoff D. Mindfulness for long-distance runners: an open trial using mindful sport performance enhancement (MSPE). J Clin Sport Psychol. 2009;4:357–76.
19. Bernier M, Thienot E, Codron R, Fournier JF. Mindfulness and acceptance approaches in sport performance. J Clin Sport Psychol. 2009;4:320–33.
20. Gross M, Moore ZE, Gardner FL, Wolanin AT, Marks DR, Pess RA. An empirical examination comparing the Mindfulness-Acceptance-Commitment (MAC) approach and psychological skills training (PST) for the mental health and sport performance of student athletes. Int J Sport Exerc Psychol. 2016;16(4):431–51.
21. Thompson RW, Kaufman KA, De Petrillo LA, Glass CR, Arnkoff DB. One year follow-up of mindful sport performance enhancement (MSPE) with archers, golfers, and runners. J Clin Sport Psychol. 2011;5:99–116.
22. Wolanin AT. Mindfulness-acceptance-commitment (MAC) based performance enhancement for Division I collegiate athletes: a preliminary investigation. Dis Abstr Int B. 2005;65(7):3735–84.
23. Kabat-Zinn J. Wherever you go, there you are: mindfulness meditation in everyday life. New York: Hyperion; 1994.
24. Kabat-Zinn J. Full catastrophe living: using the wisdom of your body and mind to face stress, pain, and illness. New York: Bantam Books; 2013.
25. Wolanin AT, Gross M, Hong E. Depression in athletes: prevalence and risk factors. Curr Sport Med Rep. 2015;14(1):56–60.
26. Brewer BW. Self-identity and specific vulnerability to depressed mood. J Pers. 1993;61(3):343–64.
27. Brewer BW, Petrie TA. A comparison between injured and uninjured football players on selected psychosocial variables. Acad Athl J. 1995;10:11–8.
28. Hammond T, Gialloreto C, Kubas H, Davis H. The prevalence of failure based depression among elite athletes. Clin J Sport Med. 2013;23(4):273–7.
29. National Collegiate Athletic Association (NCAA). In: Brown G, editors. Mind, body, and sport: understanding and supporting student-athlete mental wellness. Indianapolis, IN; NCAA; 2014.
30. Windhorst, B. Cavaliers coach Tyronn Lue says he's being treated for anxiety. 2018. Website. http://www.espn.com/nba/story/_/id/23659954/cleveland-cavaliers-coach-tyronn-lue-reveals-being-treated-anxiety. Accessed 11 Jan 2018.
31. Bishop SR. What do we really know about mindfulness-based stress reduction? Psychosom Med. 2002;64(1):71–83.
32. Creswell JD, Lindsay EK. How does mindfulness training affect health? A mindfulness stress buffering account. Curr Dir Psychol Sci. 2014;23(6):401–7.
33. Eberth J, Sedlmeier P. The effects of mindfulness meditation: a meta-analysis. Mindfulness. 2012;3(3):174–89.
34. Glass CR, Spears CA, Perskaudas R, Kaufman KA. Mindful sport performance enhancement: randomized controlled trial of a mental training program with collegiate athletes. J Clin Sport Psychol. 2019;13:609–28.

35. Scholefield R, Firsick D, Lawrence L, Miller M. Athlete mindfulness: the development and evaluation of a mindfulness based training program for promoting mental health and wellbeing in student athletes. Lecture presented at: NCAA Convention, Indianapolis, IN; 2018.
36. Hayes SC, Strosahl KD, Wilson KG. Acceptance and commitment therapy: an experiential approach to behavior change. New York: Guilford Press; 1999.
37. Hayes SC, Luoma JB, Bond FW, Masuda A, Lillis J. Acceptance and commitment therapy: model, processes and outcomes. Behav Res Ther. 2006;44(1):1–25.
38. Hayes SC, Strosahl KD, Wilson KG. Acceptance and commitment therapy: the process and practice of mindful change. 2nd ed. New York: Guilford Press; 2012.
39. Wenzlaff RM, Wegner DM. Thought suppression. Annu Rev Psychol. 2000;51:59–91.
40. Killingsworth MA, Gilbert DT. A wandering mind is an unhappy mind. Science. 2010;330:932.
41. Klinger E, Cox WM. Dimensions of thought flow in everyday life. Imagin Cogn Pers. 1987;7(2):105–28.
42. Brown KW, Ryan RM, Creswell JD. Mindfulness: theoretical foundations and evidence for its salutary effects. Psychol Inq. 2007;18(4):211–37.
43. Weinsten N, Brown KW, Ryan RM. A multi-method examination of the effects of mindfulness on stress attribution, coping, and emotional well-being. J Res Pers. 2009;43(3):374–85.
44. Kaufman KA, Glass CR, Pineau TR. Mindful sport performance enhancement: mental training for athletes and coaches. Washington, DC: American Psychological Association; 2018.
45. Harris R. ACT made simple: an easy-to-read primer on acceptance and commitment therapy. Oakland: New Harbinger; 2009.
46. Hayes SC, Wilson KW, Gifford EV, Follette VM, Strosahl K. Experiential avoidance and behavioral disorders: a functional dimensional approach to diagnosis and treatment. J Consult Clin Psychol. 1996;64(6):1152–68.
47. Chawla N, Ostafin B. Experiential avoidance as a functional dimensional approach to psychopathology: an empirical review. J Clin Psychol. 2007;63(9):871–90.
48. Kashdan TB, Barrios V, Forsyth JP, Steger MF. Experiential avoidance as a generalized psychological vulnerability: comparisons with coping and emotion regulation strategies. Behav Res Ther. 2006;44(9):1301–20.
49. Mankad A, Gordon S, Wallman K. Perceptions of emotional climate among injured athletes. J Clin Sport Psychol. 2009;3:1–14.
50. Watson JC. College student-athletes' attitudes towards help-seeking behavior and expectations of counseling services. J Coll Stud Dev. 2005;46(4):442–9.
51. Barnard JD. Student-athletes' perceptions of mental illness and attitudes toward help-seeking. J Coll Stud Psychother. 2016;30(3):161–75.

Chapter 20
Administering Mental Health: Societal, Coaching, and Legislative Approaches to Mental Health

Emily Kroshus and Brian Hainline

Introduction

Although mental health is being increasingly recognized as an important issue in the sport setting (e.g., [1, 2]), it is still infrequently addressed at an organizational level [3]. One reason may be because the prevalence of mental illness is under-recognized [4], potentially due to the overlap between some symptoms of mental illness and "good athlete" traits, or conflation of physical functioning with the absence of mental illness. Estimates of the prevalence of mental illness among athletes vary by sport (e.g., team, individual), age group and level of competition (e.g., pre-college, college, professional/elite), illness or disorder (e.g., depression, anxiety, eating disorder), and the means of measurement (e.g., clinically relevant symptoms, clinically diagnosed disorder) [5]. However, estimates tend to be relatively similar to same-age nonathlete peers [6, 7], meaning that at least one-quarter of athletes will likely experience challenges related to mental illness [8, 9].

While reducing the health burden of mental illness is important, so too is increasing positive psychological functioning, including subjective well-being [10]. Mental health is increasingly being conceptualized using a dual-factor model, in which subjective well-being and mental illness are viewed as on separate but related continuums rather than opposite ends of the same continuum [11, 12]. Thus, in addition

E. Kroshus (✉)
Seattle Children's Research Institute, Center for Child Health, Behavior and Development, Seattle, WA, USA

University of Washington, Department of Pediatrics, Seattle, WA, USA
e-mail: ekroshus@uw.edu

B. Hainline
Indiana University School of Medicine, Indianapolis, IN, USA

New York University School of Medicine, New York, NY, USA
e-mail: bhainline@ncaa.org

© Springer Nature Switzerland AG 2020
E. Hong, A. L. Rao (eds.), *Mental Health in the Athlete*,
https://doi.org/10.1007/978-3-030-44754-0_20

to reducing the burden of mental illness, some sports organizations are also focusing on the importance of fostering positive psychological functioning [1]. Despite relatively similar prevalence of mental illness among athletes and nonathletes, athletes experience a unique set of risk and potentially protective factors for the onset of mental illness and different factors that may facilitate or constrain early detection and appropriate management [7, 13, 14]. Similarly, sport settings can present both unique challenges and opportunities for the promotion of positive psychological functioning and subjective well-being.

Strategies for reducing the health burden of mental illness can be broadly grouped into categories of primary prevention (e.g., reduce risk factors for onset of mental illness), secondary prevention (e.g., early detection), and tertiary prevention (e.g., ensure appropriate management of mental illness). When discussing primary prevention of mental illness in the sport environment, it is important to emphasize the range of factors that may influence whether an individual will experience mental illness. These include immutable factors like their underlying biological vulnerability to mental illness [15, 16], which may interact with early life experiences to produce a unique risk profile [17]. However, even after the early life period, and while recognizing individual variability, environmental stressors and learned coping behaviors can influence the manifestation of mental illness [18]. Athletes experience unique stressors (e.g., related to athletic performance, time demands of sport, coaching and parental pressures, injury, transition from sport) but also have the potential to learn positive coping skills within the context of the repeated challenges of sport [19].

Secondary and tertiary prevention are also critical for reducing the health burden of mental illness as untreated mental illness can progress to worsened symptomology [20]. Many mental illnesses are never identified or treated, and when individuals do seek care, adherence to treatment is low [21]. Adolescence and emerging adulthood are the time of onset for many types of mental illness [22], making contexts within which these individuals live, learn, work, and play, which is of critical importance for early detection and facilitation of care seeking.

There are unique barriers to care seeking among athletes [23]. These include perceived stigma by others in the sport environment (e.g., coaches, teammates) and a perception that mental health help seeking will negatively impact athletic performance [7, 13, 14]. However, athletes also can theoretically benefit from the engagement of others in the sport environment in mental health promotion efforts. Stakeholders within sport environments, including coaches, sports medicine personnel, and organizational administrators, can help create sport environments that destigmatize/support mental health care seeking [19, 24]. They also can help facilitate the identification of potentially symptomatic athletes who could benefit from care seeking, either directly [19, 24, 25] or through screening initiatives [26, 27]. Tertiary prevention or care provision to athletes who are struggling with mental health problems is a critical final step in reducing the health burden of mental illness. To be optimally efficacious, this care should be from licensed mental health providers with cultural competence engaging with athletes [1]. Stakeholders in sport settings (e.g., coaches, primary medical providers, athletic trainers, administrators) can help provide access to these individuals, either directly or through information provision to athletes. Communication with sport settings can help facilitate care seeking to appropriate individuals. This can include ensuring that all sport stakeholders have access to the organization's mental health management plan. It could also include encouraging integration between mental healthcare providers and sport stakeholders to increase familiarity, for example, through an annual meeting.

Conceptual Framework

This chapter is framed using a social ecological model, in which the individual is viewed as nested within the context of interpersonal, organizational, policy, and societal levels of influence [28]. For this chapter, "individual" will be operationalized as the individual athlete among whom mental health optimization is the focus. However, this same framework could be used to think about influences on the behaviors of coaches, bystander teammates, or other stakeholders involved in mental health promotion efforts. The specific individual behaviors of focus will be care seeking and care adherence. At the interpersonal level, we will focus on coaches, as they play a central role in shaping team environments and influencing other stakeholders with the sport setting. However, we will also briefly discuss the role of other important interpersonal relationships that can influence individual care seeking and care adherence behaviors. At the organizational level, we will focus on school-level policies and initiatives, as well as school-level implementation of policies and initiatives mandated legislatively. At a policy level, we will focus on legislation and best practice guidelines of large sport governing bodies (e.g., NCAA, other college sports organizations, large single-sport governing bodies, and high school sport governing bodies). For each level of the social ecological model, our discussion will consider a continuum of prevention inclusive of primary, secondary, and tertiary prevention.

Coaching and Mental Health

Attend to Unhealthy Mental and Physical Stressors

While recognizing the centrality of risk factors outside of the sport context on an individual athlete mental health, coaches can nonetheless play an important role in primary prevention through their coaching practices. One key way is by attending to stressors associated with risk of symptomatology of mental illness. This includes chronic stressors (e.g., monitoring training loads and recovery that may contribute to overtraining and eliminating abusive coaching practices) [6, 29, 30] and acute stressors (e.g., injury) [6, 16, 31, 32]. Coaches can also attend to factors predictive of burnout (physical and emotional exhaustion and sport devaluation) by providing opportunities for connection with others, autonomous decision-making, and a sense of competence [33]. Such coaching practices must be developmentally appropriate, recognizing that what qualifies as healthy sport-related physical and psychosocial demands will vary between athletes and be patterned by age [10, 34]. For example, among younger (e.g., pre-secondary school) athletes, there is a growing focus on the developmental appropriateness of keeping sport fun, reducing achievement-related pressure, and limiting physical demands by reducing early specialization and promoting multisport participation [35].

Coaches also need to communicate about developmentally appropriate training to parents to assure parent buy-in. Parents help select the sport environment for this child and then can either amplify or counteract coaching practices designed to support sport participation that is physically and emotionally appropriate from a developmental perspective [36]. This means that in addition to themselves implementing healthy coaching practices, coaches should communicate with parents to enlist their support in reinforcing (or at least not undermining) these practices. Drawing on integrated theories for behavior change that emphasize the importance of expected outcomes, norms, and skills on behavior [37], such communication could involve sharing with parents the expected benefits of such practices, the approval of such practices by leading sports professionals and organizations, and specific and actionable strategies for their own behavior (e.g., tips for a positive discussion with their child on the way home from a loss).

Help Athletes Learn Positive Coping Skills

Sport can be used as a context within which coaches can help foster positive psychosocial development among athletes [38], in part by helping athletes learn how to respond to stressors in healthy and functional ways [19, 39]. This includes helping athletes learn skills predictive of resilience [40], such as psychological flexibility [41] and self-compassion [42]. This means adapting to situational demands (e.g., recognizing that everything might not always go as planned and being willing to change course), shifting perspectives, and making decisions about how to act while balancing competing desires and staying consistent with one's values [41].

Coaches can also help foster a process-oriented mindset, in which effort and improvement are emphasized and achievement or outcomes are de-emphasized [43]. Such mindset has been associated with improved ability to manage stressors and increased likelihood of post-traumatic growth [44]. The repeated challenges and almost inevitable losses inherent with sport participation provide a laboratory in which coaches can model, instigate, and reinforce healthy coping practices consistent with psychological flexibility, self-compassion, and a process-oriented mindset. For example, this could mean modeling responding flexibly to unexpected challenges in the sport setting (e.g., a travel delay to a game). This could also mean providing positive reinforcement when observing athletes who are performing desired coping behaviors (e.g., focusing on effort and planning steps to learn from a loss). It is also useful for minimizing performance-related anxiety [45], reducing attrition from sport [46], and optimizing the positive psychological experiences of sport participants [47].

Training for coaches can help with developing the ability to implement such positive coaching practices [48]; however, such educational practices are rarely if ever required for coaches. Helping athletes develop such positive coping skills cannot be considered sufficient in isolation to prevent mental illness among individuals with underlying vulnerability. However, it can nonetheless help reduce the impact of potential environmental triggers. More broadly, among all athletes regardless of their vulnerability to mental illness, developing positive coping skills can help optimize their subjective well-being in response to the inevitable challenges of sport. These skills also have the potential to be generalized off the sports field to help with coping in other domains [19] and after athletes have transitioned away from competitive sport [49].

Encourage Appropriate Care Seeking

The frequent and repeated contact that coaches have with athletes means they are often in a position to notice athletes who are struggling. Not all coaches feel confident in responding appropriately if they believe an athlete is experiencing a mental illness [50], meaning that there is scope to improve knowledge translation to coaches about symptom identification. Because of the possibility of athlete-specific presentation of symptoms (e.g., as manifested in athletic performance) and confounding between "good athlete" traits and symptoms of mental illness (e.g., perfectionism), sport-specific education about identification of mental illness is important. This can include information about sport-specific potentially triggering events, such as injury [6, 16, 31, 32] or retirement [7], and chronic stressors such as high training loads [6, 29].

Such education should emphasize that the coach's role is not to make a diagnosis but rather to ensure that potentially symptomatic athletes seek further evaluation from a licensed mental health care provider [1]. Theoretic models that explain whether coaches intervene to support care seeking among athletes suspected of experiencing a mental disorder point to the importance of mental health literacy, perceived stigma, and self-efficacy as key factors in explaining behavior [50–52]. A small but growing number of educational interventions have found efficacy in shifting one or more of these cognitions among coaches [53–55].

A key reason why athletes do not seek mental health care is the perception of stigma associated with such health-seeking behavior [14]. Coaches have the potential to help shape team cultures supportive of care seeking, and coach education can help support coaches in this process. Coaches can engage in direct verbal communication to their team about the importance of care seeking, starting long before there is a specific concern about mental illness. Coaches can also attend to the indirect or informal messages they are sending about mental health/mental health care seeking, for example, through their choice of language, which may unintentionally stigmatize mental health concerns. To help support desired coach behaviors, specific guidance should be provided to coaches within the context of education programming about how to communicate effectively about mental health, such as utilizing analogies to physical health (e.g., mental health concerns should be as easily addressed as a sprained ankle) and emphasizing the interplay of physical and mental health – both for well-being and for performance.

Once a coach has identified that an athlete may benefit from further evaluation or care, a trusting coach-athlete relationship can be leveraged to encourage care seeking from a licensed mental health provider. To do so, coaches need to know that care should be provided by a licensed mental health professional and be aware of appropriate individuals within a given organizational setting or community from whom care could be sought. Although athletes may choose to seek care elsewhere after consultation with their family and in consideration of financial considerations (e.g., insurance), it is important that all initial recommendations are appropriate. Additionally, coaches can help encourage adherence to the ongoing care-seeking process. This can include continuing to normalize and destigmatize care seeking and providing emotional support as appropriate within the context of the coach-athlete relationship. The response of collegiate track and field coaches to student-athletes suffering with depression suggests that coaches may require additional support to engage in optimal secondary and tertiary preventive behaviors. One-third (33%) of coaches provided student-athletes with information about campus resources, one-quarter (24%) encouraged the student-athlete to seek health care, and one-fifth (21%) alerted a member of the team's medical staff [51]. Fewer engaged in emotionally supportive communication, such as showing support (15%), sharing from personal experience (3%), attempting to remove stigma or normalize (3%), or asking if they want to talk (3%) [51]. Such coaching behaviors should be addressed by coaching education related to mental health.

Organizational Practices and Mental Health

Provide Evidence-Based Education to Coaches

One key way that organizations can influence athlete mental health is through the education that they provide to coaches. As discussed above, coaches can engage in behaviors related to primary, secondary, and tertiary prevention, but they require support in delivering these behaviors. Critically, such education should be evidence-based and efficacious [56]. At present, there are several programs that meet such threshold, largely developed and evaluated in Australia. The most commonly used educational intervention is Mental Health First Aid [57]. This two-day program teaches strategies for responding to emergent and non-emergent mental health issues, increasing mental health literacy, self-efficacy, and helping behaviors [58]. Adapted versions have been used in Australian sport settings, with similarly positive results [54, 55].

A less time-consuming intervention is the mental health in sport (MHS) workshop for coaches and support staff in elite sport settings, which is focused on increasing knowledge of mental illness signs and symptoms and confidence in helping an athlete who is experiencing a mental health problem [53]. Additional interventions, typically focused on increasing mental health literacy, have been targeted at coaches [53, 54, 56, 59]; however, there is a need for additional work evaluating these interventions, with a focus on unbiased approaches to measurement and determining clinical impact [56]. Other sports organizations, such as the NCAA, provide education for coaches based on established theoretic models (e.g., addressing mental health literacy, stigma, and self-efficacy) [60]; however, evaluation work is ongoing. There is an ongoing need for health education professionals to work collaboratively with stakeholders in the sport setting and for mental health providers and epidemiologists/biostatisticians to develop and evaluate needed educational materials for coaches. This can include evaluating whether intervention used in other countries or levels of sport translates to different sporting contexts.

Attend to Organizational Incentives

Target behaviors can be viewed within the scope of expectancies and function for coaches, thereby increasing the incentive of delivering appropriate coach education [37]. Organizational resource allocation, priorities, and the outcomes or behaviors that are rewarded can communicate to coaches whether mental health is viewed as an organizational priority. For example, if coaches are going to engage in coaching practices that are developmentally appropriate but less focused on short-term athletic achievement, they need to be confident that their organization values more than just wins and losses. Sports organizations should also attend to structural decisions made at the organizational level that can impact the extent to which coaches can engage in coaching practices supportive of athlete mental health. There may also be scope for sports organizations to provide guidance to coaches about how coaching time is allocated and whether some practice time is allocated to intentionally teaching positive psychosocial skills. Such intentional structuring of time allocation in sport settings has been associated with better youth developmental outcomes [61].

Consider Universal Screening

Some sports organizations may also be able to help screen athletes for symptoms of mental illness. However, consistent with guidance from the US Preventive Services Task Force, screening should occur only if accompanied with systems that subsequently allow for accurate diagnosis, effective treatment, and appropriate follow-up [62]. In implementing screening, organizations must also attend to the need for confidentiality in the data collection process. Screening practices may not be appropriate for all sports organizations, but should be considered by sports organizations that have integration of medical care and athletics, such as collegiate sports programs [26, 27]. One strategy for screening is for it to be conducted universally, for example, as part of the pre-participation exam [26, 27]. However, temporal changes in depression symptoms across season in collegiate athletes [63] suggest potential utility of screening at multiple time points, not just on entry. Although screening for mental illness using questionnaire-based tools has benefits in terms of relative ease of implementation and potential for each, there are nonetheless challenges. Existing questionnaire-based screening tools have been developed for a general population and not athletes [26]. Consequently, their sensitivity and specificity may be limited due to factors such as potentially confounding between mental health symptoms and symptoms of other athlete-specific health issues such as overtraining syndrome [5, 64]. The possibility that screeners are inaccurate or temporally unstable raises concern that screening could have unintended negative consequences as a result of complacency (e.g., ignoring behavioral factors that could modify risk or continued monitoring), as has been observed related to screening for other health issues such as cardiovascular disease [65].

Establish and Rehearse a Mental Health Protocol

Another key way that sports organizations can help facilitate secondary and tertiary prevention of mental illness is by having a mental health protocol for emergency and nonemergency situations [26]. This protocol should clearly outline the responsibilities of different stakeholders and describe pathways for referral in both emergency and nonemergency situations. For mental health protocols to be useful to coaches and other stakeholders in the sport environment, it needs to be communicated to and rehearsed by all relevant stakeholders. Among high school coaches, those who were aware of their school's mental health protocol had greater confidence in their ability to respond appropriately to support an athlete believed to be struggling with mental illness [50]. This protocol can also help with tertiary prevention, ensuring that referrals are made to licensed mental health providers and including guidance for stakeholders in the sport environment on the importance of supporting care-seeking adherence.

Attend to Staffing

Other ways that some sports organizations can foster secondary and tertiary prevention are through staffing decisions and the types of behaviors they encourage among existing healthcare professionals who work with their athletes. Additional research is needed to understand the conditions under which coaches are able to implement positive coaching practices. In sports organizations that employ or consult with sports medicine physicians who provide care for a range of health issues, efforts can be made to encourage a more holistic focus on athlete well-being. Injury can function as a trigger for worsening symptomatology of mental illness [31]; however, physicians providing injury care in sports medicine settings infrequently screen for or discuss psychological issues potentially related to or emergent at the time of injury [26]. Communication with sports medicine physicians about increasing the integration of mental health care with injury care, even if just for purpose of screening, may be useful in sport settings that work with dedicated sports medicine professionals [23].

Individuals providing screening and initial consultations should be appropriately trained and licensed. Some sports organizations (e.g., large collegiate athletics programs or elite/professional sports teams) may have the budget to employ dedicated mental health professionals. Having sufficient professional staffing to meet athlete demand for mental health care helps ensure that symptomatic athletes receive attention as needed. Hiring dedicated staff to work with athletes (as opposed to making referrals for athletes to community or general campus mental health care providers) means that care providers can be selected in part based on their expertise working with athletes. Cultural competence of mental health care providers is an important factor in treatment adherence in general [66]; within the context of athletics, cultural competence working with athletes is a unique consideration that intersects with the need for the healthcare provider to be culturally competent in other regards (e.g., attending to the athlete's additional identities related to race/ethnicity, gender, and sexual orientation).

Policy and Mental Health

Although sports organizations may choose to independently implement practices related to supporting athlete mental health, guidance from sport governing bodies can help with the reach of such practices. In this section, we will discuss both legislation (e.g., policy that is voted upon and approved as mandatory by a governing body such as state high school athletics associations or the NCAA) and best practice guidance provided by such governing bodies. Given the challenges related to passing legislation and then assuring compliance at the organizational level, governing bodies may choose to provide instructions to sports organizations in the form of best practice guidance. Legislation, if passed, may be broad (e.g., "provide education"), while best practice guidance can be more flexibly responsive to an evolving evidence base, recommending specific programs, practices, and protocols to sports organizations. This is the approach the NCAA has taken, working to pass legislation where possible while using inter-association documents to recommend consensus best practices to member institutions. In the United States, of the ten sports with the highest participation rates, we were unable to find formal policies of the respective national governing bodies (NGBs) related to the prevention, identification, or management of mental health concerns. However, USA Track & Field has a psychological services subcommittee with responsibilities that include mental health education for members [67]. This lack of policy-level guidance related to mental health may reflect a missed opportunity for agenda setting by leading sports organizations. The NCAA provides a model related to policy-level approaches to mental health promotion that other sports organizations may seek to adapt.

Provide Guidance Related to Coach Training

Sport governing bodies can require or recommend that coaches complete specific trainings. Such directives could theoretically be extended to include completing evidence-based training related to how they can support athlete mental health. Nearly all NGBs in the United States require that national coaches complete the SafeSport training (https://safesport.org/), an online training from the US Center for SafeSport that is focused on ending abuse in sport (e.g., bullying, harassment, hazing, physical abuse, emotional abuse, and sexual misconduct and abuse). At present, we are not aware of policies requiring coach training explicitly focused on mental illness prevention, identification, and management at any level of sport. Critically, prior evidence suggests that even when coach education is required in sport settings, there will often be variable implementation [50]. Thus, any required training related to athlete welfare, whether SafeSport or otherwise, will be exceedingly difficult to mandate or enforce at the local, grassroots level because of the minimal requirements for coach certification in the United States. While not required of coaches, the NCAA does include annual coach education about mental health as part of its best practice guidance to member institutions. Groups involved in developing educational materials about mental health for coaches should attend to dissemination and implementation throughout the program development and evaluation process. This can include working with sport governing bodies to determine how to make materials fit the needs of member organizations and how they are most easily disseminated and implemented within existing communication channels. One key strategy to facilitate implementation may be making evidence-based programming easily available to organizations, rather than making broad mandates without specific actionable support. Requiring or suggesting education without providing guidance about what is appropriate is a strategy for variable choice to materials and lack of effectiveness [68].

Provide Guidance Related to Screening

Sport governing bodies can also play a role in secondary prevention through the requirements or guidance that they provide to member organizations related to screening. In their best practice guidance, the NCAA recommends that institutions screen athletes as part of the PPE. As new screening tools are developed and validated, such best practice guidance should evolve to communicate updated recommendations and actionable strategies to member organizations. Similar guidance about screening may be more challenging, or in some cases inappropriate, for other sport governing bodies with less direct coordination with healthcare providers for athletes. However, there may be opportunity for interdisciplinary collaboration, for example, sport governing bodies working with medical and mental health organizations to make recommendations about the inclusion of mental health screening as part of standardized PPEs.

Provide Guidance Related to Mental Health Protocols

Sport governing bodies can require or provide guidance to member organizations related to having and rehearsing mental health action plan. This is of critical importance for appropriate response to emergency mental health situations and can also help facilitate appropriate response to nonemergency mental health concerns. This is one element of the NCAA's best practice guidance [1] but to our knowledge is not common practice among other sport governing bodies. Efforts to support implementation of such protocols may include providing concrete examples of policies that have been useful in different types of sports organizations.

Provide Guidance Related to Staffing

Finally, sport governing bodies can play an important role in tertiary prevention by providing guidance and resources related to staffing. One element of the NCAA's best practice guidance is the recommendation that all mental health care be provided by a licensed mental health professional. Depending on the size and nature of the sports organizations under the governing body's purview, recommendations could potentially also be made about the importance of adequate staffing to meet athlete referral needs and about the benefits of culturally competent mental health care providers.

Conclusion

While there are many factors that impact athlete mental health, most centrally their underlying biological propensity to mental illness and early life exposures, environmental factors, and learned behaviors in the sport environment has the potential to make a difference. Framed by a social ecological model, the present chapter focused on ways in which coaches, sports organizations, and sport governing bodies can positively impact athlete mental health. This includes working to help prevent, identify, and help facilitate care seeking for mental illness and by helping to promote positive psychological functioning. Although individual coaches, organizations, and sport governing bodies may be engaging in practices supportive of athlete mental health, there is a need for improvement to ensure the reach of evidence-based practices. There are several key areas of need for research and programming to support such efforts.

One key need is to evaluate educational programming related to mental health promotion in a diversity of sport settings, building on the important program development and evaluation work being conducted in Australia. Such programming may be effective in other cultural contexts, or it may require adaptation. Recommendations that coaches and other sport stakeholders complete education are limited in their scope for impact if effective programming is not available. There is also a critical need to validate existing screening tools for symptoms of mental illness to ensure appropriateness for athletes. Such work may point to the need to develop and validate athlete-appropriate measures, or it may provide confidence in the utility of existing measures.

Finally, where policy and sport governing body guidance for organizations related to mental health exist, there is a need for implementation studies to understand (1) reach and fidelity of implementation and (2) barriers and facilitators to successful implementation. Such efforts can be used to develop strategies for implementation of support for organizations and/or coaches. Given the prevalence of mental illness among athletes, the potential harms associated with untreated mental illness, and the potential benefits of positive psychological functioning, supporting athlete mental health should be a priority of sports organizations and sport governing bodies. As research, program development, and program evaluation work related to mental health continue to evolve, such efforts should be framed by a social ecological model. This means recognizing that a range of stakeholder individuals and organizations play a key role in supporting athlete well-being and that all need to be engaged in shaping sport cultures supportive of mental health.

References

1. Mental Health Best Practices [Internet]. NCAA; 2016. Available from: https://www.ncaa.org/sites/default/files/HS_Mental-Health-Best-Practices_20160317.pdf.
2. Australia's Winning Edge 2012–2022 [Internet]. Australian Sport Commission. 2012 [cited 2018 Jul 30]. Available from: https://www.ausport.gov.au/__data/assets/pdf_file/0011/509852/Australias_Winning_Edge.pdf.
3. Liddle SK, Deane FP, Vella SA. Addressing mental health through sport: a review of sporting organizations' websites. Early Interv Psychiatry. 2017;11(2):93–103.
4. Reardon CL, Factor RM. Sport psychiatry: a systematic review of diagnosis and medical treatment of mental illness in athletes. Sports Med Auckl NZ. 2010;40(11):961–80.
5. Schuch FB. Depression in athletes or increased depressive symptoms in athletes? Curr Sports Med Rep. 2015;14(3):244.

6. Armstrong S, Burcin M, Bjerke W, Early J. Depression in student athletes: a particularly at-risk group? A systematic review of the literature. PTHMS Fac Publ [Internet]. 2015;7(2). Available from: http://digitalcommons.sacredheart.edu/pthms_fac/176
7. Rice SM, Purcell R, De Silva S, Mawren D, McGorry PD, Parker AG. The mental health of elite athletes: a narrative systematic review. Sports Med Auckl NZ. 2016;46(9):1333–53.
8. Ibrahim AK, Kelly SJ, Adams CE, Glazebrook C. A systematic review of studies of depression prevalence in university students. J Psychiatr Res. 2013;47(3):391–400.
9. Merikangas KR, He J-P, Burstein M, Swanson SA, Avenevoli S, Cui L, et al. Lifetime prevalence of mental disorders in U.S. adolescents: results from the National Comorbidity Survey Replication–Adolescent Supplement (NCS-A). J Am Acad Child Adolesc Psychiatry. 2010;49(10):980–9.
10. Fraser-Thomas JL, Côté J, Deakin J. Youth sport programs: an avenue to foster positive youth development. Phys Educ Sport Pedagogy. 2005;10(1):19–40.
11. Suldo SM, Shaffer EJ. Looking beyond psychopathology: the dual-factor model of mental health in youth. Sch Psychol Rev. 2008;37(1):52–68.
12. Keyes CLM, Dhingra SS, Simoes EJ. Change in level of positive mental health as a predictor of future risk of mental illness. Am J Public Health. 2010;100(12):2366–71.
13. Bauman NJ. The stigma of mental health in athletes. are mental toughness and mental health seen as contradictory in elite sport? Br J Sports Med. 2016;50(3):135–6.
14. Watson JC. College student-athletes' attitudes toward help-seeking behavior and expectations of counseling services. J Coll Stud Dev. 2005;46(4):442–9.
15. Dunn EC, Brown RC, Dai Y, Rosand J, Nugent NR, Amstadter AB, et al. Genetic determinants of depression: recent findings and future directions. Harv Rev Psychiatry. 2015;23(1):1–18.
16. Lichtenstein P, Yip BH, Björk C, Pawitan Y, Cannon TD, Sullivan PF, et al. Common genetic determinants of schizophrenia and bipolar disorder in Swedish families: a population-based study. Lancet Lond Engl. 2009;373(9659):234–9.
17. Heim C, Binder EB. Current research trends in early life stress and depression: review of human studies on sensitive periods, gene-environment interactions, and epigenetics. Exp Neurol. 2012;233(1):102–11.
18. Belsky J, Pluess M. Beyond diathesis stress: differential susceptibility to environmental influences. Psychol Bull. 2009;135(6):885–908.
19. Kroshus E. Stigma, coping skills, and psychological help seeking among collegiate athletes. Athl Train Sports Health Care. 2017;9(6):254–62.
20. Kessler RC, Berglund PA, Bruce ML, Koch JR, Laska EM, Leaf PJ, et al. The prevalence and correlates of untreated serious mental illness. Health Serv Res. 2001;36(6 Pt 1):987–1007.
21. Krivoy A, Balicer RD, Feldman B, Hoshen M, Zalsman G, Weizman A, et al. The impact of age and gender on adherence to antidepressants: a 4-year population-based cohort study. Psychopharmacology (Berl). 2015;232(18):3385–90.
22. McGorry PD, Purcell R, Goldstone S, Amminger GP. Age of onset and timing of treatment for mental and substance use disorders: implications for preventive intervention strategies and models of care. Curr Opin Psychiatry. 2011;24(4):301–6.
23. Sudano LE, Collins G, Miles CM. Reducing barriers to mental health care for student-athletes: an integrated care model. Fam Syst Health J Collab Fam Healthc. 2017;35(1):77–84.
24. Brown GT, Hainline B, Wilfert M, editors. Mind, body and sport. Understanding and supporting student-athlete mental wellness [Internet]. Indianapolis: IN: NCAA; 2015 [cited 2018 Jul 30]. Available from: https://www.naspa.org/images/uploads/events/Mind_Body_and_Sport.pdf
25. Neal TL, Diamond AB, Goldman S, Klossner D, Morse ED, Pajak DE, et al. Inter-association recommendations for developing a plan to recognize and refer student-athletes with psychological concerns at the collegiate level: an executive summary of a consensus statement. J Athl Train. 2013;48(5):716–20.
26. Rao AL, Hong ES. Understanding depression and suicide in college athletes: emerging concepts and future directions. Br J Sports Med. 2016;50(3):136–7.

27. Trojian T. Depression is under-recognised in the sport setting: time for primary care sports medicine to be proactive and screen widely for depression symptoms. Br J Sports Med. 2016;50(3):137–9.
28. Bronfenbrenner U. Toward an experimental ecology of human development. Am Psychol. 1977;32(7):513–31.
29. Nixdorf I, Frank R, Beckmann J. An explorative study on major stressors and its connection to depression and chronic stress among German elite athletes. Adv Phys Educ. 2015;5:255–62.
30. Hwang S, Choi Y. Data mining in the exploration of stressors among NCAA student athletes. Psychol Rep. 2016;119(3):787–803.
31. Putukian M. The psychological response to injury in student athletes: a narrative review with a focus on mental health. Br J Sports Med. 2016;50(3):145–8.
32. Prinz B, Dvořák J, Junge A. Symptoms and risk factors of depression during and after the football career of elite female players. BMJ Open Sport — Exerc Med [Internet]. 2016;2(1). Available from: https://www.ncbi.nlm.nih.gov/pmc/articles/PMC5117078/
33. Lonsdale C, Hodge K, Rose E. Athlete burnout in elite sport: a self-determination perspective. J Sports Sci. 2009;27(8):785–95.
34. Patel DR, Pratt HD, Greydanus DE. Pediatric neurodevelopment and sports participation. When are children ready to play sports? Pediatr Clin North Am. 2002;49(3):505–31, v – vi.
35. Myer GD, Jayanthi N, DiFiori JP, Faigenbaum AD, Kiefer AW, Logerstedt D, et al. Sports specialization, Part II: Alternative solutions to early sport specialization in youth athletes. Sports Health. 2016;8(1):65–73.
36. Fraser-Thomas J, Côté J. Understanding adolescents' positive and negative developmental experiences in sport. Sport Psychol. 2009;23(1):3–23.
37. Montaño DE, Kasprzyk D. Theory of reasoned action, theory of planned behavior, and the integrated behavioral model. In: Health behavior: theory, research, and practice. 5th ed. San Francisco, CA, US: Jossey-Bass; 2015. p. 95–124.
38. Turnnidge J, Evans M, Vierimaa M, Allan V, Côté J, Holt NL. Coaching for positive youth development. In: Positive youth development through sport. 2nd ed: Routledge. England, United Kingdom: Abingdon-on-Thames; 2016. p. 137–50.
39. Raedeke TD, Smith AL. Coping resources and athlete burnout: an examination of stress mediated and moderation hypotheses. J Sport Exerc Psychol. 2004;26(4):525–41.
40. Wagstaff CRD, Hings RF, Larner RJ, Fletcher D. Psychological resilience moderates the relationship between organizational stressor frequency and burnout in athletes and coaches. Sport Psychol [Internet]. 2018 [cited 2018 Jul 30]; Available from: https://researchportal.port.ac.uk/portal/en/publications/psychological-resilience-moderates-the-relationship-between-organizational-stressor-frequency-and-burnout-in-athletes-and-coaches(336c122c-e080-4d07-b63d-d14ca0b123d7)/export.html
41. Kashdan TB. Psychological flexibility as a fundamental aspect of health. Clin Psychol Rev. 2010;30(7):865–78.
42. Neff KD, McGehee P. Self-compassion and psychological resilience among adolescents and young adults. Self Identity. 2010;9(3):225–40.
43. Duda J, Balaguer I. Coach-created motivational climate. In: Social psychology in sport. Champaign, IL: Human Kinetics; 2007. p. 117–30.
44. Aspinwall LG. Future-oriented thinking, proactive coping, and the management of potential threats to health and well-being. In: The Oxford handbook of stress, health, and coping. New York, NY: Oxford University Press; 2011. p. 334–65. (Oxford library of psychology).
45. Smith RE, Smoll FL, Cumming SP. Effects of a motivational climate intervention for coaches on young athletes' sport performance anxiety. J Sport Exerc Psychol. 2007;29(1):39–59.
46. Keegan RJ, Harwood CG, Spray CM, Lavallee D. A qualitative investigation of the motivational climate in elite sport. Psychol Sport Exer. 2014;15(1):97–107.
47. Bortoli L, Bertollo M, Comani S, Robazza C. Competence, achievement goals, motivational climate, and pleasant psychobiosocial states in youth sport. J Sports Sci. 2011;29(2):171–80.

48. Smoll FL, Smith RE, Cumming SP. Effects of a motivational climate intervention for coaches on changes in young athletes' achievement goal orientations. J Clin Sport Psychol. 2007;1(1):23–46.

49. Bernes KB, McKnight KM, Gunn T, Chorney D, Orr DT, Bardick AD. Life after sport: athletic career transition and transferable skills. 2009 [cited 2018 Jul 30]; Available from: https://www.uleth.ca/dspace/handle/10133/1175

50. Kroshus E, Coppel D, Chrisman SPD, Herring S. Coach support of high school student-athletes struggling with anxiety or depression. J Clin Sport Psychol. (In press).

51. Hegarty EM, Weight E, Rigester-Mihalik JK. Who is coaching the coach? Knowledge of depression and attitudes toward continuing education in coaches. BML Open Sport Exerc Med. 2018;4(e000339):1–7.

52. Mazzer KR, Rickwood DJ. Teachers' and coaches' role perceptions for supporting young people's mental health: multiple group path analyses. Aust J Psychol. 2014;67(1):10–9.

53. Sebbens J, Hassmén P, Crisp D, Wensley K. Mental Health in Sport (MHS): improving the early intervention knowledge and confidence of elite sport staff. Front Psychol [Internet]. 2016;7. Available from: https://www.ncbi.nlm.nih.gov/pmc/articles/PMC4919340/

54. Bapat S, Jorm A, Lawrence K. Evaluation of a mental health literacy training program for junior sporting clubs. Australas Psychiatry Bull R Aust N Z Coll Psychiatr. 2009;17(6):475–9.

55. Anderson R, Pierce D. Assumptions associated with mental health literacy training – Insights from initiatives in rural Australia. Adv Ment Health. 2012;10:258–67.

56. Breslin G, Shannon S, Haughey T, Donnelly P, Leavey G. A systematic review of interventions to increase awareness of mental health and well-being in athletes, coaches and officials. Syst Rev. 2017;6(1):177.

57. Kitchener BA, Jorm AF. Mental health first aid training for the public: evaluation of effects on knowledge, attitudes and helping behavior. BMC Psychiatry. 2002;2:10.

58. Hadlaczky G, Hökby S, Mkrtchian A, Carli V, Wasserman D. Mental Health First Aid is an effective public health intervention for improving knowledge, attitudes, and behaviour: a meta-analysis. Int Rev Psychiatry Abingdon Engl. 2014;26(4):467–75.

59. Pierce D, Liaw S-T, Dobell J, Anderson R. Australian rural football club leaders as mental health advocates: an investigation of the impact of the Coach the Coach project. Int J Ment Health Syst. 2010;4(1):10.

60. Mental Health Educational Resources [Internet]. NCAA.org - The Official Site of the NCAA. 2016 [cited 2018 Jul 30]. Available from: http://www.ncaa.org/sport-science-institute/mental-health-educational-resources

61. Bean C, Forneris T. Examining the importance of intentionally structuring the youth sport context to facilitate positive youth development. J Appl Sport Psychol. 2016;28(4):410–25.

62. Screening for Depression in Adults: U.S. Preventive Services Task Force Recommendation Statement. Ann Intern Med. 2009;151(11):784.

63. McGuire LC, Ingram YM, Sachs ML, Tierney RT. Temporal changes in depression symptoms in male and female collegiate student-athletes. J Clin Sport Psychol. 2017;11(4):337–51.

64. Bär K-J, Markser VZ. Sport specificity of mental disorders: the issue of sport psychiatry. Eur Arch Psychiatry Clin Neurosci. 2013;263(2):205–10.

65. Nielsen J, Clemmensen T, Yssing C. Getting access to what goes on in people's heads?: reflections on the think-aloud technique. In: Proceedings of the Second Nordic Conference on Human-computer Interaction [Internet]. New York, NY: ACM; 2002. p. 101–10. (NordiCHI '02). Available from: http://doi.acm.org/10.1145/572020.572033.

66. Bhui K, Warfa N, Edonya P, McKenzie K, Bhugra D. Cultural competence in mental health care: a review of model evaluations. BMC Health Serv Res. 2007;7:15.

67. USA Track & Field - Committees [Internet]. [cited 2018 Jul 30]. Available from: http://www.usatf.org/About/Committees.aspx

68. Kroshus E, Garnett BR, Baugh CM, Calzo JP. Social norms theory and concussion education. Health Educ Res. 2015;30(6):1004–13.

Chapter 21
Sport Psychology and Performance Psychology: Contributions to the Mental Health of Athletes

David B. Coppel

History of Expanding Domains and Roles

Sport psychology's history and evolution have been chronicled and discussed in sport and exercise psychology textbooks [1, 2], edited topic-oriented books [3–5], and scientific articles [6–9]. The history often begins with Triplett's [10] research on competitor and audience effects (social facilitation) on cyclists' performances. Temporally, this is followed by Coleman Griffith's laboratory-based research which included how psychological factors influence sport performance, including psychomotor learning, personality, and motivation. Interview data from top athletes yielded qualities and actions associated with success and produced further research into personality, arousal, achievement motivation, anxiety effects, aggression, and team cohesion. The field of applied sport psychology emerged as clinical psychological-based interventions, and cognitive-behavioral approaches were extrapolated to and developed for athletes and sport performance enhancement [11, 12]. Research in the psychophysiological factors in exercise (e.g., adherence, exercise physiology, biomechanics) was added to sport psychology's focus on psychological factors involved in competition and high performance or elite athletes, and the field was described as "sport and exercise psychology." This expansion now allowed for a more comprehensive exploration of the mind and body factors associated with maximal/optimal performance and the skills needed to obtain that result and how exercise activities impact people's mood and general well-being. The expanded sport psychology research approaches and methodologies provided information on important dimensions of optimal sport performance such as motivation, self-confidence and self-efficacy [13, 14], anxiety [15, 16], measurement and psychometric assessments [17], and interventions [3, 5, 40]. Interventions such as relaxation breathing,

D. B. Coppel (✉)
Department of Neurological Surgery, University of Washington, Seattle, WA, USA
e-mail: dcoppel@uw.edu

© Springer Nature Switzerland AG 2020
E. Hong, A. L. Rao (eds.), *Mental Health in the Athlete*,
https://doi.org/10.1007/978-3-030-44754-0_21

visualization and imagery, goal setting, and cognitive-behavioral strategies have emerged as the tools in sport psychology skill training; evolving versions of cognitive-behavioral approaches [18] and data from neuroscience and cognitive science have further expanded the sport and performance psychology field [19–22]. Over the last two decades, sport and exercise psychology concepts and interventions have been applied to other domains involving high performance, such as the performing arts [16, 23], the military [24], and medical arenas [25–27]. Sport psychologists also have increasing participation as part of the sports medicine team, working with team physicians and other medical providers [28]. Sport psychologists utilize their training and experience to provide an important and unique contribution to the sports medicine team in dealing with injuries; they can address the factors (e.g., stress) that may influence the risk of injuries, as well as the psychological reactions of being injured and dealing with recovery from sports injury [29, 30].

What Is the Field of Sport Psychology? Origins and Descriptions and Definitions

The field of sport psychology's diverse origins has allowed for a wide range of activities in practitioners and researchers. Contributions from kinesiology, physical education, and clinical and counseling psychology have helped to grow and define the field. Historically, sport and exercise psychology was defined as the scientific study of people and their behaviors in sport and exercise activities and the practical application of that knowledge [31]; more specifically, understanding how psychological factors affect physical performance and understanding how sports and exercise participation affects development, health, and well-being are the main foci. Weinberg and Gould further describe two categories: (1) clinical sport psychologists, who have training in psychology and are licensed as psychologists, as treating those athletes with severe emotional disorders and (2) educational sport psychologists who, in contrast, are described as having training in sport and exercise science, physical education, and/or kinesiology. Educational sport psychologists, seen as "mental coaches," educate athletes about psychological skills and may be involved with anxiety management. This dichotomous categorization clearly created conflict and confusion within the field. Sport psychology programs had developed within clinical/counseling psychology training programs and within kinesiology department programs, which created dual practitioner tracks in the field and some professional challenges. Clinically trained providers were said to know the clinical issues but not sport; kinesiology trained providers were said to know sport, but not be aware of clinical or emotional issues in the athlete. While these issues still exist in some forms, there is more acknowledgment that providers can have knowledge bases in both areas and greater awareness of the need to practice within your area of expertise (i.e., the ethical issue of scope of practice). Non-psychologist life coaches, performance consultants, and mental coaches, all with varied training, are often depicted as sport psychology providers, further adding to consumer confusion.

Other efforts to categorize and define the varying tracks in the field, some based on training and/or academic degree and some based on the professional activity, have been made. Van Raalte and Brewer [3] split up the field in the following structure: (1) performance enhancement (e.g., including goal setting, cognitive strategies, imagery training), (2) promoting well-being (e.g., exercise initiation and maintenance, exercise as therapy for mental health, teaching life skills through sport), and (3) clinical issues (e.g., psychopathology, measurement). Gardner and Moore [18] expand the model of sport psychology from enhancement of performance to personal development and psychological well-being of the athlete. They use the term "applied sport psychology" to refer to the application of scientific sport psychology principles with athletes, which reflects the performance enhancement interventions from cognitive-behavioral literature and psychological skills training. Clinical sport psychology reflects a comprehensive approach of professional psychological practice, which integrates assessment, case conceptualization, and intervention. The scope of practice for Gardner and Moore may include being able to assess the presence of clinical disorders, subclinical psychological barriers to change, performance skill development and dysfunction, issues related to career termination, psychological responses to injury, perfectionism, anxiety, depression, and interpersonal and intrapersonal functioning. Touching on the aforementioned conflict, they further articulate the *misconception* in the field that performance concerns can be differentiated as those due to major psychopathology or those due to insufficient mental skills and thus determine that a clinically trained psychologist is needed for the former and those trained in exercise science can consult with the latter. The issue of being able to assess the presence of a clinical disorder (or subclinical disorder) emphasizes the need for clinical or counseling training as a foundation for sport psychology consultation.

Aoyagi and Portenga [32], describing the sport psychology field, make a distinction between sport and performance psychology (with the focus on performance enhancement) and psychotherapy with athletes. Herzog and Hays's [33] article entitled "Therapist or Mental Skills Coach?" discusses these distinction and implications. They describe how sport psychologists function in different roles; as a therapist, they are dealing with diagnosed or diagnosable emotional or mental disorders and helping to reduce symptomatology and improve overall functioning; as a mental skills coach, they are making the "assumption that the client has sufficient mental strength to be able to profit from and educational focus on particular skills that will enhance performance." They cite a number of articles in which the initial focus concerned performance issues, but the sport psychology consultation and intervention involved or evolved into counseling [34]; McCann's [35] article described that at the Olympics, "everything is performance issue," but a reading of the issues cited included primarily clinical issues (e.g., suicidal ideation, depression), adjustment issues, or interpersonal conflict; while distractions and performance pressures were also included, the majority of issues appear more clinical in nature. In a similar vein, Moore and Bonagura [36] indicate that for clinical sport psychologists (defined earlier), "the intervention target is not performance." Performance is seen as an outcome, and the targets of intervention are the athlete's "psychological processes," which when modified or expanded will lead to enhanced performance in sports and possibly improved well-being.

Portenga, Aoyagi, and Cohen [8] discuss the issues of who is a sport psychologist and what is sport psychology and provide a definition of sport psychology and included it as a subfield of performance psychology; this conceptualization emphasizes the "purpose of the work" or "end goal" and not the intervention type. They propose that this emphasis will obviate some of the aforementioned dichotomies which emerged over time in the field; these include mental skills or mental health, kinesiology or psychology, and clinical or performance. "If an activity is psychological in nature, with the goal of helping people consistently perform in the upper range of their abilities, it is logical to view it as an application of performance psychology." Connecting to Hays [37] and her expansion of sport psychology to other high-performance populations, Portenga et al. define sport psychology as an "application of psychological principles of human performance in helping athletes consistently perform in the upper range of their capabilities and more thoroughly enjoy the sport performance process." Sport psychology training should allow the practitioner to be knowledgeable in what mental and emotional skills and abilities are associated with high performance, as well as have an understanding of the knowledge, skills, and abilities that could inhibit consistent excellent performances.

The American Psychological Association (APA) Division 47 (Society for Sport, Exercise, and Performance Psychology) has had evolving definitions of exercise and sport psychology over the last two decades. Exercise and sport psychology is seen as the "scientific study of the psychological factors that are associated with participation and performance in sport, exercise and other types of physical activity" (http://www.apadivisions.org/division-47/about/resources/what-is.aspx). Paralleling other views of the field, Division 47 describes that sport psychologists are interested in two main areas: (1) "helping athletes use psychological principles to achieve optimal mental health and to improve performance (performance enhancement), and (2) understanding how participation in sport, exercise and physical activity affects an individual's psychological development, health and well-being throughout the lifespan." While acknowledging the diversity and multidisciplinary aspect of sport psychology field, APA Proficiency in Sport Psychology is seen as a postgraduate specialization after a doctoral degree in one of the primary areas of psychology, involving training in psychological skills of athletes and the well-being of athletes, systemic issues within sports organizations, and the developmental and social aspects of sports participation; this specialized training is in addition to the clinical competencies required for licensure as a psychologist. It should be noted that individuals graduating with a doctoral degree in sport psychology from a department of sports science and/or kinesiology do not meet the criteria for licensure as a psychologist (or to use that designation as it is regulated by state law).

In defining the "practice" of sport psychology (often referred to as applied sport psychology), APA Division 47 focuses on the application of psychological principles of human performance to help athletes consistently perform well (peak performance) and feel positive about the performance process; the focus can be on developing and enhancing the cognitive, emotional, behavioral, and psychophysiological skills that are associated with high-level performances, as well as modifying or reducing those factors that play a detrimental role in performance. APA Division 47 provides a long list of potential applied sport psychology intervention areas with athletes. Some examples include psychological skills training; goal setting; visualization or imagery interventions; cognitive-behavioral self-regulation techniques; concentration and attentional control strategies; athletic injury and rehabilitation; career transitions; team cohesion and team building; development of self-confidence, self-esteem, and competence; and coach education. Some applied sport psychologists may also provide services to specific clinical groups such as athletes with eating disorders, substance abuse, depression or suicidality, sexual identity issues, or trauma reactions.

While the American Psychological Association (i.e., Division 47) is the major professional organization for sport psychologists, the Association for Applied Sport Psychology (AASP) is an "international, multi-disciplinary professional organization for sport psychology consultants and professionals who work with athletes, coaches, non-sports performers (dancers, musicians), business professionals, and tactical occupations (military, firefighters, police) to enhance their performance from a psychological standpoint" (http://www.appliedsportpsych. org). This organization has a diverse group of members including psychologists (clinically and counseling-trained), sport scientists, social workers, and various types of mental performance coaches. AASP initially developed a certification process that evaluated an individual's education, training, and experiences and, if accepted, would designate the individual an AASP-certified consultant; recently, the certification process was revised to include a mandatory examination, revised coursework/educational experience and mentoring requirements, and updated continuing education requirements. The current certification process leads to the Certified Mental Performance Consultant (CMPC) designation, which was felt to more clearly describe the focus of services provided; this certification allows for appropriately trained, non-licensed (as psychologists) providers working with athletes and other non-sport groups to have some designation within the field. AASP's certification effort places the emphasis on "mental performance" and expands to include non-sport domains. Interestingly, AASP's certification efforts have emerged at a time when NCAA guidelines (Mental Health Best Practices) recommend intercollegiate athletic departments to utilize *licensed* practitioners who are qualified to provide mental health services; the document recognizes certification by AASP and encourages ongoing continuing education for those professional without formal training, but ultimately, AASP certification is not equivalent to licensure by a state. More specifically, the Best Practices document acknowledges that some athletic departments employ or contract with individual trained and focused on performance enhancement, but "unless they are licensed practitioners who are qualified to provide mental health services, they should not provide mental health care to student-athletes." This can become complicated when a performance issue presentation is revealed to be due to, or strongly influenced by, an emotional/clinical issue or factor; for example, the role of anxiety or mood difficulties/disorders on sport or school performance is well-researched

[38], and some form of assessment and intervention may be indicated. In some cases, performance enhancement practitioners may be focused on the topography of the athlete's performance and not have the training/skill to assess or explore for contributory or underlying factors. Some see competency in sport psychology as beginning with being a skilled and capable clinical or counseling psychologist [39]. Other practitioners feel that the athlete's issue or issues are so tied to their sport performance that addressing this directly will have a positive effect on other issues, if they exist; also, many athletes find it easier to discuss sport performance concerns than other mental health symptoms, which is more comfortable in the short run due to stigma and other factors but may result in mental health issues not being addressed or fully evaluated, creating more difficulties in the long run.

Summary

The field of sport psychology, and performance psychology as an overarching term, is one of diversity and widening applications. While the range found in the training and education of "sport psychology" practitioners is positive for the expansion of the field, it continues to be a target for consumer confusion and professional territorial conflict. Certification and licensure provide some indication of training and levels of competency in the field and may, over time, help this confusion to a degree. However, mental health issues and addressing the psychological factors that affect athletes' performance and functioning, on and off the field, may be best responded to by clinically or counseling-trained sport psychologists. Performance-enhancement-focused providers may play an important role if the initial presentation is as a performance concern, but sorting out the potential psychological factors associated with the concern is within the scope of practice of a clinically or counseling-trained psychologist. While the perceived dichotomy between clinical- and performance-focused practitioners may continue to exist, it is far more relevant to focus on approaches to best support the athlete in their sport performance, overall well-being, and mental health. Further, inclusion of sport psychologists within the multi- or interdisciplinary approach in sports medicine affords opportunities to provide added value and a unique contribution in discussions regarding athletes' mental and related medical health, as sports medicine physicians vary in their knowledge, training, and experience with psychological factors and mental health issues. Being seen as part of the sports medicine team from the outset may help to further destigmatize seeking mental health resources. Sports-related physical injuries that involve a substantial amount of time in recovery or rehab (away from training and the team) can alter the athlete's sense of identity or sport trajectory for the season and beyond. These situations often involve a psychological "injury" at a clinical or subclinical level and declining performance and functioning in non-sports activities and should be addressed by appropriate mental health providers.

References

1. Weinberg R, Gould D. Foundations of sport and exercise psychology. 4th ed. Champaign, IL: Human Kinetics; 2007.
2. Weinberg R, Gould D. Foundations of sport and exercise psychology. 6th ed. Champaign, IL: Human Kinetics; 2015.
3. Van Raalte J, Brewer B. Exploring sport and exercise psychology. 3rd ed. Washington, DC: American Psychological Association; 2014.
4. Papaioannou AG, Hackfort D, editors. Routledge companion to sport and exercise psychology: global perspectives and fundamental concepts. London and New York: Routledge/Taylor and Frances Group; 2015.
5. Murphy S. Sport psychology interventions. Champaign, IL: Human Kinetics; 1995.
6. Barker JB, Neil R, Fletcher D. Using sport and performance psychology in the management of change. J Chang Manag. 2016;16(1):1–7. https://doi.org/10.1080/14697017.2016.1137149.
7. Kornspan A. History of sports performance. In: Murphy S, editor. The Oxford handbook of sport and performance psychology. New York, NY: Oxford University Press; 2012. p. 3–23.
8. Portenga S, Aoyagi M, Cohen A. Helping to build a profession: a working definition of sport and performance psychology. J Sport Psychol Action. 2017;8(1):47–59. https://doi.org/10.108 0/21520704.2016.1227413.
9. Tod D, Hutter R, Eubank M. Professional development for sport psychology practice. Curr Opin Psychol. 2017;16:133–7.
10. Triplett N. The dynamogenic factors in pacemaking and competition. Am J Psychol. 1898;9:507–33.
11. Straub W, Williams J, editors. Cognitive sport psychology. Lansing, NY: Sports Sciences Associates; 1984.
12. May J, Asken M, editors. Sport psychology: the psychological health of the athlete. New York: PMA Publishing; 1987.
13. Vealey R. Conceptualization of sport-confidence and competitive orientation: preliminary investigation and instrument development. J Sport Psychol. 1986;8:221–46.
14. Feltz D, Short S, Sullivan. Self-efficacy in sport. Champaign, IL: Human Kinetics; 2008.
15. Hackfort D, Schwenkmezger P. Anxiety. In: Singer R, Murphey M, Tennant L, editors. Handbook of research in sport psychology. New York: Macmillan; 1993.
16. Hays K, editor. Performance psychology in action. Washington, DC: American Psychological Association; 2009.
17. Razon S, Tenenbaum G. Measurement in sport and exercise psychology. In: Van Raalte J, Brewer B, editors. Exploring sport and exercise psychology. 3rd ed. Washington, DC: American Psychological Association; 2014. p. 279–310.
18. Gardner F, Moore Z. Clinical sport psychology. Champaign, IL: Human Kinetics; 2006.
19. Moran A. The psychology of concentration in sport performers: a cognitive analysis. East Sussex: Psychology Press; 1996.
20. Beliock S. Beyond the playing field: sport psychology meets embodied cognition. Int Rev Sport Exerc Psychol. 2008;I(1):19–30.
21. Zaichowsky L. Psychophysiology and neuroscience in sport: introduction to the special issue. J Clin Sport Psychol. 2012;6(1):1–5.
22. Furley P, Wood G. Working memory, attentional control, and expertise in sports: a review of current literature and directions for future research. J Appl Res Mem Cogn. 2016;5(4):415–25.
23. Cotterill S. Preparing for performance: strategies adopted across performance domains. Sports Psychol. 2015;29:158–70.
24. DeWiggins S, Hite B, Alston V. Personal performance plan: application of mental skills training to real-world military tasks. J Appl Sport Psychol. 2010;22(4):458–73.
25. Causer J, Vickers J, Snelgrove R, Arsenault G, Harvey A. Quiet eye training improves surgical knot-tying performance. Surgery. 2014;156(5):1089–96.

26. Cocks M, Moulton C, Luu S, Cil T. What surgeons can learn from athletes: mental practice in sports and surgery. J Surg Educ. 2014;71(2):262–9.
27. Rao A, Tait J, Alijani A. Systematic review and meta-analysis of the role of mental training in the acquisition of technical skills in surgery. Am J Surg. 2015;210(3):545–53.
28. Coppel D. Psychological aspects of sports medicine. Curr Phys Med Rehabil Rep. 2015;3(1):36–42.
29. Coppel D. The role of sport psychology and psychiatry. In: Madden C, Putukian M, McCarty E, Young C, editors. Netter's sports medicine. 2nd ed. Philadelphia, PA: Elsevier Publishing; 2018. p. 173–9.
30. Herring SA, Kibler WB, Putukian M, Coppel D, et al. Psychological issues related to illness and injury in athletes and the team physician: a consensus statement (2016 update). Med Sci Sport Exerc. 2017;49:1043.
31. Gill D. Psychological dynamics of sport and exercise. Champaign, IL: Human Kinetics; 2000.
32. Aoyagi M, Portenga S. The role of positive ethics and virtues in the context of sport and performance psychology service delivery. Prof Psychol Res Pract. 2010;41(3):253–9.
33. Herzog T, Hays K. Therapist or mental skills coach? How to decide. Sport Psychol. 2012;26:486–99.
34. Meyers A, Whelan J, Murphy S. Cognitive behavioral strategies in athletic performance enhancement. Prog Behav Modif. 1995;30:137–64.
35. McCann S. At the Olympics, everything is a performance issue. Int J Sport Exerc Psychol. 2008;6(3):267–76.
36. Moore Z, Bonagura K. Current opinion in clinical sport psychology: from athletic performance to psychological well-being. Curr Opin Psychol. 2017;16:176–9.
37. Hays K. The psychology of performance in sport and other domains. In: The Oxford handbook of sport and performance psychology. Oxford, UK: Oxford University Press; 2012. p. 24–45.
38. Ford J, Ildefanso K, Jones M, Arvinen-Barrow M. Sport-related anxiety: current insights. Open Access J Sports Med. 2017;8:205–12.
39. Sullivan J, Coppel D, Maniar S, Minniti A. Sport psychologists. In: Sternberg R, editor. Career paths in psychology. 3rd ed; 2017. p. 273–89.
40. Murphy S. The sport psych handbook. Champaign, IL: Human Kinetics; 2005.

Chapter 22
Exercise as a Prescription for Mental Health

Vicki R. Nelson and Irfan M. Asif

Introduction

Mental health complaints present a significant burden to the healthcare system. In the United States, one in five adults experience a mental health disorder each year with 64.8% seeking treatment [1]. Long-term adherence to traditional pharmacologic and psychiatric therapies is poor; the time commitment, cost, and pharmacologic side effects of therapy can be substantial. Physical activity as an alternative or adjuvant strategy to promote mental health and treat mental illness shows comparable outcomes in depression and anxiety treatment, without negative side effects.

Regular exercise provides numerous health benefits but is also an effective strategy for promoting mental health. Participation in regular physical activity can prevent and treat common disorders such as depression, anxiety, and ADHD, promotes better sleep, and improves memory and mood. Exercise can improve one's sense of well-being and can be a powerful technique to promote and maintain mental health. Providing a clear, succinct prescription for exercise tailored to the patient's individual needs, health concerns, and fitness allows a physician to promote physical activity as an effective treatment option for mental illness.

Effects of Physical Activity

Many mechanisms have been proposed describing how physical activity improves mental health and treats mental illness. The positive effects are likely multifactorial with contributions from physiologic and psychologic mechanisms.

V. R. Nelson (✉) · I. M. Asif
Prisma Health - Upstate and University of South Carolina School of Medicine – Greenville, Greenville, SC, USA
e-mail: Vicki.Nelson@PrismaHealth.org; IAsif@uab.edu

© Springer Nature Switzerland AG 2020
E. Hong, A. L. Rao (eds.), *Mental Health in the Athlete*,
https://doi.org/10.1007/978-3-030-44754-0_22

Physiology

During physical activity, important neurotransmitters including dopamine, serotonin, and norepinephrine are upregulated, mimicking the effects of common pharmacotherapy in mood and anxiety disorders [2]. Endorphin release during exercise also has an acute energizing and beneficial effect on mood and cognition.

Physical activity causes sympathetic activation, which mimics symptoms experienced by patients during anxiety or panic. While this may initially exacerbate symptoms, tolerance can be developed through feedback mechanisms. Modulation of cortisol release through the hypothalamic-pituitary-adrenal (HPA) axis is one potential mechanism. In the acute setting, cortisol is a stress hormone. Regular physical activity can reduce stress through negative feedback, resulting in a reduction in pituitary stimulation and lower baseline cortisol levels [3, 4].

Animal studies evaluating the impact of exercise upon physiological parameters have demonstrated cellular changes in the brain including increased cell regeneration, new cell formation, volume increases in the hippocampus, increased brain vasculature, and improved oxidative capacity [5–7]. Finally, regular exercise may even modulate genetic factors and regulate gene expression including several important trophic factors such as insulin-like growth factor (IGF-1) and vascular endothelial growth factor (VEGF) [8]. While these findings have not been established in humans, they provide potentially important areas for further investigation.

Psychology

Similar to cognitive behavioral therapy, physical activity may break the cycle of negative thoughts contributing to depression or distract from anxiety-provoking stimuli. In depression, behavior is often characterized by passivity and social isolation. Participating actively in exercise requires a behavior change affecting thought patterns and emotions. Physical activity provides an avenue for patients to participate in positive thought patterns and provide strategies for self-confidence and self-control.

The regular investment in one's mind and body through physical activity, as well as improved functional abilities, can foster a sense of self-worth, well-being, and achievement. These qualities can help promote mental wellness and improve resilience. Short periods of exercise in the morning and early afternoon can help to regulate sleep patterns and improve energy. For patients struggling with sleep disturbances and fatigue, this may be invaluable.

Exercise and Depression

Major depression is one of the most common mental disorders in the United States with an estimated 16 million adults experiencing at least one episode of major depression in the past year [9].

Depression has a high comorbidity with other mental and physical disorders, most notably anxiety disorders and cardiovascular disease, contributing to morbidity and complicating treatment.

Regular physical activity can reduce the risk of developing clinical depression and reduces depressive symptoms [10, 11]. Exercise is a safe and often effective strategy for both the treatment and prevention of clinical depression alone or in conjunction with traditional therapies.

In the treatment of major depression, regular physical activity has a moderate to large effect on the reduction of depressive symptoms, showing comparable outcomes with cognitive behavioral therapy or antidepressant pharmacotherapy [12–17]. Participation in regular physical activity over several weeks can be effective in cases of depression resistant to pharmacotherapy [18]. In individuals who continue actively exercising long-term, the risk of recurrent depressive episodes is significantly reduced and more patients experience full remission [19].

Interactions with Medical Therapy

Current antidepressant medications such as selective serotonin reuptake inhibitors (SSRIs) or serotonin-norepinephrine reuptake inhibitors (SNRIs) are generally well tolerated with exercise. Tricyclic antidepressants and monoamine oxidase inhibitors (MAOIs) can cause increased heart rate and lower blood pressure and may induce muscle cramping, dry mouth, or increased sweating, all of which could make exercise more difficult. Monitoring medication tolerance and side effects should be considered before recommending an exercise program.

Contraindications

Patients that are underweight or have a comorbid eating disorder should not be prescribed exercise for depression until these concerns have been addressed. Participation in a supervised cardiac rehabilitation program may be appropriate for patients with comorbid cardiovascular disease or reactive depression following acute coronary events or open-heart procedures.

Special Considerations

For many suffering with mood disorders, the thought of finding time or motivation to exercise can be particularly overwhelming. Providing a clear, simple prescription for physical activity with an agreed-upon time commitment can help overcome this challenge.

Exercise and Anxiety

Anxiety disorders including generalized anxiety disorder, panic disorder, and post-traumatic stress disorder are among the most common mental health disorders. The prevalence in the United States is around 18%, with females 60% more likely to experience an anxiety disorder. Participating in regular physical activity can reduce the symptoms of anxiety in chronic anxiety disorders as well as intermittent feelings of acute anxiety.

Exercise is at least as effective as standard medical treatment (pharmacotherapy or cognitive behavioral therapy) for anxiety [20]. Even a single episode of moderate-intensity physical activity can lead to a reduction in anxiety symptoms. This effect is more robust in females, sedentary individuals, and individuals older than 25 years [21]. Participation in regular physical activity over weeks to months produces a cumulative reduction in anxiety symptoms in healthy individuals as well as, to a lesser degree, those with physical or mental illnesses [22]. Limited evidence suggests that physical activity may also be beneficial in treatment and prevention of PTSD [23, 24].

Interactions with Medical Therapy

Antidepressant medications (e.g., SSRIs) used to treat anxiety disorders do not hinder participation in physical activity. Beta blockers, used for situational anxiety, may limit physical capacity to some degree due to suppression of maximal heart rate but present no risk of adverse events. This effect is minimized with beta-1-selective blockade and is of minimal consequence in the non-elite athlete [25]. Benzodiazepines may contribute to a raising or lowering of blood pressure and function as a central nervous system relaxant. This does not prevent participation in physical activity, but it may be prudent to monitor the patient's tolerance on this medication for a short time prior to initiating a physical activity program.

Contraindications

There are no contraindications to physical activity in physically well patients with anxiety.

For patients whose symptoms mimic cardiac pathology, such as chest pains or palpitations, a medical evaluation should be completed prior to initiating a physical activity program. Electrocardiogram or thyroid hormone testing could be considered. If the etiology of the patients' symptoms is unclear, consultation with a cardiologist may be pursued. It is important to remain cognizant that patients with anxiety symptoms may become more anxious with repeated examinations, testing, or uncertainty in their providers.

Special Considerations

Initiating a physical activity program may initially exacerbate anxiety symptoms. Activation of the sympathetic nervous system resulting in elevated heart rate, sweating, and breathlessness may mimic anxiety or panic reactions. Counseling patients about this phenomenon in advance can help patients overcome these symptoms and successfully participate in physical activity. Particularly in sedentary patients, initiating programs with low-intensity activities to facilitate acclimation and tolerance should be considered.

For individuals who exercise regularly, being forced to modify or cut down on their activity, such as following an injury, may increase symptoms of anxiety. Consider providing alternative options for physical activity in these settings.

Prescribing Exercise for Mental Health

The Exercise Prescription

Recommendations for an aerobic exercise program should address frequency, intensity, time, and type of physical activity (FITT Framework). For general health promotion, inclusion of aerobic, strength, and mobility exercise should be included in a complete exercise program.

Frequency In the treatment of depression and anxiety, a frequency of at least 3 days per week is recommended. A single episode of moderate to vigorous physical activity can improve sleep, cognition, and anxiety symptoms on the same day [26]. However, effects become larger with regular performance and benefits are acquired after days to weeks of consistent physical activity.

Intensity Moderate-intensity physical activity is safe, appropriate, and best for most people. This should be encouraged in patients who can tolerate moderate intensity. In the case of anxiety, lighter-intensity exercise and strength or flexibility training can improve symptoms, minimize sympathetic effects, and should be considered in patients resistant to higher-intensity activity. When counseling patients new to exercise, moderate-intensity activities such as a brisk walk or jog may be described that they should be able to carry on a conversation, but not sing, during activity. Alternatively, a goal of 40–50% of the patient's maximal heart rate (220 minus age) can be utilized in unconditioned individuals with a goal to gradually increase to 70% of maximum over 1–2 months as fitness improves.

Time Episodes of no less than 20 minutes should be recommended. Greater benefit is achieved with 30–45 minutes of activity [27].

Type Many types of activities are appropriate and beneficial. Regular walking is beneficial, easy, and cost-effective for previously inactive patients. Other activities such as bicycling, water aerobics, swimming, dancing, or tennis could be pursued. The patient's enjoyment and compliance with the activity over a period of time are more important than the particular activity selected.

Duration Most mental health benefits from physical activity require consistent participation over 8–10 weeks [28, 29]. Particularly when treating anxiety disorders, the type or intensity of physical activity is not as essential as regular participation, and activity should be tailored to facilitate compliance.

Mind-Body Exercises The practice of mindfulness, controlled breathing, and emphasis on the mind-body connection in alternative exercise practices such as yoga, meditation, qigong, or tai chi may be helpful to individuals with mental illness, particularly anxiety disorders [30–33]. Including mindfulness components of exercise such as a focusing on the rhythm of breathing or a walking cadence can help to refocus cognitive awareness and disrupt negative thought processes [34]. Evidence is currently limited to support these activities as effective treatments; however, the risk of negative effects is low, and they could be considered as adjunctive therapies.

Prescription for Mental Health

The 2008 Physical Activity Guidelines for Americans recommends 150 minutes of moderate to vigorous intensity physical activity per week [35]. This recommendation is likely sufficient to receive the mental health benefits of consistent physical activity. However, even lighter intensity or shorter durations can benefit mental health. A prescription of at least 20 minutes of moderate-intensity aerobic activity 3 days per week for 8 weeks can be appropriate in those who are not physically active. To obtain maximal benefit, activity should be gradually increased in time, intensity, and/or frequency to meet guidelines for aerobic activity and strength training introduced. For treatment of mental illness, titration up to 45–60 minutes of moderate to vigorous physical activity 3–5 days per week over a 10-week period may be required to obtain benefit.

Summary

Physical activity is a cost-effective, low-risk intervention that can be utilized to prevent and treat mental illness and improve mental well-being. The 2008 Physical Activity Guidelines for Americans recommended 150–300 minutes per week (500–1000 MET-minutes) of moderate-intensity physical activity for adults, which is sufficient to obtain the mental health benefits [26, 35]. Unfortunately, half of the US adult population does not meet this recommendation, and nearly one-third report participating in no physical activity [26]. For these patients, even modest improvements in physical activity could provide physical and mental health benefits. Furthermore, mindfulness-based exercise practices can offer an alternative modality to enhance mood and maintain mental health.

References

1. National Institute of Mental Health. Mental illness statistics. https://www.nimh.nih.gov/health/statistics/mental-illness.shtml. Accessed 23 July 2018.
2. Meeusen R. Exercise and the brain. Insight in new therapeutic modalities. Ann Transplant. 2005;10:49–51.
3. Stranahan AM, Lee K, Mattson MP. Central mechanisms of HPA axis regulation by voluntary exercise. NeuroMolecular Med. 2008;10:118–27.
4. Pereira AC, Huddleston DE, Brickman AM, Sosunov AA, Hen R, et al. An in vivo correlate of exercise-induced neurogenesis in the adult dentate gyrus. Proc Natl Acad Sci USA. 2007;104:5638–43.
5. Björnebekk A, Mathé AA, Brené S. The antidepressant effect of running is associated with increased hippocampal cell proliferation. Int J Neuropsychopharmacol. 2005;8:357–68.
6. van Praag H, Christie BR, Sejnowski TJ, Gage FH. Running enhances neurogenesis, learning, and long-term potentiation in mice. Proc Natl Acad Sci USA. 1999;96:13427–31.
7. Dishman RK, Berthoud HR, Booth FW, Cotman CW, Edgerton VR, Fleshner MR, et al. Neurobiology of exercise. Obesity. 2006;14:345–56.
8. Duman RS. Neurotrophic factors and regulation of mood: role of exercise, diet and metabolism. Neurobiol Aging. 2005;26(suppl 1):88–93.
9. Center for Behavioral Health Statistics and Quality. Key substance use and mental health indicators in the United States: Results from the 2015 National Survey on Drug Use and Health. HHS Publication No. SMA 16–4984, NSDUH Series H-51. Rockville, MD: Substance Abuse and Mental Health Services; 2016. https://www.samhsa.gov/data/sites/default/files/NSDUH-FFR1–2015/NSDUH-FFR1–2015/NSDUH-FFR1–2015.pdf. Accessed 6 July 2018.
10. Franz SI, Hamilton GV. Effects of exercise upon the retardation in condition of depression. Am J Psychiatr. 1905;62:239–56. Published online 2006.
11. McCann IL, Holmes DS. Influence of aerobic exercise on depression. J Pers Soc Psychol. 1984;46:1142–7.
12. Park SH, Han KS, Kang CB. Effects of exercise programs on depressive symptoms, quality of life, and self-esteem in older people: a systematic review of randomized controlled trials. Appl Nurs Res. 2014;27(4):219–26.
13. Cooney GM, Dwan K, Greig CA, et al. Exercise for depression. Cochrane Database Syst Rev. 2013;(9):Cd004366.
14. Robertson R, Robertson A, Jepson R, Maxwell M. Walking for depression or depressive symptoms: a systematic review and meta-analysis. Ment Health Phys Act. 2012;5(1):66–75.
15. Josefsson T, Lindwall M, Archer T. Physical exercise intervention in depressive disorders: meta-analysis and systematic review. Scand J Med Sci Sports. 2014;24(2):259–72.
16. Schuch FB, Vancampfort D, Richards J, Rosenbaum S, Ward PB, Stubbs B. Exercise as a treatment for depression: a meta-analysis adjusting for publication bias. J Psychiatr Res. 2016;77:42–51.
17. Farah WH, Alsawas M, Mainou M, et al. Non-pharmacological treatment of depression: a systematic review and evidence map. Evid Based Med. 2016;21(6):214–21.

18. Trivedi MH, Greer TL, Granneman BD, Chambliss HO, Alexander J. Exercise as an augmentation strategy for treatment of major depression. J Psychiatr Pract. 2006;12:205–13.
19. Harris AHS, Cronkite R, Moos R. Physical activity, exercise coping and depression in a 10-year cohort study of depressed patients. J Affect Disord. 2006;93:79–85.
20. Wegner M, Helmich I, Machado S, Nardi AE, Arias-Carrion O, Budde H. Effects of exercise on anxiety and depression disorders: review of meta-analyses and neurobiological mechanisms. CNS Neurol Disord Drug Targets. 2014;13(6):1002–14.
21. Bartley CA, Hay M, Bloch MH. Meta-analysis: aerobic exercise for the treatment of anxiety disorders. Prog Neuro-Psychopharmacol Biol Psychiatry. 2013;45(2):34–9.
22. Gordon BR, McDowell CP, Lyons M, Herring MP. The effects of resistance exercise training on anxiety: a meta-analysis and meta-regression analysis of randomized controlled trials. Sports Med. 2017;47(12):2521–32.
23. Whitworth JW, Ciccolo JT. Exercise and post-traumatic stress disorder in military veterans: a systematic review. Mil Med. 2016;181(9):953–60.
24. Sciarrino NA, DeLucia C, O'Brien K, McAdams K. Assessing the effectiveness of yoga as a complementary and alternative treatment for post-traumatic stress disorder: a review and synthesis. J Altern Complement Med. 2017;23(10):747–55.
25. Fagard R, Staessen J, Thijs L, Amery A. Influence of antihypertensive drugs on exercise capacity. Drugs. 1993;24(Supp 2):32–6.
26. Physical Activity Guidelines Advisory Committee. Physical activity guidelines advisory committee scientific report, 2018. Washington, DC: U.S. Department of Health and Human Services; 2018.
27. Martinsen EW, Hoffart A, Solberg. Aerobic and non-aerobic exercise in the treatment of anxiety disorders. Stress Med. 1989;5:115–20.
28. Craft LL, Landers DM. The effect of exercise on clinical depression and depression resulting from mental illness. A meta-analysis. J Sport Exerc Psychol. 1998;20:339–57.
29. Dunn AL, Trivedi MH, O'Neal HA. Physical activity dose response effects on outcomes of depression and anxiety. Med Sci Sports Exerc. 2001;33:587–97.
30. Cramer H, Lauche R, Langhorst J, Dobos G. Yoga for depression: a systematic review and meta-analysis. Depress Anxiety. 2013;30(11):1068–83.
31. Li AW, Goldsmith CA. The effects of yoga on anxiety and stress. Altern Med Rev. 2012;17(1):21–35.
32. Wang F, Lee EK, Wu T, Benson H, Fricchione G, et al. The effects of tai chi on depression, anxiety, and psychological well-being: a systematic review and meta-analysis. Int J Behav Med. 2014;21(4):605–17.
33. Orme-Johnson DW, Barnes VA. Effects of the transcendental meditation technique on trait anxiety: a meta-analysis of randomized controlled trials. J Altern Complement Med. 2014;20(5):330–41.
34. Bahrke MS, Morgan WP. Anxiety reduction following exercise and meditation. Cogn Ther Res. 1978;4:323–33.
35. Physical Activity Guidelines Advisory Committee. Physical activity guidelines for Americans, 2008. Washington, DC: U.S. Department of Health and Human Services; 2008.

Chapter 23
The Role of Sleep in Psychological Well-Being in Athletes

Chad Asplund and Cindy J. Chang

Introduction

Sleep is a complex process in which our body undertakes a number of essential activities, including brain rest, regeneration, memory formation, and physical recovery. Many people, including athletes, have sleep difficulties or simply do not get enough sleep. Travel or the timing of competition often contributes to sleep issues among athletes. Poor sleep can also be a sign of a mental health disorder or can exacerbate existing mental health conditions.

While athletes can have a comparable quantity of sleep to nonathletes, significant differences have been observed in the quality of sleep [1]. In college students, there is a high prevalence of common mental disorders comorbid with sleep disorders; those who experienced poor sleep quality had nearly a 2.4-fold higher odds of depression, anxiety, and somatoform disorder than those students with good sleep quality [2]. In athletes, the prevalence of poor sleep quality with high levels of daytime sleepiness is as high as 50–83% [3]. Poor sleep quality, insomnia, and excessive daytime sleepiness have also been shown in elite athletes with disabilities [4]. Elite athletes experience worse sleep prior to an important competition, with over 70% reporting problems falling asleep, an increased intensity of worry symptoms 4 days before competition, and deterioration in sleep quality [5]. Sleep *quantity* among college athletes deteriorated prior to competition due to anxiety [6, 8, 9].

C. Asplund
Department of Orthopaedics and Family Medicine, Mayo Clinic, Minneapolis, MN, USA
e-mail: asplund.chad@mayo.edu

C. J. Chang (✉)
Departments of Orthopaedics and Family & Community Medicine, University of California, San Francisco, San Francisco, CA, USA
e-mail: cindy.chang@ucsf.edu

© Springer Nature Switzerland AG 2020
E. Hong, A. L. Rao (eds.), *Mental Health in the Athlete*,
https://doi.org/10.1007/978-3-030-44754-0_23

There is no known psychiatric condition in which sleep is not disturbed. This is true of depression, anxiety, post-traumatic stress disorder (PTSD), schizophrenia, and bipolar disorder [10]. Interestingly, fMRI studies demonstrate that blocking sleep in otherwise healthy people can demonstrate neurological patterns of brain activity very similar to those found in psychiatric conditions [11]. Many of the brain regions impacted by psychiatric mood disorders are the same regions impacted by poor sleep [10]. However, improved sleep quantity and quality can improve the symptoms of depression, anxiety, and bipolar disorder [12], which is why having good sleep habits or improving existing sleep habits is so important for the mental health of athletes.

Why Do We Sleep?

Sleep is an important component of the daily routine. Most people spend up to one-third of their time sleeping. Everyone needs sleep, but its true biological purpose remains somewhat of a mystery. There are several theories as to why we need sleep. The *inactivity theory* proposes that organisms sleep at night to protect themselves from danger. The *energy conservation theory* suggests that the primary function of sleep is to reduce an individual's energy demand and expenditure during part of the day or night, especially at times when it is least efficient to search for food. The *restorative theory* proposes that sleep is necessary for the body to repair and rejuvenate itself. Finally, the *brain plasticity theory* suggests that sleep is important for the organization and the structure of the brain [13, 14].

Recently, researchers have proposed the "synaptic pruning" theory as a purpose of sleep. During the day, our brains build connections with other parts of the brain. During sleep, important connections are strengthened and the nonessential ones are pruned. Sleep is an opportunity to clear the brain of clutter and waste [15]. Mendelsohn found that poor sleep results in poor clearance of metabolites, such beta-amyloid, which may be associative with an increase in movement disorders and memory issues and possibly an increase in other mental health issues as well [16]. This lack of clearance caused by poor sleep increases the activity in genes that cause inflammation; inflammation within the brain, in fact, has been linked to depression [17]. Finally, sleep dysfunction and poor metabolite clearance have been linked to serotonergic dysfunction [18], which is clearly associated with depression and anxiety. Poor sleep thus impairs the metabolic and hormonal function of the brain, which may lead to mental illness.

Normal Sleep Architecture

Sleep architecture is defined as the composite structure of sleep. It is composed of rapid eye movement (REM) sleep and non-REM (NREM) sleep. The sleep stages represent polysomnographic changes corresponding to changes in brain activity as the brain transitions from wakefulness, light sleep, deep sleep, and then REM sleep. People will typically pass through three NREM sleep stages before beginning REM sleep. In total, NREM sleep accounts for approximately 75–80% of total sleep in the average adult and is divided into substages N1, N2, and N3 [19].

N1 sleep describes the stage where the body transitions from wakefulness to sleep. Stage N2 is an intermediate phase comprising the largest percentage (50%) of the total night's sleep. While N1 and N2 are characterized as *light sleep*, N3 is typically referred to as *slow wave* or *deep sleep*. Finally, REM sleep is divided into phasic REM and tonic REM. Phasic REM is where there are bursts of rapid eye movement, while tonic REM exists between phasic bursts in which low muscle tone is constant [20].

Typically, sleep occurs in multiple cycles throughout the night with fairly typical patterns of NREM and REM sleep, with each cycle lasting approximately 90 min. Most people will require five complete sleep cycles to awaken feeling refreshed and restored; however, there can be much variability in individual needs [21].

Although the exact reason is unclear, the amount of time spent in the different sleep stages appears to relate to people's mental health. Those who suffer from depression have been shown to have more REM sleep [22], enter REM earlier, and have an increase in the frequency of rapid eye movements [23]. For people with schizophrenia, there can be a delay in reaching both deep sleep and REM sleep [23]. Similarly, people who suffer from anxiety may spend less time in deep sleep [24].

Medication Effects on Sleep Architecture

Medications, specifically those that target the central nervous system (CNS), cardiovascular system, or respiratory system, can adversely affect sleep architecture. Commonly prescribed CNS medications include benzodiazepines, non-benzodiazepine receptor agonists (NBRA), anti-seizure medications, antidepressants, and stimulant medications.

Benzodiazepines and NBRA reduce the amount of stage 1 sleep and may moderately reduce REM sleep at higher doses [25]. Seizure medications such as phenobarbital or carbamazepine inhibit CNS activity, whereas other drugs such as gabapentin enhance GABA activity. Carbamazepine increases deep sleep and reduces REM sleep. Phenobarbital increases light sleep but decreases deep sleep [26].

Antidepressant medications include tricyclic antidepressants (TCA), selective serotonin reuptake inhibitors (SSRIs), and serotonin antagonist and reuptake inhibitors (SARIs) and are known to affect sleep architecture. All antidepressant medications across the classes suppress REM sleep, except SARIs. SARIs such as trazodone increase deep sleep, while SSRIs appear to increase light sleep [27].

Nonsteroidal anti-inflammatory drugs (NSAIDS) and acetaminophen should be the medication of choice for analgesia, as neither has been shown to alter sleep architecture [28]. Narcotic analgesics can decrease deep sleep and as doses increase can also cause decreased REM sleep [29].

Stimulant medications have profound effects on sleep architecture. Amphetamines, dextroamphetamines, methylphenidate, and modafinil all lead to increased light sleep and decreased deep sleep and REM sleep [30, 31]. However, with discontinuation of these stimulant medications, there may be increased sleepiness and a rebound in REM sleep [31]. Over-the-counter decongestants such as pseudoephedrine have not been specifically studied but could disrupt sleep in a manner similarly to the stimulant medications.

Beta-blockers, especially propranolol or metoprolol, will suppress REM sleep [27]. Alpha-blockers increase the percentage of very light sleep while also suppressing REM sleep [32]. Methylxanthines, such as theophylline, increase light sleep, but don't alter the remainder of the sleep architecture. Glucocorticoids have not been widely studied for their effect on sleep, but many patients who take steroids for pulmonary complaints experience decreased REM sleep and increased awakening after sleep onset [33].

The Anatomy of Sleep

There are several structures in the brain that are involved in sleep as well as emotional regulation. Within the hypothalamus lies the suprachiasmatic nucleus (SCN), which receives information about light exposure directly from the eyes. Sleep-promoting cells within the hypothalamus and brainstem secrete gamma-aminobutyric acid (GABA), which acts to reduce the activity of arousal centers in the brain. The pineal gland receives signals from the SCN and increases the endogenous production of the hormone melatonin. The cyclical rise and fall of melatonin is critical for matching the body's circadian rhythm to the external lightness and darkness. During the daytime, the thalamus relays information from the senses to the cerebral cortex. During most of sleep, the thalamus is quiet but increases activity during REM sleep, which contributes to the sensations observed during dream sleep. The amygdala, which is involved in processing emotions, also becomes increasingly active during REM sleep.

It is the amygdala that serves as a main link between sleep and mental health conditions. The amygdala is the integrative center for emotions, emotional behavior, motivation, and fear. Walker and colleagues found that sleep deprivation amplified the emotional reactivity of the amygdala by up to 60%, which enhanced the brain's response to negative emotional stimuli [11]. Additionally, in Japan it was found that decreased sleep of only 5 h per night for 5 days causes the same dysregulation of the amygdala as total sleep deprivation [34].

Common Sleep Disorders and Their Association/Effect on Psychological Well-Being in Athletes

Sleep-wake disorders, as defined per the *Diagnostic and Statistical Manual of Mental Disorders, Fifth Edition (DSM-5)*, comprise 11 diagnostic groups including insomnia disorder, breathing-related sleep disorders, circadian rhythm sleep-wake disorders, substance-/medication-induced sleep disorder, non–rapid eye movement (NREM) sleep arousal disorders (sleepwalking), rapid eye movement (REM) sleep behavior disorder, and restless legs syndrome. Only two of these disorders have been studied specifically in athletes, and these will be discussed in more detail. Sleep disorders can coexist with other medical and psychiatric disorders and may not be mutually exacerbating. It is important to rule out a sleep disorder regardless of possible mental or other medical problems that may also be present, although these coexisting medical conditions, mental disorders, and sleep disorders are interactive.

Insomnia

The major criteria for a diagnosis of insomnia disorder (DSM-5) include the following:

1. Difficulty initiating or maintaining sleep or early-morning awakening that leads to dissatisfaction with sleep quantity or quality.
2. Resulting sleep disturbance leads to impairment in social, occupational, educational, academic, behavioral, or other important areas of functioning, as well as causing significant distress.
3. Patients experience insomnia even with adequate opportunity to sleep, at least three nights per week and for at least 3 months.
4. Insomnia is not explained by presence of other mental or medical conditions and is not associated with another sleep disorder.

The main characteristic of insomnia related to another mental disorder is the presence of insomnia that is judged to be temporally or causally related to another mental disorder.

Much has been studied on insomnia and sleep disruption and their effect on athletic performance and little of its effect on mental health. Symptoms associated with insomnia can include lack of concentration, irritability, and depression. Yearly psychological evaluations of elite athletes assessed for insomnia symptoms found ongoing sleep problems in 21.5%, with difficulty falling asleep and nocturnal waking reported more often in women and daytime somnolence significantly greater in younger athletes 17 years old and younger [35].

There has long been robust evidence linking decreases in both the quality and duration of sleep to the detriment of overall health including impaired cognitive functioning and judgment, mood problems, and somatic symptoms [36, 37], as well as an increase in perceived physical exertion and decrease in pain tolerance [36, 38]. Motivation, focus, memory, and learning can also be impaired. In a large study of college students, over 60% were categorized as poor-quality sleepers and reported significantly more problems with physical and psychological health. The students surveyed also reported frequently taking prescription, over the counter, and recreational psychoactive drugs to alter sleep/wakefulness [39].

Because sleep deprivation may cause or modulate acute and chronic pain and pain may disturb sleep by inducing arousals during sleep, these two issues can augment each other, and a continuous cycle can develop [40]. Sleep loss is associated with an increase in both sympathetic activity and catecholamine levels and, over time, may lead to altered stress system responsiveness, similar to that seen in mood disorders [41]. In athletes already experiencing pain from injuries or surgeries, sleep may play an important role in pain perception and mental and physical recovery. Sleep deprivation is also a risk factor for illicit substance and alcohol use, violence-related behaviors, and motor vehicle accidents [42, 43, 44].

Athletes diagnosed with overtraining syndrome showed decreased sleep quality, leading to the conclusion that worsened sleep was a trigger [45]. In nearly 50% of elite Gaelic athletes who were categorized as poor sleepers, there was a significant relationship with lower general health, increased stress, and increased confusion [46]. Elite volleyball players with poor sleep quality reported higher scores for confusion and, if they lost their game, were more likely to demonstrate higher tension [47]. Seventy percent of athletes who had disrupted sleep prior to a competition had negative moods of fatigue and tension.

Obstructive Sleep Apnea-Hypopnea (OSA)

For persons with OSA, during an apnea episode, the individual stops breathing for a short period of time. Snoring is a common feature, and this can progress to loud disruptive snoring with arousals associated with partial or complete airflow obstruction. This results in forced awakening that disrupts the individual's sleep, reduces total sleep time, and negatively impacts overall sleep health. Because of the frequent awakenings and non-restorative sleep, daytime symptoms can include morning headache, dry mouth, irritability, fatigue, and sleepiness. With the restriction of airflow, baroreceptor modulation of sympathetic nerve activity is impaired, and this dysregulation can exacerbate hypertension and other cardio-metabolic disorders [48–50]. OSA has been linked to hypertension as well as cognitive impairment and mood disorder [51], but there are few studies looking at the prevalence in athletes.

The diagnosis of obstructive sleep apnea can be made by polysomnography alone when there are more than 15 respiratory events an hour, regardless of symptoms (DSM-5). Using this criterion stresses the importance of diagnosing and treating OSA, which can cause and worsen medical disorders such as hypertension, diabetes, substance use, and anxiety.

Physical characteristics of athletes in certain sports such as American football and rugby may predispose them to OSA. One-half of elite rugby and cricket athletes were poor sleepers (Pittsburgh Sleep Quality Index or PSQI >5), and daytime sleepiness was clinically significant (Epworth Sleepiness Scale or ESS score of ≥10) in 28% of athletes. Over 1/3 defined themselves as snorers, and 8% reported having a witnessed apneic episode (Swinbourne 2016). Collegiate American football players exhibit several risk factors for OSA, including large neck circumference and high body mass index, and the prevalence of sleep-disordered breathing among collegiate football players is estimated to be 8% [52]. The rate of OSA in professional American football players exceeds the population with a 5- to 11-fold increase in risk, with a prevalence ranging from 14% to 19%, compared to the general US population prevalence estimated at 2–5% [50, 53, 54, 55]. In retired NFL players, sleep-disordered breathing was present in 52% [56].

While OSA has also been linked to cognitive impairment and mood disorder [51], there are no known studies looking at the specific effect of OSA on psychological well-being in athletes. In a large study of Veterans Health Administration beneficiaries, those diagnosed with OSA had a significantly greater prevalence ($P < 0.0001$) of mood disorders, anxiety, post-traumatic stress disorder, psychosis, and dementia compared with patients not diagnosed with sleep apnea [55]. High rates of depression in people with OSA in both community (17%) and clinical populations (21–41%) have been shown, and one large cohort study identified OSA as a risk factor for depression [57]. Symptoms common to both OSA and depression include sleepiness and fatigue, and there have been varied results in controlled trials on the effectiveness of OSA treatment in reducing depressive symptoms. However, these associations in the general population suggest that athletes should be evaluated for OSA if they have mood disorders and coincident symptoms that may indicate sleep-disordered breathing.

The Specifics of Optimal Sleep for Athletes

Sleep and Athletic Performance

Most people, including athletes, require 7–9 h or more of sleep per night depending on their training volume. The average sleep cycle is approximately 90 min in length, so most people require five sleep cycles per night or 35 sleep cycles per week [21]. Sleep is very important for recovery from sport. The natural increase in growth hormone occurs at approximately one o'clock in the morning, and in order to maximize the level of growth hormone, athletes must be in deep sleep at the time of its secretion. Therefore, if athletes are not in bed by 11:30 pm, they may miss their best opportunity for recovery.

Athletes will often worry about poor sleep before a big event; however, research shows that neither endurance nor strength is significantly diminished by one night of poor sleep [58, 59]. However, consistent sleep deprivation or repeated bouts of sleep decrement (prolonged periods of time without sleep or repeated nights of poor sleep) will result in decreased strength [60], endurance [61], and perceived level of exertion [62] and an increased rate of injury [63]. The best sleep strategy for athletes is to consistently strive for a minimum of five sleep cycles or 7.5 h of sleep every night.

Extending sleep has also been shown to improve mood in elite athletes [64, 65]. Sleep education and optimization programs have led to significant improvements in self-reported total sleep time, sleep efficiency, fatigue, and vigor in athletes [66, 67]. In athletes who frequently experience pain as a result of injury, appropriate pain management and adequate sleep are likely to be very important for athletes from both a pain and sleep perspective [40].

How Can Athletes Improve Their Sleep?

The prevention of sleep disorders and poor sleep habits starts with identifying and eliminating risk factors and behaviors that would reduce the quantity and quality of sleep, establishing and maintaining a regular sleep routine, and ensuring adequate sleep duration depending on age and hours of training each day. Parents, healthcare providers, and coaching staff should discourage the use of computers and other tech devices before bedtime, as these may perpetuate sleep deficiency and disrupt circadian rhythms, which can have adverse impacts on athletic performance [68]. Excessive worry and anxiety related to training, competition, academics, or personal relationships may cause significant emotional reactions that decrease sleep quality.

While athletes are often advised to not exercise prior to bedtime due to potential overstimulation, evening exercise (2–4 h before bed) has not been associated with worse sleep [69, 70]. In fact, high volumes of exercise are related to improved sleep and psychological functioning. Adolescent athletes who trained almost 18 h a week (versus 4.5 h a week for the control group) reported better sleep patterns including higher sleep quality, shortened sleep-onset latency, and fewer awakenings after sleep onset. They also reported less tiredness and increased concentration during the day and significantly lower anxiety and fewer depressive symptoms [71].

Insomnia

High-quality research, while not specific for athletes, has established that insomnia-specific cognitive behavioral therapy (CBT) is first-line treatment for sustained improvements in sleep in those with insomnia alone or insomnia comorbid with other conditions [72, 73]. A large sample of Australian athletes found that 59% of team sport athletes had no strategy to overcome poor sleep compared with individual athletes, 32.7%, who utilized simple relaxation and reading techniques [7].

Diet may influence the central nervous system by regulating the production of serotonin and melatonin, specifically through manipulation of their precursor amino acid, L-tryptophan. Melatonin doses as low as 1 g can improve sleep latency and subjective sleep quality [74, 75]. Meanwhile, a review of multiple studies concluded that diets high in carbohydrate may result in shorter sleep latencies, diets high in protein may result in improved sleep quality, and diets high in fat may negatively influence total sleep time [75].

Double-blinded placebo-controlled studies exploring sleep medications' influence on reliable measures of athletes' mental status and physical performance are lacking. Benzodiazepines may help to improve sleep yet not ideal for the

competitive athlete because of its hangover effect [76]. Non-benzodiazepine hypnotics include zolpidem and eszopiclone; both improve sleep latency, and the latter
also improves maintenance of sleep [77, 78]. Besides increasing total sleep, no
impairment on measures of psychomotor and physical performance was noted for
zolpidem, and in university volleyball athletes, even arousal was improved compared to placebo indicating improved nocturnal sleep [79].

Although melatonin is the first choice by psychiatrists for the treatment of insomnia in athletes [80], research investigating the use of melatonin for primary insomnia demonstrates inconclusive results. Melatonin did not improve sleep quality in
athletes [81]. One metanalysis reported a reduction in sleep-onset latency of only
7.2 min, although it does appear safe for short-term use [82]. Others have reported
that melatonin produces significant improvement in sleep onset and increases subjective quality of life [83], although side effects such as headaches, nausea, daytime
sleepiness, dizziness, and vivid dreams and nightmares have been reported [84].
Because melatonin is a supplement and not regulated by the FDA, elite athletes risk
testing positive if drug tested. The prescription medication ramelteon, a melatonin
receptor agonist, would eliminate this concern, but it carries a longer half-life and
may have a hangover effect, and it has also not been studied in athletes [85].
Antihistamines and other first-generation antihistamines are also touted as over-the-
counter sleep medications; however, there is an absence of efficacy in the treatment
of sleep-onset insomnia [86]. Also, despite minimal evidence of adverse events in
excess of placebo, adverse anticholinergic properties (dry mouth, urinary retention)
and a quicker onset of tolerance and longer duration of action than benzodiazepines
have been reported.

Obstructive Sleep Apnea (OSA)

The primary treatment for OSA is continuous positive airway pressure (CPAP), a
mask that fits over the nose and/or mouth that transmits air into the airway to help
keep it open during sleep. Compliance, however, is poor. Various behavioral therapies are also used, particularly in patients unable to tolerate or benefit from CPAP
or who have mild OSA. The principal purpose of these measures is to reduce risk
factors that may underlie or exacerbate the disorder. These interventions include
oral appliances to reposition the lower jaw and tongue, positional therapy to stay out
of the supine position, weight loss, reduction of alcohol and tobacco use, upper
airway surgeries, and hypoglossal nerve stimulation [87]. No studies of these have
been performed specifically in athletes.

Summary

Sleep plays an important role in the psychological well-being of athletes. Regardless
of the actual theory of why humans need to sleep, studies have demonstrated that
psychological symptoms and even mental health conditions can occur or become

exacerbated in the setting of poor sleep quality and quantity. Most telling is the fact that there is no known psychiatric condition where sleep is normal. Because the same brain regions are impacted by mood disorders and poor sleep, it is not surprising that blocking sleep in otherwise healthy people can demonstrate neurological patterns of brain activity similar to those found in psychiatric conditions.

Optimizing sleep in athletes first starts with sleep education, including the identification and elimination of risk factors and behaviors that would reduce the quantity and adversely affect the quality of sleep. While not specific for athletes, insomnia-specific cognitive behavioral therapy (CBT) is first-line treatment in those with insomnia alone or insomnia comorbid with other conditions. Meanwhile, athletes may also turn to medications to improve sleep. Despite melatonin being identified as a safe first choice by psychiatrists for the treatment of insomnia in athletes, research has demonstrated inconclusive results. Melatonin is also not regulated by the FDA, and its purity may be questionable; therefore, elite athletes enrolled in a drug testing program must use this over-the-counter (OTC) supplement with extreme caution.

References

1. Leeder J, Glaister M, Pizzoferro K, Dawson J, Pedlar C. Sleep duration and quality in elite athletes measured using wristwatch actigraphy. J Sports Sci. 2012;30(6):541–5.
2. Byrd KL, Gelaye B, Tadesse MG, Williams MA, Lemma S, Berhane Y. Sleep disturbances and common mental disorders in college students. Health Behav Policy Rev. 2014;1(3):229–37.
3. Drew M, Vlahovich N, Hughes D, Appaneal R, Burke LM, Lundy B, Rogers M, Toomey M, Watts D, Lovell G, Praet S. Prevalence of illness, poor mental health and sleep quality and low energy availability prior to the 2016 Summer Olympic Games. Br J Sports Med. 2018;52(1):47–53.
4. Swinbourne R, Gill N, Vaile J, Smart D. Prevalence of poor sleep quality, sleepiness and obstructive sleep apnoea risk factors in athletes. Eur J Sport Sci. 2016;16(7):850–8.
5. Silva A, Queiroz SS, Winckler C, Vital R, Sousa RA, Fagundes V, Tufik S, de Mello MT. Sleep quality evaluation, chronotype, sleepiness and anxiety of Paralympic Brazilian athletes: Beijing 2008 Paralympic Games. Br J Sports Med. 2012;46:150–4. https://doi.org/10.1136/bjsm.2010.077016.
6. Samuel DA, Patricio AJ, Camila VS, Tomas H-V, Cristobal MC, Rodolfo PR, et al. Quality of sleep, drowsiness and insomnia in elite Paralympic athletes in Chile. Nutr Hosp [Internet]. 2015;32(6):2832–7. Available at: http://scielo.isciii.es/scielo.php?script=sci_arttext&pid=S0212-16112015001200063&lng=es. https://doi.org/10.3305/nh.2015.32.6.9893
7. Juliff LE, Halson SL, Peiffer JJ. Understanding sleep disturbance in athletes prior to important competitions. J Sci Med Sport. 2015;18(1):13–8.
8. Ehrlenspiel F, Erlacher D, Ziegler M. Changes in subjective sleep quality before a competition and their relation to competitive anxiety. Behav Sleep Med. 2016;10:1–4.
9. Savis JC, Eliot JF, Gansneder B, Rotella RJ. A subjective means of assessing college athletes' sleep: a modification of the morningness/eveningness questionnaire. Int J Sport Psychol. 1997;28(2):157–70.
10. Walker M. Why we sleep: unlocking the power of sleep and dreams. New York: Scribner; 2017.
11. Gujar N, Yoo SS, Hu P, et al. Sleep deprivation amplifies reactivity of brain reward networks, biasing the appraisal of positive emotional experiences. J Neurosci. 2011;31:4466–74. https://doi.org/10.1523/JNEUROSCI.3220-10.2011, pmid:21430147.

12. Harvey A, Murray G, Chandler RA, et al. Sleep disturbance as transdiagnostic: consideration of neurobiological mechanisms. Clin Psychol Rev. 2011;31:225–35.
13. Frank MG. The mystery of sleep function: current perspectives and future directions. Rev Neurosci. 2006;17:375–92.
14. Siegel JM. Clues to the functions of mammalian sleep. Nature. 2005;437:1264–71.
15. Xie L, Kang H, Xu Q, Chen MJ, Liao Y, Thiyagarajan M, et al. Sleep drives metabolite clearance from the adult brain. Science. 2013;342:373–7. https://doi.org/10.1126/science.1241224.
16. Mendelsohn AR, Larrick JW. Sleep facilitates clearance of metabolites from the brain: glymphatic function in aging and neurodegenerative diseases. Rejuvenation Res. 2013;16:518–23. https://doi.org/10.1089/rej.2013.1530.
17. Berk M, Williams LJ, Jacka FN, O'Neil A, Pasco JA, Moylan S, Allen NB, Stuart AL, Hayley AC, Byrne ML, Maes M. So depression is an inflammatory disease, but where does the inflammation come from? BMC Med. 2013;11:200.
18. Wilson H, Giordano B, Turkheimer FE, et al. Serotonergic dysfunction is linked to sleep problems in Parkinson's disease. Neuroimage Clin. 2018;18:630–7.
19. Berry RB, Albertario CL, Harding SM, et al for the American Academy of Sleep Medicine. The AASM manual for the scoring of sleep and associated events: rules, terminology and technical specifications, version 2.5, www.aasmnet.org, American Academy of Sleep Medicine, Darien, IL 2018.
20. Ohayon MM, Carskadon MA, Guilleminault C, Vitiello MV. Meta-analysis of quantitative sleep parameters from childhood to old age in healthy individuals: developing normative sleep values across the human lifespan. Sleep. 2004;27:1255.
21. Littlehale N. Sleep: the myth of 8 hours, the power of naps…and a new plan to recharge your body and mind. UK: New York, Penguin; 2016.
22. Medina AB, Lechuga DA, Escandón OS, Moctezuma JV. Update of sleep alterations in depression. Sleep Sci. 2014;7(3):165–9. https://doi.org/10.1016/j.slsci.2014.09.015.
23. Monti JM, Monti D. Sleep disturbance in schizophrenia. Int Rev Psychiatry. 2005;17(4):247–53.
24. Monti JM, Monti D. Sleep disturbance in generalized anxiety disorder and its treatment. Sleep Med Rev. 2000;4:263–76.
25. Kilduff TS, Mendelson WB. Mechanisms of action and pharmacologic effects. In: Kryger MH, Roth T, Dement WC, editors. Principles and practices of sleep medicine. 6th ed. St Louis: Elsevier Saunders; 2016. p. 424.
26. Buysse DJ, Tyagi S. Clinical pharmacology of other drugs used as hypnotics. In: Kryger MH, Roth T, Dement WC, editors. Principles and Practices of Sleep Medicine. 6th ed. St Louis: Elsevier Saunders; 2016. p. 432.
27. Schweitzer PK. Drugs that disturb sleep and wakefulness. In: Principles and practice of sleep medicine. 4th ed. Philadelphia: Saunders; 2005. p. 499.
28. Murphy PJ, Badia P, Myers BL, et al. Nonsteroidal anti-inflammatory drugs affect normal sleep patterns in humans. Physiol Behav. 1994;55:1063.
29. Dimsdale JE, Norman D, DeJardin D, Wallace MS. The effect of opioids on sleep architecture. J Clin Sleep Med. 2007;3:33.
30. O'Malley MB, Gleeson SK, Weir ID. Wake-promoting medications: Efficacy and adverse effects. In: Kryger MH, Roth T, Dement WC, editors. Principles and Practices of Sleep Medicine. 5th ed. St. Louis: Elsevier Saunders; 2011. p. 527.
31. Roehrs TA, Randall S, Harris E, et al. Twelve months of nightly zolpidem does not lead to rebound insomnia or withdrawal symptoms: a prospective placebo-controlled study. J Psychopharmacol. 2012;26:1088.
32. Spiegel R, DeVos JE. Central effects of guanfacine and clonidine during wakefulness and sleep in healthy subjects. Br J Clin Pharmacol. 1980;10(Suppl 1):165S.
33. Gillin JC, Jacobs LS, Fram DH, Snyder F. Acute effect of a glucocorticoid on normal human sleep. Nature. 1972;237:398.
34. Motomura Y, Kitamura S, Oba K, et al. Sleep debt elicits negative emotional reaction through diminished amygdala-anterior cingulate functional connectivity. PLoS One. 2013;8(2):e56578.

35. Schaal K, Tafflet M, Nassif H, Thibault V, Pichard C, Alcotte M, Guillet T, El Helou N, Berthelot G, Simon S, Toussaint JF. Psychological balance in high level athletes: gender-based differences and sport-specific patterns. PLoS One. 2011;6(5):e19007.
36. Venter R. Sleep performance for recovery. Contin Med Educ. 2008;26(7):331–3.
37. Fullagar HHK, Skorski S, Duffield R, et al. Sports Med. 2015;45:161. https://doi.org/10.1007/s40279-014-0260-0
38. Haack M, Mullington JM. Sustained sleep restriction reduces emotional and physical well being. Pain. 2005;15(119):56–64.
39. Lund HG, Reider BD, Whiting AB, Prichard JR. Sleep patterns and predictors of disturbed sleep in a large population of college students. J Adolesc Health. 2010;46(2):124–32.
40. Lautenbacher S, Kundermann B, Krieg JC. Sleep deprivation and pain perception. Sleep Med Rev. 2006;10(5):357–69.
41. Meerlo P, Sgolfo A, Sucheki D. Restricted and disturbed sleep: effects on autonomic function, neuroendocrine stress systems and stress responsivity. Sleep Med Rev. 2008;12(3):197–201.
42. Paiva T, Gaspar T, Matos MG. Mutual relations between sleep deprivation, sleep stealers and risk behaviors in adolescents. Sleep Science (Sao Paolo, Brazil). 2016;9(1):7–13.
43. Hildenbrand AK, Daly BP, Nicholls E, Brooks-Holliday S, Kloss JD. Increased risk for school violence-related behaviors among adolescents with insufficient sleep. J Sch Health. 2013;83(6):408–14.
44. Taylor DJ, Bramoweth AD. Patterns and consequences of inadequate sleep in college students: substance use and motor vehicle accidents. J Adolesc Health. 2010;46(6):610–2.
45. Cadegiani FA, Kater CE. Body composition, metabolism, sleep, psychological and eating patterns of overtraining syndrome: results of the EROS study (EROS-PROFILE). J Sports Sci. 2018;36(16):1902–10.
46. Biggins M, Cahalan R, Comyns T, Purtill H, O'Sullivan K. Poor sleep is related to lower general health, stress and increased confusion in elite Gaelic athletes. Phys Sports Med. 2018;46(1):14–20.
47. Andrade A, Bevilacqua GG, Coimbra DR, Periera FS, Brandt R. Sleep quality, mood, and performance: a study of elite Brazilian volleyball athletes. J Sports Sci Med. 2018;15(4):601–5.
48. Lastella M, Lovell GP, Sargent C. Athlete's precompetitive sleep behavior and its relationship with subsequent precompetitive mood and performance. Eur J Sports Sci. 2014;14(Supp 1):S123–30.
49. Buell JL, Calland D, Hanks F, Johnston B, Pester B, et al. Presence of metabolic syndrome in football linemen. J Athl Train. 2008;43:608–16.
50. Rogers AJ, Xia K, Soe K, Sexias A, Sogade F, Hutchinson B, Vieira D, McFarlane SI, Jean-Louis G. Obstructive sleep apnea among players in the national football league: a scoping review. J Sleep Disord Ther. 2017;6(5):278.
51. Emsellem HA, Murtagh KE. Sleep apnea and sports performance. Clin Sports Med. 2005;24(2):329–41.
52. Dobrosielski DA, Nichols D, Ford J, Watts A, Wilder JN, Douglass-Burton T. Estimating the prevalence of sleep-disordered breathing among collegiate football players. Respir Care. 2016;61:1144–50. https://doi.org/10.4187/respcare.04520.
53. George CF, Kab V, Levy AM. Increased prevalence of sleep-disordered breathing among professional football players. N Engl J Med. 2003;348:367–8.
54. Rice TB, Dunn RE, Lincoln AE, Tucker AM, Vogel RA, Heyer RA, Yates AP, Wilson PW, Pellmen EJ, Allen TW, Newman AB. Sleep-disordered breathing in the National Football League. Sleep. 2010;33(6):819–24.
55. Sharafkhaneh A, Giray N, Richardson P, Young T, Hirshkowitz M. Association of psychiatric disorders and sleep apnea in a large cohort. Sleep. 2005;28(11):1405–11.
56. Albuquerque FN, Kuniyoshi FH, Calvin AD, Sierra-Johnson J, Romero-Corral A, Lopez-Jimenez F, George CF, Rapoport DM, Vogel RA, Khandheria B, Goldman ME. Sleep-disordered breathing, hypertension, and obesity in retired National Football League players. J Am Coll Cardiol. 2010;56(17):1432–3.

57. Harris M, Glozier N, Ratnavadivel R, Grunstein RR. Obstructive sleep apnea and depression. Sleep Med Rev. 2009;13(6):437–44.
58. Reilly T, Edwards B. Altered sleep-wake cycles and physical performance in athletes. Physiol Behav. 2007;90(2–3):274–84.
59. Daanen HA, van Ling S, Tan TK. Subjective ratings and performance in the heat and after sleep deprivation. Aviat Space Environ Med. 2013;84(7):701–7.
60. Blumert PA, Crum AJ, Emsting M, Volek JS, Hollander DB, Hall EE, et al. The acute effects of twenty-four hours of sleep loss on the performance of national caliber male collegiate weight-lifters. J Strength Cond Res. 2007;21(4):1146–54.
61. Rae DE, Chin T, Dikgomo K, Hill L, McKune AJ, Kohn TA, et al. One night of partial sleep deprivation impairs recovery from a single exercise training session. Eur J Appl Physiol. 2017;117(4):699–712.
62. Simpson NS, Gibbs EL, Matheson GO. Optimizing sleep to maximize performance: implications and recommendations for elite athletes. Scand J Sports Med. 2016;27(3):266–74.
63. Milewski MD, Skaggs DL, Bishop GA, Pace JL, Ibrahim DA, Wren TA, et al. Chronic lack of sleep is associated with increased sports injuries in adolescent athletes. J Pediatr Ortho. 2014;34(2):129–33.
64. Mah CD. Extended sleep and the effects on mood and athletic performance in collegiate swimmers. Baltimore, MD (2008) Annual Meeting of the Associated Professional Sleep Societies.
65. Mah CD, Mah KE, Kezirian EJ, Dement WC. The effect of sleep extension on the athletic performance of collegiate basketball players. Sleep. 2011;34(7):943–50.
66. van Ryswyk E, Weeks R, Bandick L, O'Keefe M, Vakulin A, Catcheside P, et al. A novel sleep optimization programme to improve athletes' well being and performance. Eur J Sport Sci. 2017;17(2):144–51.
67. Simpson NS, Gibbs EL, Matheson GO. Optimizing sleep to maximize performance: implications and recommendations for elite athletes. Scand J Med Sci Sporst. 2017;27(3):266–74.
68. Chang AM, Aeschbach D, Duffy JF, Czeisler CA. Evening use of light-emitting ereaders negatively affects sleep, circadian timing, and next morning alertness. Proc Natl Acad Sci U S A. 2015;112(4):1232–7.
69. Myllymäki T, Kyröläinen H, Savolainen K, Hokka L, Jakonen R, Juuti T, et al. Effects of vigorous late-night exercise on sleep quality and cardiac autonomic activity. J Sleep Res. 2011;20(1 Pt 2):146–53. https://doi.org/10.1111/j.1365-2869.2010.00874.x.
70. Buman MP, Winkler EA, Kurka JM, Hekler EB, Baldwin CM, Owen N, Ainsworth BE, Healy GN, Gardiner PA. Reallocating time to sleep, sedentary behaviors, or active behaviors: associations with cardiovascular disease risk biomarkers, NHANES 2005–2006. Am J Epidemiol. 2014;179:323–34. https://doi.org/10.1093/aje/kwt292.
71. Brand S, Gerber M, Beck J, Hatzinger M, Puhse J, Holsboer-Trachsler E. High exercise levels are related to favorable sleep patterns and psychological functioning in adolescents: a comparison of athletes and controls. J Adolesc Health. 2010;46(2):133–41.
72. Anderson KN. Insomnia and cognitive behavioral therapy – how to assess your patient and why it should be a standard part of care. J Thorac Dis. 2018;10(Suppl 1):S94–S012.
73. Taylor DJ, Pruiksma KE. Cognitive and behavioral therapy for insomnia (CBT-I) in psychiatric populations: a systemic review. Int Rev Psychiatry. 2014;26(2):205–13.
74. Silber BY, Schmitt JA. Effects of tryptophan loading on human cognition, mood, and sleep. Neurosci Behav Rev. 2010;34(3):387–407.
75. Halson SL. Sleep in elite athletes and nutritional interventions to enhance sleep. Sports Med. 2014;44(Suppl 1):S13–23.
76. Grobler LA, Schwellnus MP, Trichard C, Calder S, Noakes T, Derman W. Comparative effects of zopiclone and loprazolam on psychomotor and physical performance in active individuals. Clin J Sport Med. 2000;10(2):123–8.
77. Dündar Y, Boland A, Strobl J, et al. Newer hypnotic drugs for the short-term management of insomnia: a systematic review and economic evaluation. Health Technol Assess. 2004;8:iii–x. 1–125.

78. Morin CM, Vallières A, Guay B, Ivers H, Savard J, Mérette C, et al. Cognitive behavioral therapy, singly and combined with medication, for persistent insomnia: a randomized controlled trial. JAMA. 2009;301:2005–15. https://doi.org/10.1001/jama.2009.682.
79. Ito SU, Kanbayashi T, Takemura T, et al. Acute effects of zolpidem on daytime alertness, psychomotor and physical performance. Neurosci Res. 2007;59:309–13.
80. Reardon CL. The sports psychiatrist and psychiatric medication. International Review of Psychiatry. 2016;28(6):606–13.
81. Atkinson G, Buckley P, Edwards B, Reilly T, Waterhouse J. Are there hangover-effects on physical performance when melatonin is ingested by athletes before nocturnal sleep? Int J Sports Med. 2001;22(3):232–4.
82. Buscemi N, Vandermeer B, Friesen C, Bialy L, Tubman M, et al. The efficacy and safety of drug treatments for chronic insomnia in adults: a meta-analysis of RCTs. J Gen Intern Med. 2007;22:1335–50.
83. Kloss JD, Nash CO, Horsey SE, Taylor DJ. The delivery of behavioral sleep medicine to college students. J Ad Health. 2011;48:553–61.
84. Zisapel N. New perspectives on the role of melatonin in human sleep, circadian rhythms and their regulation. Br J Pharmacol. 2018;175:3190–9.
85. Atkin T, Comai S, Gobbi G. Drugs for insomnia beyond benzodiazepines: pharmacology, clinical applications, and discovery. Pharmacol Rev. 2018;70:197–245. https://doi.org/10.1124/pr.117.014381.
86. Sateia MJ, Buysse DJ, Krystal AD, Neubauer DN, Heald JL. Clinical practice guideline for the pharmacologic treatment of chronic insomnia in adults: an American Academy of sleep medicine clinical practice guideline. J Clin Sleep Med. 2017;13(2):307–49.
87. Sutherland K, Almeida FR, de Chazal P, Cistulli PA. Prediction in obstructive sleep apnoea: diagnosis, comorbidity risk, and treatment outcomes. Expert Rev Respir Med. 2018;12(4):293–307.

Index

A

Acceptance, 239–241
Action-based strategies, 228
Alcohol
  and anxiety/daytime sleepiness, 107
  and athletic performance, 107
  epidemiology and pattern of, 104
  and medication, 108
  and weight gain, 107, 108
  social and legal context of, 104, 105
Alcohol abuse, 19
Alcohol use disorders identification test
    (AUDIT), 19
Amenorrhea, 132, 133, 136
Amygdala, 280
Anabolic-androgenic steroid (AAS), 118, 119
Anabolic steroids, 115
Anabolic Steroids Control Act, 120
Anterior cruciate ligament (ACL) injury, 30
Antidepressant medications, 279
Anti-doping organizations (ADOs), 62
Anxiety, 16, 107, 109
  concussion, 152–154
  DSM-5 criteria for, 16
  exercise and, 272
    contraindications, 272
    interactions with medical therapy, 272
    sympathetic nervous system,
      activation of, 273
  mental health screening, 15, 16
  psychiatric disorders, 60
  sport participation, 193, 194
    cognitive appraisal, 194
    environmental demands, 194
    stress response, 195
  young athletes, 193–195

Anxiety/mood clinical profiles, 150
Anxiety-related behaviors, 213
Appetite suppression, 82
Applied sport psychology, 263
Aripiprazole, 64
Astrocytes, 216, 217
Athlete Fear Avoidance Questionnaire
    (AFAQ), 18
Athletes, 1
Athletic culture, 1, 168, 169
  bullying in, 166, 167
  hazing, 166
Athletic Milieu Direct Questionnaire
    (AMDQ), 17
Athletic performance, 283, 284
Attentional shift, 237
Attention deficit/hyperactivity disorder
    (ADHD), 27, 61–63
  abuse considerations, 81, 82
  adult considerations, 81
  athlete, 72
  co-morbidities, 71, 72
  definition, 69
  diagnosis, 70, 71
  doping considerations, 77
  epidemiology, 70
  ergogenic effects, 76
  medical risks
    cardiovascular considerations, 74, 75
    concussion, 75, 76
    hyperthermia, 75
  monitoring, 76
  non-competitive athletic activities, 78
  Olympic/International Federation
    Athletes, 78
  pathophysiology, 70

© Springer Nature Switzerland AG 2020
E. Hong, A. L. Rao (eds.), *Mental Health in the Athlete*,
https://doi.org/10.1007/978-3-030-44754-0

Attention deficit/hyperactivity
        disorder (ADHD) (*cont.*)
    pediatric considerations, 78, 81
    physician considerations, 82
    sport/competition-level specific
        considerations
        college athletes, 77
        professional athletes, 78–80
    treatments
        behavioral/psychosocial, 73
        psychosocial, 73, 74
    young athletes, 198, 199
Autonomy, 227

B
Behavioral basis, 167, 168
Behavioral deficits, TBI
    anxiety-related behaviors, 213
    astrocytes, 216, 217
    cell death, 215
    depression-like behavior, 212, 213
    microglial activation, 216
    neurotransmitter dysfunction, 217, 218
    post-traumatic headache, 213, 214
    repetitive mild TBI, 214
    sleep disturbances, 213
    traumatic axonal injury, 215
Behavioral/psychosocial therapy, 73
Behavioral responses, 96, 97
Benzodiazepines, 61, 279, 284
β-Amyloid precursor protein (APP), 215
Beta-blockers, 280
Binge eating disorder (BED), 63
Bipolar disorder, 63, 64
Bone mineral density (BMD), female athlete
        triad, 133–135
Brief Eating Disorders in Athletes
        Questionnaire (BEDA-Q), 17
Bullying, 43
    athletic culture, 166, 167
    epidemiology of, 170, 171
    impact of, 172, 173
    prevention, 175
    recognition of, 171, 172
    risk factors for, 171
    treatment, 173, 174
Burnout, 197
Buspirone, 60

C
Cannabis abuse, 104
Cannabis Use Disorders Identification
        Test-Revised (CUDIT-R), 20, 106

Career termination, depression, 30, 31
Carriage, 88
Cell death, 215
Chronic traumatic encephalopathy
        (CTE), 155–157
Coaching and mental health
    care seeking, encouraging, 249, 250
    mental and physical stressors, 247, 248
    positive coping skills, 248, 249
Coaching support, 45
Cognitive appraisal, 194
Cognitive behavioral therapy (CBT), 33, 284
Cognitive defusion, 235–237
Cognitive difficulties, 158
Cognitive distortions, 33
Cognitive response, 96, 97
Collegiate athletes, 25, 26, 75, 87, 88, 97, 98,
        122, 129, 154, 156, 173, 185, 194,
        206, 252
Co-morbid psychiatric disorders, 118, 119
Competence, 227
Compulsive exercise test (CET), 206
Conceptual framework, 247
Concussion, 44, 149, 211
    ADHD, 75, 76
    anxiety/mood profile, 152–154, 158–160
    clinical profiles and mental health issues,
        150, 151
    concurrent psychological and profiles,
        157, 158
    CTE effect, 156, 157
    depression, 154, 155
    functional neurological and somatic
        symptom disorders, 155, 156
    malingering, 155
    mental health symptoms, etiology of,
        151, 152
    and suicide, 156
Conduct disorder (CD), 199, 200
Counseling, 105, 111
Cyberbullying, 170, 182, 183
Cycle, 120

D
Daytime sleepiness, 107
Deadly weapon, 88
Delayed menarche, 132
Depression, 3, 8, 12, 109, 212, 213, 217
    concussion, 154, 155
    exercise and, 270, 271
        contraindications, 271
        interactions with medical therapy, 271
        suffering with mood disorders, 271
    mental health screening, 13–15

prevalence, 26, 27
psychiatric disorders, 59, 60
risk factors, 27
    athletic performance, level of, 28
    career termination, 30, 31
    injury, 28–30
    performance, 31, 32
    sport, type of, 28
social media, 183, 184
sport participation, 196
symptoms, social desirability and
        underreporting, 32
treatment approaches, 32, 33
young athletes, 196
Disordered eating, 128, 131–132, 134, 143,
        203, 206, 207
Doping, 116
Down-stream signaling, 218
Drive for leanness, 203, 204
Drive for muscularity, 203, 204
Drive for thinness, 203
DSM 5 major depressive disorder, 14

E
Eating Disorder Examination (EDE), 17
Eating disorders, 63, 127, 130, 136, 141, 206, 207
    mental health screening, 16, 17
Education, 121
Emotional response, 95, 96
Energy conservation theory, 278
Engagement, 88
Ethnicity, 43
Exercise, 81, 269
    addiction, 204, 205
    and anxiety, 272
        contraindications, 272
        interactions with medical therapy, 272
        sympathetic nervous system,
            activation of, 273
    and depression, 270, 271
        contraindications, 271
        interactions with medical therapy, 271
        suffering with mood disorders, 271
    exercise prescription
        duration, 274
        frequency, 273
        intensity, 273
        mind-body exercises, 274
        time, 273
        types, 274
    mental health, prescription for, 274
Exercise Addiction Inventory (EAI), 206
Exercise prescription
    duration, 274

frequency, 273
intensity, 273
mind-body exercises, 274
time, 273
types, 274

F
Facebook, 181
Facial allodynia, 214
Fear avoidance, 17, 18
Fear-Avoidance Beliefs Questionnaire
        (FAB-Q), 18
Female athlete screening tool (FAST), 17
Female athlete triad, 127
    clearance and return-to-play guidelines, 139
    cumulative risk assessment tool, 135
    epidemiology, 129, 130
    follow-up, 138
    low bone mineral density, 133–135
    low energy availability, 130–132
    menstrual dysfunction, 132, 133
    prevention, 142, 143
    recovery from, 140
    return-to-play guidelines, 138–140
    screening, 135, 136
    spectrum of, 128
    terminology, 128, 129
    treatment, 136–138
Fighting, risk-taking behaviors, 88, 89
Financial distress, 44
Financial gain, 46
Fluoxetine, 63
Functional neurological disorder, 155, 156

G
Gambling, risk-taking behaviors, 89
Gamma-aminobutyric acid (GABA), 215
Gender differences, depression, 27
Generalized anxiety disorder– 7 index
        (GAD-7), 16
Goldman's dilemma, 204

H
Harassment, 182, 183
Hazing, 43, 167
    athletic culture, 166
    epidemiology of, 169, 170
    impact of, 172, 173
    prevention, 175
    recognition of, 171, 172
    risk factors for, 170
    treatment, 173, 174

HeadSpace, 239
Healthcare providers, role of, 98
High mental toughness, 97
High risk sexual behaviors, 89, 90
Human growth hormone (HGH)., 115
Hyperthermia, 75
Hypothalamic amenorrhea, 132
Hysteria, 157

I
Illness and injury, rehabilitation/recovery
    from, 96, 97
Impaired axonal transport (IAT), 215
Inactivity theory, 278
Inflammation, 216
Informal mindfulness exercises, 239
Injury
    depression, 28–30
    psychological and sociocultural risk factors
        for, 95, 96
    and rehabilitation/recovery
        from, 96, 97
Insomnia, 60, 61, 281, 282, 284, 285
Instagram, 182
International Olympic Committee, 78
Interpersonal engagement, social media,
    184, 185

K
Knowledge-based strategies, 227, 228

L
Lamotrigine, 64
Life event stress, 95
Lisdexamfetamine, 63
Lithium, 64
Litigating abuse, 174
Low energy availability (EA), female athlete
    triad, 130–132

M
Major depressive episode, 14
Male Athlete Triad, 141
Malingering, concussion, 155
Marijuana, 82
    and athletic performance, 108
    and sleep quality, 108
Melatonin, 61, 285
Menstrual dysfunction, 132, 133
Mental coaches, 262
Mental edge, 232

Mental health, 1–2, 245
    barriers to, 4, 5
    coaching and
        care seeking, encouraging, 249, 250
        mental and physical stressors, 247, 248
        positive coping skills, 248, 249
    culture change, 6
    determinants of, 191, 192
        physical activity, 192
        self-esteem and sport, 193
        sport culture, 192, 193
    facilitators to, 5
    institutions and organizations, 5
    mental illness, 3
    vs. mental toughness, 3, 4
    organizational practices and
        coach training, guidance
            providance, 254
        evidence-based education, 250, 251
        organizational incentives, 251
        policy and, 253, 254
        protocol, establish and rehearse, 252
        protocols, guidance providance, 255
        screening, guidance providance,
            254, 255
        staffing, attend to, 252, 253
        staffing, guidance providance, 255
        universal screening, 251, 252
    rules and guidelines, 6
    stigma, 2, 3, 6, 7
        awareness, 7, 8
        culture, 7
        research, 9
        response, 8
        support, 8, 9
    studies, 2
Mental Health First Aid, 250
Mental health partners (MHP), 52
Mental health screening, 11, 12
    alcohol abuse, 19
    anxiety disorders, 15, 16
    depression, 13–15
    drug use, 19, 20
    eating disorder, 16, 17
    injured athlete, 17, 18
    mechanics, 12
    substance abuse, 18, 19
Mental health in sport (MHS), 251
Mental health treatment engagement, 224
    negative outcomes, 225, 226
    stereotypical beliefs, 224, 225
    stigma and shame, 225
Mental illness, 1, 3, 25, 245, 246
Mental performance, 265
Mental stressors, 247, 248

Mental toughness, 3, 4
Microglial activation, 216
Mind-body exercises, 274
Mindfulness, 231–233
    acceptance, 239–241
    cognitive defusion, 235–237
    present moment awareness, 238, 239
    and sport-related stress, 233–235
Mirtazapine, 59
Monoamine oxidase inhibitors (MAOIs), 271
Mood disturbance, 18
Motivational model, effective treatment
        engagement, 226
    action-based strategies, 228
    knowledge-based strategies, 227, 228
    relationship-based strategies, 226, 227

N
National Comorbidity Survey-Adolescent
        Supplement (NCS-A), 196
National Institute for Alcohol Abuse and
        Alcoholism (NIAAA), 106
Negative predictive value (NPV), 19
Neurotransmitter dysfunction, 217, 218
Non-benzodiazepine receptor agonists
        (NBRA), 279
Non-competitive athletic activities, 78
Non-REM (NREM) sleep, 278
Non-steroidal anti-inflammatory drugs
        (NSAIDS), 279
Nutrition, 63

O
Observing mind, 236
Obstructive sleep apnea hypopnea (OSA), 282,
        283, 285
Oligomenorrhea, 132
Olympic/International Federation Athletes, 78
Oppositional defiant disorder (ODD), 199, 200
Optimal sleep
    athletic improvement, 284
    athletic performance, 283, 284
    insomnia, 284, 285
    OSA, 285
Organizational incentives, 251
Organizational practices
    coach training, guidance providance, 254
    and evidence-based education, 250, 251
    organizational incentives, 251
    policy and, 253, 254
    protocol, establish and rehearse, 252
    protocols, guidance providance, 255
    screening, guidance providance, 254, 255

    staffing, attend to, 252, 253
    staffing, guidance providance, 255
    universal screening, 251, 252
Overreaching (OR) syndrome, 197
Overtraining syndrome (OTS), 197, 282

P
Para-athletes, 141
Parental support, 46
Pathological exercise, 205, 206
    disordered eating, eating disorders,
        screening for, 206, 207
    exercise addiction, exploring increased
        rates of, 204, 205
    prevalence, 204
Patient Health Questionnaire 9-item
        (PHQ-9), 13, 154
Peak performance, 226, 227
Performance-enhancing drug (PED), 44, 115,
        263, 264
    AAS and co-morbid psychiatric disorders,
        118, 119
    adverse systemic effects, 116
    legal issues and sources, 119, 120
    positive test, potential fallout from, 122
    prohibition and testing, 116
    psychological and psychiatric effects, 119
    and risk-taking behavior, 119
    subculture and at-risk or using athlete,
        120, 121
    use, abuse, and dependence, 118
Performance psychology, 264
Photophobia, 214
Physical activity
    mental health determinants, 192
    physiology, 270
Physical stressors, 247, 248
Pinterest, 182
Polysubstance abuse, 119
Positive coping skills, 248, 249
Possession, 88
Post-traumatic amnesia, 211
Post-traumatic headache, 213, 214
Professional athletes, 78–80
Psychiatric disorders, 57
    anxiety, 60
    attention-deficit/hyperactivity
        disorder, 61–63
    bipolar disorder, 63, 64
    depression, 59, 60
    eating disorders, 63
    insomnia, 60, 61
    medications, 57, 58
    variables, 58

Psychological processes, 263
Psychological response
    illness and injury, injury and rehabilitation/
        recovery from, 96, 97
    injury, psychological and sociocultural risk
        factors for, 95, 96
    prevention, 97, 98
    team physicians and healthcare providers,
        role of, 98
Psychological skills, 262, 263, 265
Psychological well-being, 280, 281
    insomnia, 281, 282
    OSA, 282, 283
    overtraining syndrome, 282
Psychosocial interventions, 73, 74
Psychotherapy, 63
Psychotic disorders, 64
Psychotropic medications, 33

R
Race, 43
Rapid eye movement (REM) sleep, 278
Rehabilitation, 18
Relatedness, 227
Relationship-based strategies, 226, 227
Relative energy deficiency in sport
        (RED-S), 129
Repetitive mild TBI, 214
Resiliency, 97
Restorative theory, 278
Retirement and end of career, 45
Return-to-play guidelines, female athlete
        triad, 138–140
Risk-taking behaviors
    deadly weapon, possession and
        carriage of, 88
    defining, 86
    driving while intoxicated, 87, 88
    fighting, 88, 89
    gambling, 89
    high risk sexual behaviors, 89, 90
    limitations, 91
    riding with intoxicated driver, 87
    seatbelt omission, 87
    study context and quality, 86
    tobacco use, 90, 91

S
Seatbelt, risk-taking behaviors, 87
Second impact syndrome (SIS), 155

Selective serotonin reuptake inhibitors
        (SSRIs), 59
Self-determination theory (SDT), 224, 227
Self-esteem, mental health determinants, 193
Serotonin-norepinephrine reuptake inhibitors
        (SNRIs), 59, 271
Sexual assault, 14
Sexual misconduct, 44
Sexually transmitted infections (STIs), 85
Shame, 225
Sleep, 277–279
    anatomy of, 280
    deprivation, 282
    disruptions, 211
    disturbances, 213
    medication effects, 279, 280
    psychiatric condition, 278
    quality of, 277
Sleep disorders, 280, 281
    insomnia, 281, 282
    OSA, 282, 283
    overtraining syndrome, 282
Sleep-promoting cells, 280
Sleep quality, 184
Sleep-wake disorders, 280
Snapchat, 182
Social desirability, 32
Social ecological model, 247
Social media and mental health, 42, 181, 182
    benefits of, 185, 186
    cyberbullying and harassment, 182, 183
    depression, 183, 184
    interpersonal engagement, 184, 185
    policies, 186
    sleep quality, 184
Social networking, 181, 183–185
Social stigma, 224, 225
Social structure, 45
Somatic symptom disorders, 155, 156
Sport anxiety scale (SAS), 16
Sport culture, mental health determinants,
        192, 193
Sport participation, 192
    anxiety, 193, 194
        cognitive appraisal, 194
        environmental demands, 194
        stress response, 195
    burnout, 197
    depression, 196
    OTS, 197
Sport psychology, 231, 232, 261, 262
    AASP certification, 265

field of, 262–265
  practice of, 264
Sport-related stress, 233–235
Sport, type of, 28
Sports culture, 3
Sports medicine, 51, 223, 225, 262
State-Trait Anxiety Inventory (STAI), 16
Stereotypical beliefs, 224, 225
Stigma, 2, 3, 57, 225
  awareness, 7, 8
  culture, 7
  research, 9
  response, 8
  support, 8, 9
Stimulants, 61, 73, 280
Stress fracture, 109
  affiliate medical and team personnel, 110
  overcoming barriers, 110, 111
  pre-screening, 110
Stress response, 195
Student-athletes, 182, 186
Substance abuse, 18, 19, 103, 214
  clinical recommendations, 109
  interventions, 105, 106
  mental health, observations related to, 109
  research studies related to, 106
    alcohol and anxiety/daytime
      sleepiness, 107
    alcohol and athletic performance, 107
    alcohol and medication, 108
    alcohol and weight gain, 107, 108
    marijuana and athletic
      performance, 108
    marijuana and sleep quality, 108
    withdrawal symptoms, benefits of use
      from, 108
  screening for, 106
  social and legal context of, 104, 105
Sudden deaths, 74
Suffocation, 41
Suicide, 39, 40
  cause of death, 41
  in college athletes, 47
  concussion and, 156
  defining, 40
  in high school athletes, 46, 47
  management strategies, 48, 49
    ask and assess, 50, 51
    danger, removing, 51
    empathize, 50
    LEARN approach, 49
    look, 50

method of death, 41
  in professional athletes, 48
  rates of, 41
  risk factors for, 41–45
  scope of, 40
  supports, 45, 46
Suprachiasmatic nucleus (SCN), 280
Supraventricular arrhythmias, 59
Synaptic pruning theory, 278

T
Therapeutic use exemption
  (TUE), 62, 78
Tobacco use, 90, 91
Transtheoretical model (TTM), 228
Traumatic axonal injury, 215
Traumatic brain injury (TBI), 211, 212
  behavioral deficits
    anxiety-related behaviors, 213
    astrocytes, 216, 217
    cell death, 215
    depression-like behavior, 212, 213
    microglial activation, 216
    neurotransmitter dysfunction,
      217, 218
    post-traumatic headache, 213, 214
    repetitive mild TBI, 214
    sleep disturbances, 213
    traumatic axonal injury, 215
  behavioral outcomes, 212
Tricyclic antidepressants, 59
Twitter, 185

U
Unites States Preventative Services Taskforce
  (USPSTF), 13

V
Ventricular arrhythmias, 59
Vestibular dysfunction, 158
Violence, 167, 171, 175
Vitamin D deficiency, 137

W
World Anti-Doping Agency (WADA),
  59, 62, 73
Well-being of athletes, 232–234, 242
Women's Sports Foundation (WSF), 192

Y
Young athletes
    ADHD, 198, 199
    anxiety, 193–195
    burnout, 197
    conduct and ODD, 199, 200
    depression, 196
    OR and OTS, 197
    parents and coaches, resources for, 200

Youth Risk Behavior Surveillance system
        (YRBSS), 86
Youth Risk Behavioral Survey, 85
YouTube, 182

Z
Ziprasidone, 64

Printed in the United States
by Baker & Taylor Publisher Services